ESSENTIALS
OF CLINICAL
GERIATRICS

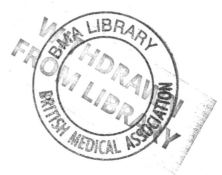

NOTICE

Medicine is an ever-changing science. As new research and clinical experience broaden our knowledge, changes in treatment and drug therapy are required. The authors and the publisher of this work have checked with sources believed to be reliable in their efforts to provide information that is complete and generally in accord with the standards accepted at the time of publication. However, in view of the possibility of human error or changes in medical sciences, neither the authors nor the publisher nor any other party who has been involved in the preparation or publication of this work warrants that the information contained herein is in every respect accurate or complete, and they disclaim all responsibility for any errors or omissions or for the results obtained from use of the information contained in this work. Readers are encouraged to confirm the information contained herein with other sources. For example and in particular, readers are advised to check the product information sheet included in the package of each drug they plan to administer to be certain that the information contained in this work is accurate and that changes have not been made in the recommended dose or in the contraindications for administration. This recommendation is of particular importance in connection with new or infrequently used drugs.

ESSENTIALS OF CLINICAL GERIATRICS

SIXTH EDITION

ROBERT L. KANE, MD

Professor and Minnesota Endowed Chair in Long-Term Care and Aging
School of Public Health
University of Minnesota
Minneapolis, Minnesota

JOSEPH G. OUSLANDER, MD

Director, Institute for Quality Aging
Boca Raton Community Hospital
Boca Raton, Florida
Professor of Medicine (Voluntary)
Assistant Dean for Geriatric Education
University of Miami Miller School of Medicine (UMMSM) at Florida Atlantic University
Associate Director, Division of Gerontology and Geriatric Medicine
Department of Medicine, UMMSM
Miami, Florida
Professor (Courtesy)
Christine E. Lynn College of Nursing
Florida Atlantic University

ITAMAR B. ABRASS, MD

William E. Colson Chair in Gerontology
Professor of Medicine and Division Head, Gerontology and Geriatric Medicine
University of Washington Harborview Medical Center
Seattle, Washington

BARBARA RESNICK, PHD, CRNP, FAAN, FAANP

Professor
University of Maryland School of Nursing
Sonya Gershowitz Chair in Gerontology
Baltimore, Maryland

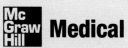 **Medical**

NEW YORK / CHICAGO / SAN FRANCISCO / LISBON / LONDON
MADRID / MEXICO CITY / MILAN / NEW DELHI / SAN JUAN
SEOUL / SINGAPORE / SYDNEY / TORONTO

The *McGraw·Hill* Companies

ESSENTIALS OF CLINICAL GERIATRICS
SIXTH EDITION

1 2 3 4 5 6 7 8 9 0   DOC/DOC   12 11 10 9 8

ISBN 978-0-07-149822-7
MHID 0-07-149822-2

This book was set in Times by International Typesetting and Composition.
The editors were James Shanahan and Christie Naglieri.
The production supervisor was Catherine Saggese.
Project management was provided by Preeti Longia Sinha of International Typesetting and Composition.
Cover Designer: Maria Scharf
Photo Credit: LWA. Caption: Female doctor assisting senior woman, smiling
RR Donnelley was printer and binder.

This book is printed on acid-free paper.

Library of Congress Cataloging-in-Publication Data

Kane, Robert L., 1940-
    Essentials of Clinical Geriatrics / Robert L.Kane, Joseph G. Ouslander, Itamar B. Abrass, Barbara Resnick.—6th. ed.
        p. ; cm.
    Includes bibliographical references and index.
    ISBN-13: 978-0-07-149822-7 (pbk. : alk. paper)
    ISBN-10: 0-07-149822-2 (pbk. : alk. paper)
    1. Clinical implications of the aging process I. Kane, Robert L., 1940- Kane, Robert L., 1940- Essentials of clinical geriatrics. 2. The geriatric patient: demography, epidemiology, and health services Utilization. 3. utilization—Evaluating the geriatric patient WT 100 E78 2009]
    RC952 .K36 2009
    618.97 22
                                                                    2008034799

CONTENTS

PART III

GENERAL MANAGEMENT STRATEGIES 333

TABLES AND FIGURES

CHAPTER FOUR

CHAPTER FIVE

CHAPTER SIX

CHAPTER SEVEN

CHAPTER EIGHT

CHAPTER NINE

CHAPTER TEN

CHAPTER ELEVEN

C H A P T E R   T W E L V E

C H A P T E R   T H I R T E E N

C H A P T E R   F O U R T E E N

C H A P T E R   F I F T E E N

CHAPTER SIXTEEN

C H A P T E R   S E V E N T E E N

PREFACE

The publication of the sixth edition of the *Essentials* marks a milestone. Not only is the field growing older (and we along with it), it is changing. The composition of geriatrics and primary care has shifted. It has become ever clearer that care for older people will not be delivered primarily by geriatricians. The goal for such care must be to make all those who will be delivering care to become more aware of the principles of geriatrics. Because nurse practitioners represent a substantial proportion of the clinical workforce responsible for caring for older people and continue to provide care to older adults across a variety of health care settings, we are pleased to welcome the contributions of Barbara Resnick, PhD, CRNP. Barbara's participation re-enforces our commitment to the interdisciplinary nature of clinical geriatrics, and to producing a book that will be widely useful, and hopefully widely used.

The five years since the last edition has seen some important changes both in the practice of geriatrics and the organization of care. Medicare Part D has been implemented. The place of managed care is still being debated. New drugs are available for many diseases including cardiovascular conditions, depression, and diabetes. Genetics is on the verge of becoming a major toll in adapting care. Pay-for performance is being tested. Transitions between care settings have become increasingly important in geriatric care. Assisted living facilities and other similar settings have increased; care for acutely ill older adults and those at the end-of-life care is now offered across a spectrum of service sites. We hope this book is helpful to geriatric care providers across all of these settings.

In response to the new sense of commitment to evidence-based practice we have added material at the end of most chapters summarizing what has been shown to be effective. Much of these conclusions rely heavily on the ACOVE project.[1] While it is important to encourage systematic practice based on evidence, it is also important to recognize that geriatrics is concerned with the whole person. At a time when people are talking about individualized care as implying genotyping, it is worth considering Groopman's distinction between clinicians who strictly follow protocols and those who attend to their patients as individuals.[2] Central to good geriatrics and a guiding principal of this book, is the ability to appreciate the evidence with regard to preventive health, and disease management, and apply this knowledge to older adults, using ethical principles and individualized care.

1. Wenger NS, Shekelle PG. Measuring medical care provided to vulnerable elders: The assessing care of vulnerable elders-3 (ACOVE-3) quality indicators. *Journal of the American Geriatrics Society.* October 2007;55(S2):S247-S487.
2. Groopman J. *How Doctors Think.* Boston: Houghton Mifflin Company; 2007.

PART I

THE AGING PATIENT AND GERIATRIC ASSESSMENT

CHAPTER 1

CLINICAL IMPLICATIONS OF THE AGING PROCESS

The care of older patients differs from that of younger patients for a number of reasons. While there continues to be a debate about the cause of these differences, it is likely that they are a combination of biological changes that occur during the course of aging, associated diseases, and attitudes and beliefs of older adults and their caregivers. Aging is defined as the time-sequential deterioration that occurs in most living beings including weakness, increased susceptibility to disease and adverse environmental conditions, loss of mobility and agility, and age-related physiological changes (Goldsmith, 2006).

It is important to distinguish life expectancy from life span. The former refers to what proportion of the possible age a person may live. The latter suggests a biological limit to how many years a species can expect to survive. In general, geriatrics has the most to contribute to improving life expectancy, but new genetic breakthroughs may ultimately affect life span as well. Another helpful distinction is between chronological aging and gerontological aging. The latter is calculated on the basis of the risk of dying, the so-called force of mortality. Thus, two people of the same chronological age may have biologically very different ages depending on their health state. Some of that propensity for death is malleable; some is simply predictable.

Perhaps one of the most intriguing challenges in medicine is to unravel the process of aging. From a medical perspective the question continues to haunt us as to whether aging is a feature of an organism's design that has evolved over time and is beneficial to the survival of species, or aging is a disease or defect that confers no survival benefit. Even more important to medical management of aging is the question of whether there are medically treatable factors that are common to the various manifestations of aging we see. Could aging treatments delay the signs and symptoms of aging such as sensory changes, musculoskeletal problems, or skin-related changes?

Nonetheless, the distinction between so-called normal aging and pathologic changes is critical to the care of older people. We wish to avoid both dismissing treatable pathology as simply a concomitant of old age and treating natural aging processes as though they were diseases. The latter is particularly dangerous because older adults are so vulnerable to iatrogenic effects.

There is growing appreciation that everyone does not age in the same way or at the same rate. The changing composition of today's older adults compared with that of a generation ago may actually reflect a bimodal shift wherein there are both more disabled people and more healthy older people. We continue to learn more and more about healthy or successful aging through hearing the stories of the growing number of centenarians. Generally the consensus is that moderation in all areas (eg, food intake, alcohol intake), regular physical activity, and an engaging social life are critical to successful aging. A recent large actuarial study (Gavrilova and Gavrilov, 2005) further suggested that environmental factors may also be relevant. Social factors can also play a strong role (Banks et al., 2006). The challenge is to recognize and appreciate aging changes while utilizing resources to prevent or halt further changes and overcome aging challenges.

CHANGES ASSOCIATED WITH "NORMAL" AGING

We have noted and appreciated the distinctions a clinician must make to attribute a finding to either the expected course of aging or the result of pathologic changes. This distinction perplexes the researcher as well. We currently lack precise knowledge of what constitutes normal aging. Much of our information comes from cross-sectional studies, which compare findings from a group of younger persons with those from a group of older individuals. Such data may reflect differences other than simply the effects of age such as those associated with lifestyle behaviors (physical activity, alcohol intake, smoking, and diet), as well as prophylactic medication management. For example, older adults in the coming century may present with less evidence of osteoporosis because of prophylactic lifelong intake of high calcium and vitamin D diets, regular physical activity, and early interventions with biphosphanates and potentially future treatments for osteoporosis. Statins can drastically affect the course of cardiovascular disease.

Many of the changes associated with aging result from gradual loss. These losses may often begin in early adulthood, but—thanks to the redundancy of most organ systems—the decrement does not become functionally significant until the loss is fairly extensive.

Based on cross-sectional comparisons of groups at different ages, most organ systems seem to lose function at about 1% a year beginning around age 30 years.

Other data suggest that the changes in people followed longitudinally are much less dramatic and certainly begin well after age 70 years.

In some organ systems, such as the kidney, a subgroup of persons appears to experience gradually declining function over time, whereas others' function remains constant. These findings suggest that the earlier theory of gradual loss must be reassessed as reflecting disease rather than aging. Given a pattern of gradual deterioration—whether from aging or disease or both—we are best advised to think in terms of thresholds.

The loss of function does not become significant until it crosses a given level. Thus the functional performance of an organ in an older person depends on two principal factors: (1) the rate of deterioration and (2) the level of performance needed. It is not surprising then to learn that most older persons will have normal laboratory values. The critical difference—in fact, the hallmark of aging—lies not in the resting level of performance but in how the organ (or organism) adapts to external stress. For example, an older person may have a normal fasting blood sugar but be unable to handle a glucose load within the normal parameters for younger subjects.

The same pattern of decreased response to stress can be seen in the performance of other endocrine systems or the cardiovascular system. An older individual may have a normal resting pulse and cardiac output but be unable to achieve an adequate increase in either with exercise.

Sometimes the changes of aging work together to produce apparently normal resting values in other ways. For example, although both glomerular filtration and renal blood flow decrease with age, many elderly persons have normal serum creatinine levels because of the concomitant decreases in lean muscle mass and creatinine production. Thus serum creatinine is not as good an indicator of renal function in the elderly as in younger persons. Knowledge of kidney function is critical in drug therapy. Therefore, it is important to get an accurate measure of kidney function. A useful formula for estimating creatinine clearance on the basis of serum creatinine values in the elderly was developed (Cockcroft and Gault, 1976). (The actual formula is provided in Chap. 14.) Table 1-1 (Schmidt, 1999) summarizes some of the pertinent changes that occur with aging. For many items, the changes begin in adulthood and proceed gradually; others may not manifest themselves until well into seniority.

THEORIES OF AGING

It is helpful to be familiar with the many theories of aging as these theories help direct the philosophy of care that is provided. If we believe that there is no way to intervene on the aging process we will likely help our older patients accept and adjust to these changes and focus on disease management. Conversely, if we believe in the potential of antiaging medicine and treatments and protocols that

TABLE 1-1   PERTINENT CHANGES THAT COMMONLY OCCUR WITH AGING

System	Common Age Changes	Implications of Changes
Cardiovascular	Atrophy of muscle fibers that line the endocardium	Increased blood pressure
	Atherosclerosis of vessels	Increased emphasis on atrial contraction with an S_4 heard
	Increased systolic blood pressure	Increased arrhythmias
	Decreased compliance of the left ventricle	Increased risk of hypotension with position change
	Decreased number of pacemaker cells	Valsalva maneuver may cause a drop in blood pressure
	Decreased sensitivity of baroreceptors	Decreased exercise tolerance
Neurologic	Decreased number of neurons and increase in size and number of neuroglial cells	Increased risk for neurological problems: cerebro-vascular accident
	Decline in nerves and nerve fibers	Parkinsonism
	Atrophy of the brain and increase in cranial dead space	Slower conduction of fibers across the synapses
	Thickened leptomeninges in spinal cord	Modest decline in short-term memory
		Alterations in gait pattern: wide based, shorter stepped, and flexed forward
		Increased risk of hemorrhage before symptoms are apparent
Respiratory	Decreased lung tissue elasticity	Decreased efficiency of ventilatory exchange
	Thoracic wall calcification	Increased susceptibility to infection and atelectasis
	Cilia atrophy	Increased risk of aspiration
	Decreased respiratory muscle strength	Decreased ventilatory response to hypoxia and hypercapnia
	Decreased partial pressure of arterial oxygen (Pao_2)	Increased sensitivity to narcotics

System	Age-Related Change	Implication
Integumentary	Loss of dermal and epidermal thickness	Thinning of skin and increased susceptibility to tearing
	Flattening of papillae	Dryness and pruritus
	Atrophy of sweat glands	Decreased sweating and ability to regulate body heat
	Decreased vascularity	Increased wrinkling and laxity of the skin
	Collagen cross-linking	Loss of fatty pads protecting bone and resulting in pain
	Elastin regression	Increased need for protection from the sun
	Loss of subcutaneous fat	Increased time for healing of wounds
	Decreased melanocytes	
	Decline in fibroblast proliferation	
Gastrointestinal	Decreased liver size	Change in intake caused by decreased appetite
	Less efficient cholesterol stabilization and absorption	Discomfort after eating related to slowed passage of food
	Fibrosis and atrophy of salivary glands	Decreased absorption of calcium and iron
	Decreased muscle tone in bowel	Alteration of drug effectiveness
	Atrophy of and decrease in number of taste buds	Increased risk of constipation, esophageal spasm, and diverticular disease
	Slowing in esophageal emptying	
	Decreased hydrochloric acid secretion	
	Decreased gastric acid secretion	
	Atrophy of the mucosal lining	
	Decreased absorption of calcium	
Urinary	Reduced renal mass	Decreased GFR
	Loss of glomeruli	Decreased sodium-conserving ability
	Decline in number of functioning nephrons	Decreased creatinine clearance
	Changes in small vessel walls	Increased BUN

TABLE 1-1 PERTINENT CHANGES THAT COMMONLY OCCUR WITH AGING (*Continued*)

SYSTEM	COMMON AGE CHANGES	IMPLICATIONS OF CHANGES
	Decreased bladder muscle tone	Decreased renal blood flow
		Altered drug clearance
		Decreased ability to dilute urine
		Decreased bladder capacity and increased residual urine
		Increased urgency
Reproductive	Atrophy and fibrosis of cervical and uterine walls	Vaginal dryness and burning and pain with intercourse
	Decreased vaginal elasticity and lubrication	Decreased seminal fluid volume and force of ejaculation
	Decreased hormones and reduced oocytes	Reduced elevation of the testes
	Decreased seminiferous tubules	Prostatic hypertrophy
	Proliferation of stromal and glandular tissue	Connective breast tissue is replaced by adipose tissue, making breast examinations easier
	Involution of mammary gland tissue	
Musculoskeletal	Decreased muscle mass	Decreased muscle strength
	Decreased myosin adenosine triphosphatase activity	Decreased bone density
		Loss of height
	Deterioration and drying of joint cartilage	Joint pain and stiffness
	Decreased bone mass and osteoblastic activity	Increased risk of fracture
		Alterations in gait and posture
Sensory: Vision	Decreased rod and cone function	Decreased visual acuity, visual fields, and light/dark adaptation
	Pigment accumulation	

System/Category	Age-Related Changes	Implications
	Decreased speed of eye movements	Increased sensitivity to glare
	Increased intraocular pressure	Increased incidence of glaucoma
	Ciliary muscle atrophy	Distorted depth perception with increased falls
	Increased lens size and yellowing of the lens	Less able to differentiate blues, greens, and violets
	Decreased tear secretion	Increased eye dryness and irritation
Sensory: Hearing	Loss of auditory neurons	Decreased hearing acuity and isolation (specifically, decreased ability to hear consonants)
	Loss of hearing from high to low frequency	Difficulty hearing, especially when there is background noise, or when speech is rapid
	Increased cerumen	Cerumen impaction may cause hearing loss
	Angiosclerosis of ear	
Sensory: Smell, taste, and touch	Decreased number of olfactory nerve fibers	Inability to smell noxious odors
		Decreased food intake
	Altered ability to taste sweet and salty foods; bitter and sour tastes remain	Safety risk with regard to recognizing dangers in the environment: hot water, fire alarms, or small objects that result in tripping
	Decreased sensation	
Endocrine	Decreased testosterone, GH, insulin, adrenal androgens, aldosterone, and thyroid hormone	Decreased ability to tolerate stressors such as surgery
	Decreased thermoregulation	Decreased sweating and shivering and temperature regulation
	Decreased febrile response	Lower baseline temperature; infection may not cause an elevation in temperature
	Increased nodularity and fibrosis of thyroid	Decreased insulin response, glucose tolerance
	Decreased basal metabolic rate	Decreased sensitivity of renal tubules to antidiuretic hormone
		Weight gain
		Increased incidence of thyroid disease

BUN, blood urea nitrogen; GFR, glomerular filtration rate; GH, growth hormone.

slow or eliminate many manifestations of aging (eg, statins and aspirin) we will likely approach these individuals differently.

It is now a commonly accepted notion that aging is a multifactorial process. Extended longevity is frequently associated with enhanced metabolic capacity and response to stress. The importance of genetics in the regulation of biological aging is demonstrated by the characteristic longevity of each animal species. However, heritability of life span accounts for ≤35% of its variance, whereas environmental factors account for >65% of the variance (Finch and Tanzi, 1997), and genes specifically selected to promote aging are unlikely to exist.

Several theories of aging have been promulgated and recently reviewed (Vijg and Wei, 1995; Kirkwood and Austad, 2000; Kaeberlein, 2007). These theories fall into either of three general categories: (1) accumulation of damage to informational molecules, (2) the regulation of specific genes, or (3) depletion of stem cells (Table 1-2).

Biological theories of aging focus on the belief that aging, or life span, is part of the organism's design. Researchers such as Hayflick (2007) promote the idea that genes do not drive the aging process but the general loss of molecular fidelity does. Specifically he postulates that every molecule becomes the substrate that experiences the thermodynamic instability characteristic of the aging process. Aging is thus different from disease as it occurs in every multicellular animal that reaches a fixed size at reproductive maturity, occurs in all species after reproductive maturity, and has the same universal molecular etiology, that is, thermodynamic instability.

TABLE 1-2   MAJOR THEORIES ON AGING

THEORY	MECHANISMS	MANIFESTATIONS
Accumulation of damage to informational molecules	Spontaneous mutagenesis Failure in DNA repair systems	Copying errors
	Errors in DNA, RNA, and protein synthesis	Error catastrophe
	Superoxide radicals and loss of scavenging enzymes	Oxidative cellular damage
Regulation of specific genes	Appearance of specific protein(s)	Genetically programmed senescence
Depletion of stem cells	Convergence of above mechanisms	Proliferative potential decreases

Evolution theory has been a traditional theory of aging as described by Darwin. This theory suggests that the designs of current organisms resulted from an incrementally accumulative evolutionary process. This is essentially the "survival of the fittest" premise as organisms that survived longer had more opportunity to breed and therefore propagate their particular design in the population. According to traditional Darwinian evolution theory, it is impossible for an organism to evolve in a way that reduces its life span, unless the evolution simultaneously improves the organism's ability to produce adult descendents. Human aging, however, does not improve our ability to procreate unless one emphasizes the group effect of having the old die to make room for the young. Many theories were subsequently developed to adjust the Darwinian evolution theory to correct for the changes in reproduction that occur. These include group selection theories, selfish gene theory, and evolvability theory. Evolvability theory, for example, holds that organisms can generally evolve characteristics that act to improve their ability to evolve and adapt to external circumstances by changing the genetic design of subsequent generations. If aging is a design feature, there might be increased benefit if a species could regulate life span. For example, the life spans of individual animals having the same genetic design could be adjusted to compensate for external conditions.

Damage theories are another group of theories of aging that have been propagated. These theories suggest that aging is a result of wearing out caused by damage to fundamental life processes that occur in accumulative microscopic increments such as damage to chromosomes, accumulation of poisonous by-products, nuclear radiation, or the forces of entropy. Damage theories are clearly pessimistic regarding medical intervention. For readers who seek additional information on theories of aging, please review the online resources included at the end of this chapter and the work of Goldsmith (2006) and Hayflick (2007).

DNA undergoes continuous change both in response to exogenous agents and intrinsic processes. Stability is maintained by the double-strandedness of DNA and by specific repair enzymes. It has been proposed that somatic mutagenesis, either owing to greater susceptibility to mutagenesis or deficits in repair mechanisms, is a factor in biological aging. In fact, there is a positive correlation of species longevity with DNA repair enzymes. In humans, the spontaneous mutagenesis rate is not adequate to account for the number of changes that would be necessary, and there is no evidence that a general failure in repair systems causes aging. However, limited maintenance and repair may lead to accumulation of somatic damage.

A related theory, the error catastrophe theory, proposes that errors occur in DNA, RNA, and protein synthesis, each augmenting the other and finally culminating in an error catastrophe. Translation was considered the most likely source for age-dependent errors because it was the final common pathway. However, increased translational errors have not been found in either in vivo or in vitro aging. Amino acid substitutions do not increase with age, although some enzyme activities may be altered by changes in posttranslational modification, such as glycosylation.

The major by-products of oxidative metabolism include superoxide radicals that can react with DNA, RNA, proteins, and lipids, leading to cellular damage and aging. There are several scavenging enzymes and some small molecules such as vitamins C and E that protect the cell from oxidative damage. There is no significant loss of scavenging enzymes in aging, and vitamins C and E do not increase longevity in experimental animals. However, interest in this hypothesis persists because overexpression of antioxidative enzymes retards the age-related accrual of oxidative damage and extends the maximum life span of transgenic fruit flies; moreover, caloric restriction lowers levels of oxidative stress and damage and extends the maximum life span of rodents (Finkel and Holbrook, 2000; Masoro, 2005).

One hypothesis of aging is that it is regulated by specific genes. Support for such a hypothesis has been gained mainly from yeast, nematodes, fruit flies, and models of in vitro aging. Several genes in yeast, nematodes, and fruit flies have been found to extend the species life span. They appear to reinforce the importance of metabolic capacity and stress responses in aging. By DNA microarrays, relatively few genes changed in human fibroblasts with aging, and downregulation of genes involved in control of mitosis was proposed as a possible general cause of aging (Ly et al., 2000). However, others have not shown the same gene pattern changes in other aging tissues, suggesting that different changes underlie aging in different tissues.

In adulthood, cells can be placed into one of three categories based on their replicative capacity: continuously replicating, replicating in response to a challenge, and nonreplicating. Epidermal, gastrointestinal, and hematopoietic cells are continuously renewed; the liver can regenerate in response to injury while neurons and cardiac and skeletal muscle do not regenerate.

In vitro replication is closely related to in vivo proliferation. Neurons and cardiac myocytes from adults can be maintained in culture but do not divide, whereas hepatocytes, marrow cells, endothelial cells, and fibroblasts replicate in vitro. Because they are easily obtained from skin, fibroblasts have been the most extensively studied. Although some cells continuously replicate in vivo, they have a finite replicative life. For fibroblasts in vitro, this is about 50 doublings (Hayflick, 2007). Replicative life in vitro correlates with the age of the donor, such that the older the donor, the fewer the doublings in vitro. With time in culture, doubling time decreases and ultimately stops. Several lines of evidence suggest that replicative senescence evolved to protect higher organisms from developing cancer (Campisi, 2000).

With each cell division, a portion of the terminal end of chromosomes (the telomere) is not replicated and therefore shortens. It is proposed that telomere shortening is the clock that results in the shift to a senescent pattern of gene expression and ultimately cell senescence (Fossel, 1998). Telomerase is an enzyme that acts by adding DNA bases to telomeres. Transfection of the catalytic component of this enzyme into senescent cells extends their telomeres as well as the replicative life span of the cells and induces a pattern of gene expression typical of young cells. The extent to which telomere shortening is relevant to cellular senescence and aging in vivo, however, remains unknown. In contrast, telomerase inhibitors may be potent anticancer therapies. The role of replicative senescence in aging and associated chronic disease processes is now being explored.

These experiments help define the finite life span of cells in vitro but do not themselves explain in vivo aging. However, factors associated with finite cell replication may more directly influence in vivo aging. Fibroblasts aged in vitro or obtained from older adult donors are less sensitive to a host of growth factors. Such changes occur at both the receptor and postreceptor levels. A decrease in such growth factors, a change in sensitivity to growth factors, and/or a slowing of the cell cycle may slow wound healing and thus place the older individual at greater risk for infection.

For tissues with nonreplicating cells, cell loss may lead to a permanent deficit. With aging, dopaminergic neurons are lost, thus influencing gait and balance and the susceptibility to drug side effects. With further decrements such as ischemia or viral infection, Parkinson disease may develop. Similar cell loss and/or functional deficits may occur in other neurotransmitter systems and lead to autonomic dysfunction as well as alteration in mental function and neuroendocrine control.

The immune system demonstrates similar phenomena. Lymphocytes from older adults have a diminished proliferative response to a host of mitogens. This appears to be a result of both a decrease in lymphokines and a decrease in response to extracellular signals. As the thymus involutes after puberty, levels of thymic hormones (thymosins) decrease.

Basal and stimulated interleukin-2 (IL-2) production and responsiveness also diminish with age. The latter appears to be due, at least in part, to a decreased expression of IL-2 receptors. Some immune functions can be restored by the addition of these hormones to lymphocytes in vitro, or in vivo, by their administration to aged animals. The proliferative defect can also be reversed in vitro by calcium ionophores and activators of protein kinase C, suggesting that the T-cell defect may be in transduction of extracellular signals to intracellular function. In vivo molecular mechanisms, such as those described above, contribute to physiologic deficits and altered homeostatic mechanisms that predispose older individuals to dysfunction in the face of stress and disease.

The gene for Werner syndrome, a progeric syndrome associated with the early onset of age-related changes—such as gray hair, balding, atherosclerosis, insulin resistance, and cataracts, but not Alzheimer disease—has been cloned. The gene codes for a helicase involved in DNA replication. There is great interest in understanding how a defect in just this one gene leads to the multiple abnormalities of this syndrome.

Molecular geneticists have also cloned several genes related to early-onset familial Alzheimer disease and identified susceptibility genes for the late-onset form of the disease (Tanzi et al., 1996).

A small number of families have mutations in the amyloid precursor protein located on chromosome 21. The largest number of families with early-onset familial Alzheimer disease have a mutation in a gene on chromosome 14. This gene has been named presenilin 1. A similar gene has been identified on chromosome 1 and labeled presenilin 2. The role of the presenilins in Alzheimer disease pathology is not yet known, but the identification of the three loci mentioned above has led to much excitement for the potential understanding of pathophysiologic mechanisms in this devastating disease. Similarly, the identification of apolipoprotein (apo E) alleles as risk factors for late-onset Alzheimer disease has raised interest in both the diagnosis and pathology of this disease.

Interventions that slow aging are likely to delay the onset of many important diseases including cancer, diabetes, cardiovascular diseases, and neurodegenerative diseases. Dietary restriction (DR) remains the major intervention in enhancing longevity (Reviewed in Masoro, 2005). DR is known to increase life span in yeast, worms, flies, and rodents. DR is not likely to be a successful intervention in humans. Therefore, much attention is being given to understanding the pathways that mediate DR and to the development of DR mimetics that target these pathways to enhance health and longevity without requiring reduced food consumption.

Growth hormone (GH) has received notoriety as a potential antiaging treatment, but so far has not been proven to be effective (reviewed in Perls, 2004). In rodents, reduced GH signaling, rather than increased activity, is correlated with increased longevity. In addition to reduced GH levels, reduced insulin and insulin-like growth factor-1 levels increase the life span of worms and flies. Human longevity, too, may be associated with more efficient glucose handling.

Stem cells offer hope to greatly extend the numbers and range of patients who could benefit from cell replacement therapy to treat debilitating diseases such as diabetes, Parkinson, Huntington, and Alzheimer. There is a long way to go in basic research before new therapies will be established, but clinical trials in some diseases are underway (Lovell-Badge, 2001).

Although there continue to be many theories of aging, there is some evidence to support the feasibility of antiaging medicine as we move toward the aging of the baby boomers and a new cohort of older adults. Caloric restriction, or nutritionally balanced semistarvation, when applied to mammals has been noted to increase life span as much as 50% (Antebi, 2007; Lenaerts, van Eygen, and van Fleteren, 2007). Research is focused on identifying an agent that would signal caloric restriction when it actually was not occurring and thus trick the aging system. Aging genes have been identified in mice and there is current research focused on disabling these aging genes by means of genetic engineering. In doing so, life span has been increased by 600% (Kenyon, 2002). Work continues in the area of genetics and attempts to alter aging through genetic manipulation. Research in genetics, and the interface between genetics and hormone signaling, is ongoing. This work has been informed by the study of human genetic disorders of Hutchinson-Guilford progeria and Werner syndrome, diseases in which accelerated aging occurs.

A defining feature of humans is their plasticity, or flexibility, in the range and spectrum of function, and in their ability to adapt to endogenous changes in themselves and exogenous changes in the environment. Findings from cognitive training studies in life span psychology, and use of mind plasticity interventions in individuals with early dementia, as well as physical training using a plasticity philosophy for those recovery neurological disorders such as stroke, have shown some useful outcomes. Increasingly we are finding that older adults still possess substantial reserved plasticity and even have demonstrated neurogenesis and physical and cognitive benefits to these interventions. While not a specific theory of aging, a philosophy of care of older adults that considers plasticity as an option is an important consideration and one in which future research will focus.

CLINICAL IMPLICATIONS

As we try to understand aging, we appreciate the limitations of available information. Several large studies in the United States, Israel, and Italy have followed cohorts of people longitudinally as they age. The findings thus far consistently suggest much variability to aging, despite anticipated declines in areas such as cardiovascular function; strength; and brain, bone, and muscle mass. Further there are indications that environment, behavior, and health are interrelated and can alter physical changes. For example, in Israeli older adults, normal renal function, good vision, avoiding afternoon naps, volunteer or compensated work, physical activity, and instrumental activities of daily living (IADL) independence, all correlated with improved survival. Moreover, good vision, volunteer work or work for pay, and physical activity were independently associated with continued functional independence over a 7-year period. Similar findings associated with remaining engaged in regular physical activity have been noted in the Baltimore Longitudinal Studies of Aging (http://www.grc.nia.nih.gov/branches/blsa/blsa.htm) and the Italian InChianti Study (http://www.inchiantistudy.net/).

The health-care provider must utilize the notion of variability in aging to help individuals make lifestyle and treatment choices to optimize their own aging. This is particularly true given that there are many age-related changes which occur that are lessened by medical and behavioral interventions. It has been noted that there are longitudinal changes in the rate of decline in peak Vo_2 in healthy adults. These changes are not constant across the age span in healthy persons, but accelerate markedly with each successive age decade, regardless of physical activity habits. Bone changes also occur with age and in addition to the common development of osteoporosis, persons with radiographic osteoarthritis, a common finding with age, lose bone at different rates than those with normal radiographs. This relationship varies between the site of the osteoarthritis and the site of measurement of bone mass density (BMD). Reports have shown that there tends to be significant longitudinal tissue loss for both gray and white matter even in the brains of very healthy older adults. Metabolic syndrome was noted to be a very common finding in aged Italians, and was associated with stroke and diabetes in both sexes.

Conversely, much evidence supports the benefit of lifestyle interventions, specifically diet and physical activity that will help to overcome some of the physical changes that can occur with age, and may improve overall health and quality of life. With regard to diet, repeatedly it has been noted that there are protective effects to diets low in saturated fats and high in fruits and vegetables. Likewise, engaging in regular physical activity, at least 30 minutes daily, has been noted to have not only physical but mental health benefits. Numerous resources help clinicians prescribe and motivate older adults to change prior behaviors and/or continue to engage in health-promoting activities (Table 1-3).

It is impossible to address aging without considering the psychosocial aspects that occur in addition to the more visible biological and physical changes (Rowe and Kahn, 1987). Transitions associated with aging are commonly noted around retirement, loss of a spouse or significant other, pet, home, car and ability to drive, as well as the loss of sensory function (hearing and vision), or ambulatory ability or capacity. Many fear the loss of independence with age, cognitive decline, and worry about having an acute catastrophic problem such as a hip fracture or stroke. Conversely, many older adults are quite resilient in the face of these losses and have much to teach the younger generation on how to respond to loss, optimize remaining function and ability, and adjust.

It is critical when working with older adults to be well aware of one's own beliefs with regard to theories of aging, attitudes about the aging process, and philosophies about how to age successfully. Recognizing these beliefs, clinicians must be open to evaluating their patient's beliefs and attitudes about aging and match interventions and recommendations with those beliefs. From a diagnostic perspective, this is particularly important as the older adults, who assume that with age it is normal to be short of breath, forgetful, and fatigued, may not report these symptoms as significant and thereby won't provide the health-care provider with the necessary information to facilitate a diagnosis. This requires the provider working with older adults to develop keen assessment skills and to use objective measures appropriately developed for older individuals.

Common examples of missed diagnoses occur related to cognitive impairment and depression. Older individuals, particularly those who have strong social skills and were well educated and engaged in social and professional activities throughout their life, may appear to be cognitively intact in the course of a social interaction and even a brief medical visit. However, on closer evaluation and with the use of standardized screening measures of memory, it may become evident that the individual has significantly impaired short-term memory. Functional assessment texts are particularly useful for a variety of assessments in older adults (Gallo et al., 2006) as are online resources (consultgerirn.org).

TABLE 1-3   WEB-BASED RESOURCES FOR HEALTH PROMOTION

National Guideline Clearinghouse	www.guideline.gov
Redi-Reference Clinical Guidelines Handbook	www.shop.store.yahoo.com/ pilotgearsw/redclinguide.html
Centers for Disease Control and Prevention: Healthy aging for older adults	http://www.cdc.gov/HealthyLiving/
Canadian Task Force on Preventive Health Care	www.ctfphc.org
National Cholesterol Education Program	www.nhlbi.nih.gov/about/ncep/
The Seventh Report of the Joint National Committee on Prevention, Detection, Evaluation, and Treatment of High Blood Pressure (JNC-7)	www.nhlbi.nih.gov/guidelines/ hypertension/
Agency for Healthcare Research and Quality Guidelines from the USPSTF	www.ahrq.gov/clinic/uspstfix.htm
American Academy of Family Physicians: Summary of policy recommendations for periodic health examinations	www.aafp.org/exam.xml

WEB-BASED RESOURCES RELATED TO EXERCISE FACILITATION IN OLDER ADULTS

AgePage: Exercise: Feeling fit for life	www.iamfitforlife.com/
The Exercise Assessment and Screening for You Tool	www.easyforyou.info
International Counsel on Active Aging	www.icaa.cc/
International Society for Aging and Physical Activity	http://www.isapa.org/ ISAPA_Newsletter/
National Blueprint: Increasing physical activity among adults age 50 and older	http://www.agingblueprint.org/tips.cfm

TABLE 1-3 WEB-BASED RESOURCES FOR HEALTH PROMOTION (*Continued*)

National Institute of Aging: Exercise: A guide from the National Institute of Aging	http://www.nia.nih.gov/ HealthInformation/Publications/ ExerciseGuide/
President's Council on Physical Fitness and Sports	http://www.fitness.gov/
YMCA Programs such as Active Older Adults (AOA)	http://www.ymca-austin.org/aoa.htm
The Canadian Centre for Activity and Aging's Home Support Exercise Program: Geriatrics and aging	http://www.geriatricsandaging.ca/ PDF/PDFJuly2003/ 0607homesupport.pdf
American Heart Association	http://www.americanheart.org
Fitness Past 50 Materials	http://www.fitnesspastfifty.com/ articles.html
International Council on Active Aging (ICAA)	http://www.icaa.cc/checklist.htm

A hallmark of aging is the reduced response to stress, including the stress of disease. Many symptoms of disease are not the direct effect of the disease, but rather the organism's response. Thus, the symptom intensity may be dampened by the aged body's decreased responsiveness. The presentation of illness in the geriatric patient can be thought of as a combination of dampened primary sound in the presence of background noise.

In treating an older adult, it is useful to keep in mind that an individual's ability to function depends on a combination of his or her characteristics (eg, innate capacity, motivation, pain tolerance, or fear) and the setting in which that person is expected to function. The same individual may be functional in one setting and dependent in another. Think of how well you would do if you were suddenly transported to a country where you could not speak the language or understand the customs. It is critical to allow the older adult to independently perform all activities during clinical encounters to facilitate a true assessment of capability and function. For example, observing the patient's ability to get up and down from an examination chair or table, walk into the examination room, and don and doff a shirt are critical components of the examination. Physicians and other primary health-care providers should serve as role models to encourage optimal function among older individuals. Unfortunately, caregivers, both formal and informal, may tend to provide unnecessary care for the older individual in an effort to decrease their risk of trauma or fatigue. This propagates a dependent status and can cause functional impairment and disability.

The clinician's first responsibility is to diagnose any acute clinical problems and alleviate all treatable symptoms. Once the patient's physical and psychological health has been optimized, the health-care provider has the opportunity to engage all members of the health-care team (nursing, physical and occupational therapy, social work, etc) to help the patient achieve their highest level of function and quality of life. For example, a social worker may help to identify community resources that can provide friendly visits to an older adult who is feeling isolated in the home setting.

Special consideration should be given to the older adult's physical and social environment. While multiple environmental assessments can be utilized (Gallo et al., 2006), it is also important to consider the fit between the individual and their environment. The Housing Enabler (www.enabler.nu/) is a tool that helps the clinician conduct such a comprehensive evaluation considering not only the environment and the environment risks, but the match of the person's functional abilities with that environment. Again, once evaluated the team can be utilized to identify interventions to decrease risks of falls and optimize function.

GERIATRIC SYNDROME

Because diagnoses often do not tell the whole story in geriatrics, it is more helpful to think in terms of presenting problems. One aid to recalling some of the common problems of geriatrics uses a series of Is:

- Immobility
- Instability
- Incontinence
- Intellectual impairment
- Infection
- Impairment of vision and hearing
- Irritable colon
- Isolation (depression)
- Inanition (malnutrition)
- Impecunity
- Iatrogenesis
- Insomnia
- Immune deficiency
- Impotence

The list is important for several reasons. Especially with older patients, the expression of the problem may not be a good clue to the etiology. Conversely, a problem may occur for a variety of reasons.

For example, immobility may be caused by a variety of underlying physical and emotional problems. The older individual may have sustained a fractured hip or congestive heart failure, a recent fall and fear of falling, or significant pain caused by degenerative joint disease, any or all of which may cause immobility. It is important to explore with the individual the underlying cause(s) so that appropriate interventions can be implemented. It may be necessary, for example, to alleviate patients' pain and address their fear of falling before initiating therapy or engaging the individual in a regular exercise program.

Among the list of Is is iatrogenesis, which is an all too common for older individuals. The risk of iatrogenesis increases with exposure to the care system. This includes tests, surgical intervention, and medications and treatments. In all patient interactions, the risk-benefit of any given treatment should be considered, and of course explained to the individual and their health-care proxy. Medication management in particular needs considerable and careful deliberation as older adults are well known to have marked changes in absorption, metabolism, and excretion (See Chap. 4). Even more dangerous is the careless, hasty application of clinical "labels." The patient who becomes confused and disoriented in the hospital may not be suffering from dementia. The individual who has an occasional urinary accident is not necessarily incontinent. Labeling patients as demented or incontinent is too often the first step toward their placement in a nursing home, a setting that can make such labels self-fulfilling prophecies. We must exercise great caution in applying these potent labels. They should be reserved for patients who have been carefully evaluated, lest we unnecessarily condemn countless persons to a lifetime of institutionalization.

ATYPICAL PRESENTATION OF COMMON CLINICAL PROBLEMS

One of the greatest challenges in the care of older adults is the atypical presentation of many diseases. It is not unusual for the first sign of an acute problem such as an infection (urine, respiration, or wound being the most common) to present with an atypical finding such as confusion, functional change, or a fall, rather than more typical symptoms such as urinary burning, cough, or fever. When the older individual has an underlying cognitive impairment, these changes may be very subtle and caregivers may report that "he just isn't himself today" without providing more specific clinical signs. It is not unusual for an independent and cognitively intact older individual to come into the office with complaints that they just didn't feel right or didn't feel like making their bed and on examination are in acute atrial fibrillation. Any report of this type of new or sudden change in the individual's behavior or function should be treated as an acute medical problem and a comprehensive evaluation should be done.

The first and principal task of the physician is to identify a correctable problem and correct it. No amount of rehabilitation, compassionate care, or environmental manipulation will compensate for missing a remediable diagnosis. However, diagnoses alone are usually insufficient. The elderly are the repositories of chronic disease more often cared for than cured. The process of geriatrics is thus threefold: (1) careful clinical assessment and management to identify acute and remediable problems, (2) ongoing management of underlying chronic illnesses, and (3) careful evaluation for evidence of geriatric syndromes (as per the Is above). It is only through optimal medical management of these clinical problems that the individual will be able to optimize the use of resources (eg, environmental interventions, social interactions) and achieve their highest level of health and function.

References

Antebi A. Ageing: when less is more. *Nature.* 2007 May 31;447(7144):536-537.

Banks J, Marmot M, Oldfield Z, et al. Disease and disadvantage in the United States and in England. *JAMA.* 2006;295:2037-2045.

Campisi J. Aging, chromatin, and food restriction—connecting the dots. *Science.* 2000;289(5487):2062-2063.

Cockcroft DW, Gault MH. Prediction of creatinine clearance from serum creatinine. *Nephron.* 1967;16:31-41.

Finch CE, Tanzi RE. Genetics of aging. *Science.* 1997; 278(5337):407-411.

Finkel T, Holbrook NJ. Oxidants, oxidative stress and the biology of ageing. *Nature.* 2000;408(6809):239-47.

Fossel M. Telomerase and the aging cell: implications for human health. *JAMA.* 1998;279(21):1732-1735

Gallo JJ, Bogner HR, Fulmer T, et al. *Handbook of Geriatric Assessment.* 4th ed. Rockville, MD: Aspen; 2006.

Gavrilova NS, Gavrilov LA. (2005). Living to 100 and beyond. International Symposium at the Society of Actuaries; 2006; http:// www.soa.org/research/life/research-living-to-100-and-beyond-search-for-predictors-of-exceptional-human.aspx. Last accessed August, 2008.

Goldsmith TC. (2006). Aging theories and their implications for medicine. http://www.azinet.com/aging/anti-aging_medicine.pdf. Last accessed June, 2008.

Hayflick L. Biological aging is no longer an unsolved problem. *Ann N Y Acad Sci.* 2007;1100:1-13.

Kaeberlein M. Molecular basis of ageing. *EMBO Rep.* 2007;8:907-911.

Kenyon C. Regulation of life-span by germ-line stem cells in *Caenorhabditis elegans. Science.* 2002;295:12-15.

Kirkwood TB, Austad SN. Why do we age? *Nature*. 2000;408(6809):233-238.

Lenaerts I, van Eygen S, van Fleteren J. Adult-limited dietary restriction slows gompertzian aging in *Caenorhabditis elegans*. *Ann N Y Acad Sci*. 2007 Apr;1100:442-448.

Lovell-Badge R. The future for stem cell research. *Nature*. 2001;414(6859):88-91.

Ly DH, Lockhart DJ, Lerner RA, Schultz PG. Mitotic misregulation and human aging. *Science*. 2000; 287(5462):2486-92.

Masoro EJ, Austad SN, eds. *Handbook of the Biology of Aging*. 5th ed. San Diego, CA: Academic Press; 2001.

Perls TT. Anti-aging quackery: human growth hormone and tricks of the trade: more dangerous than ever. *J Gerontol A Biol Sci Med Sci*. 2004;59:682-691.

Rowe JW, Kahn RL. Human aging: usual and successful. *Science*. 1987;237:143-149.

Schmidt K. Physiology and pathophysiology of senescence. *International Journal of vitamin and Nutrition Research*. 1999;69(3):150-153.

Tanzi RE, Kovacs DM, Kim T-W, et al. The gene defects responsible for familial Alzheimer's disease. *Neurobiol Dis*. 1996;3(16):159-168.

Vijg J, Wei JY. Understanding the biology of aging: the key to prevention and therapy. *J Am Geriatr Soc*. 1995;43:426-434.

Suggested Readings

Goldsmith TC. *The Evolution of Aging*. 2nd ed. Annapolis, MD: Azinet Press; 2006.

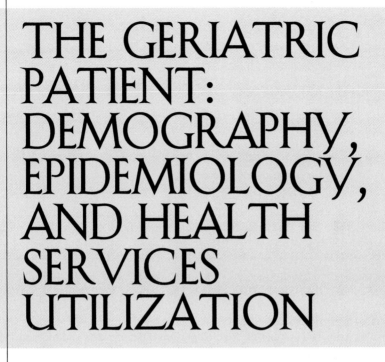

CHAPTER 2

THE GERIATRIC PATIENT: DEMOGRAPHY, EPIDEMIOLOGY, AND HEALTH SERVICES UTILIZATION

From the physician's perspective, the demographic curve strongly argues that medical practice in the future will include a great many geriatrics. Persons aged 65 years and older currently represent little more than one-third of the patients seen by a primary care physician; in 40 years, we can safely predict that at least every other adult patient will be an older person (ie, age 65 or older).

The concern so often heard about the epidemic of aging stems primarily from two factors: numbers and dollars. We hear a great deal of talk about the incipient demise of Social Security, the bankrupt status of Medicare, the death of the institution of family, and dire predictions of demographic cataclysms. There is, indeed, cause for concern but not necessarily for alarm. The message of the numbers is straightforward: we cannot go on as we have; new approaches are needed. The shape of those approaches to meeting the needs of growing numbers of elderly persons in this society will reflect societal values. The costs associated with an aging society have already stimulated major changes in the way we provide care.

There is actually some basis for optimism. Data from the National Long-term Care Survey show a decline in the rate of disability among older people. Overall, the rate of disability among older persons has decreased by 1% or more annually for last several decades. However, the growth in the aging population more than

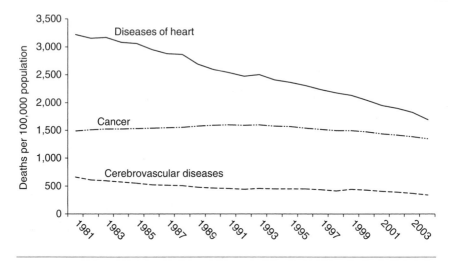

— FIGURE 2-1 — Deaths per 100,000 men, age 65 and over (age-adjusted), selected causes, 1981-2004. (Data source: The National Vital Statistics System.)

offsets this gain. The number of disabled persons aged 65 years and older in 1982 was 6.4 million. It increased to 7 million in 1994, and in 1999, the projected level of disability applied to population projections called for was about 9.3 million. It remains to be seen if this trend toward lower disability rates can be sustained, but if so, it will greatly offset the effects of an aging population. Death rates from major killers have been falling in some areas. As seen in Fig. 2-1, death in older men from heart disease has dropped precipitously, while death from cerebrovascular disease has declined somewhat, but death from cancer overall has not changed much. The pattern for women is very similar. Life expectancy at age 65 continues to increase for both men and women, and the gender gap is narrowing (Fig. 2-2).

However, aging is not the major contributor to the rapidly escalating costs of care. Although older people use a disproportionately large amount of medical care, most of the growth in costs is traceable to tremendous expansion in medical technology, both diagnostic and therapeutic. We have potent, but often, expensive tools at our disposal. In some ways, we can be said to be reaping the fruits of our success. While a substantial number of older people live to enjoy many active years, some persons who might not have survived in earlier times are now living into old age and bringing with them the chronic disease burden that would have been avoided by death.

The press for dramatic responses to the growth in the older population and its concurrent medical costs has led in two directions. Programs like managed care have been launched to serve Medicare beneficiaries in the hope that such approaches might constrain costs. To date, this promise has not been achieved.

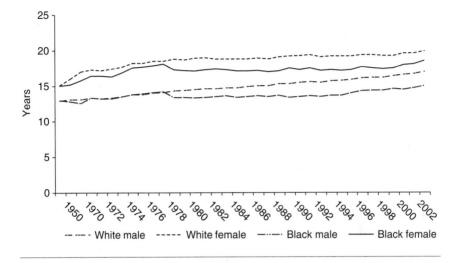

— FIGURE 2-2 —   Life expectancy at age 65 by sex and race/ethnicity, 1950-2003. (Data source: The National Vital Statistics System.)

Managed care programs face strong disincentives to enroll sick people and thus are not motivated to create programs that might attract such a clientele. Where they have taken steps to address chronic disease, they have relied on substitution to reduce the costs of hospitalizations. These substitutions have taken two forms: (1) They have cared for older persons in less expensive settings (eg, nursing homes in lieu of hospitals). (2) They have used other types of practitioners to supplement or supplant physicians (eg, nurse practitioners). There have been extensive efforts too to manage chronic diseases more effectively. Although the jury is still out on the effectiveness of disease management, there are growing doubts about it (Weingarten et al., 2002). Nonetheless, the hope persists that some variant of risk-based care could create incentives for greater efficiencies if more appropriate risk-adjusted capitation rates were developed. The second strategy has promoted rationing through the back door, by emphasizing the avoidance of futile care at the end of life. The technique for implementing this objective has been the use of advance directives. Rather than overtly limiting the availability of treatment, advance directives empower patients to authorize less care. However, as discussed in Chap. 17, advance directives may not appeal to many older persons. If such directives fail to stem the tide of end-of-life care, will more draconian strategies be employed?

Geriatricians have an important role to play in distinguishing age as a crude marker for basing care decisions from a simple indicator of where to look for better prognostic markers. For example, the difference in the course of breast cancer with age may not simply be an effect of age per se, but a difference in the distribution with age of salient genomic markers like *HER2/neu*. Thus, it would be more effective to examine the actual marker rather than relying on the gross proxy of age.

GROWTH IN NUMBERS

A look at a few trends will help to focus the problem. The numbers of older people in this country (and in the world) have been growing in both absolute and relative terms. The growth in numbers can be traced to two phenomena: (1) the advances in medical science that have improved survival rates from specific diseases and (2) the birth rate. The relative numbers of older persons is primarily the result of two birth rates: (1) the one that occurred 65 or more years ago and (2) the current one. The first one provides the people, most of whom will survive, to become old. The second means that the proportion of those who are old depends on how many were born subsequently. This ratio is critical in estimating the size of the workforce available to support an elderly population. The looming demographic crisis is based on the forecast of a large number of older persons increasing through the first half of the next century as a result of the post–World War II baby boom. That group of people, born in the late 1940s and early 1950s, will begin to reach seniority by 2010. The relative rate of growth increases with each decade over age 75 years. Indeed, many older persons are now surviving longer. It is no longer rare to encounter a centenarian; there are now over 84,000 of them. No wonder Hallmark makes "Happy 100th Birthday" greeting cards!

The impact of this projection can be better appreciated by looking at Table 2-1, which expresses the growth as a percentage of the total population. Although these forecasts can vary with the future birth and death rates, they are likely to be reasonably accurate. Thus, since the turn of the twentieth century, we have gone from a situation in which 4% of the population was aged 65 or older to a time when more than 12% has reached 65 years. By the year 2030, that older population will have almost doubled. Put another way, in 2030 there will be as many people older than 75 years as there are today who are older than 65 years. When that observation is combined with the reduction in births in the cohort behind the baby boomers, the social implications become more obvious. There will be fewer workers to support the larger older population. This demographic observation has led to several urgent recommendations: (1) redefine retirement age to recognize the increase in life expectancy and thereby reduce the ratio of retirees to workers, (2) encourage younger persons to personally save more for their retirement to avoid excessive dependency on public funds, and (3) change public programs to accrue surpluses to meet these projected drains.

Because older people use more health-care services than do younger people, there will be an even greater demand on the health-care system and a concomitant rise in total health-care costs. Because Medicare beneficiaries use more institutional

TABLE 2-1   THE ELDERLY POPULATION OF THE UNITED STATES:
             TRENDS 1900-2050

PERCENT OF THE TOTAL POPULATION							
AGE (YEARS)	1900	1940	1960	1990	2010	2030	2050
65-74	2.9	4.8	6.1	7.3	7.4	12.0	10.5
75-84	1.0	1.7	2.6	4.0	4.3	7.1	7.2
85+	0.2	0.3	0.5	1.3	2.2	2.7	5.1
65+	4.0	6.8	9.2	12.6	13.9	21.8	22.9

** US Senate Subcommittee on Aging; American Association of Retired Persons; Federal
Council on Aging; and US Administration on Aging. *Aging America: Trends and
Projections.* Washington, DC: US Department of Health and Human Services; 1991.
DHHS Publ No. (FCoA)91-28001.

services (ie, hospital and nursing home care), their health-care costs are higher
than those for younger groups. Only 12% of the population, those aged 65 years
and older, account for over one-third of health expenditures.

As seen in Table 2-2, health expenditures increase substantially with disability.
However, the rate of increase has been greater among those with less disability.

The increased number of older persons has been accompanied by a number
of changes in the way medical care is financed. Although these programs are

TABLE 2-2   AVERAGE PER CAPITA HEALTH SPENDING FOR MEDICARE
             BENEFICIARIES AGE 65 AND OVER (AGE-ADJUSTED) IN
             2003, DOLLARS BY FUNCTIONAL STATUS, 1992-2003

LIMITATIONS	1992	2003	%CHANGE 1992-2003
None	$4,257	$6,683	57%
Physical limitation only	$4,954	$7,639	54%
IADL	$8,243	$11,669	42%
1-2 ADLs	$10,533	$14,573	38%
3-6 ADLs	$24,368	$29,433	21%

Medicare Current Beneficiary Survey.
ADLs, activities of daily living; IADLs, instrumental activities of daily living.

discussed in more detail in Chap. 15, we note here that the appearance of programs such as Medicare and Medicaid, with all their shortcomings, has been associated with a growing expenditure on health care for older people and an increasing role in this area for public dollars. It is important to bear in mind that even in the face of greatly increased public financing, the elderly person still must bear a considerable share of the financial burden. In fact, in 2003, elderly persons' out-of-pocket costs for health care represented approximately 21% of their income, a figure comparable to before the passage of Medicare.

The growing number of older persons has created great consternation among forecasters. There is a sense of doom about a future in which all resources will go to support the elderly members of our society. To counter this ageist misimpression, two facts should be borne in mind: (1) The effects of technology on medical care costs dwarf the impact of an aging population. (2) The increasing numbers of older persons will be accompanied by a decrease in the proportion of those younger than 18 years. It is important to consider the overall dependency ratio. This index compares the proportion of the population younger than 18 and older than 65 years with that of persons between the ages of 18 and 64 years (the group presumed to be working to support the rest). While the relative contribution of the older population will increase impressively, the total will never be as high as it was in the mid-1960s.

The growth in the number of aged persons results from improvements in both social living conditions and medical care. Over the course of this century, we have moved from a preponderance of acute diseases (especially infections) to an era of chronic illnesses. Today at least two-thirds of all the money spent on health care goes toward chronic disease. (For older people that proportion is closer to 95%.) Medical care can be criticized for continuing to practice in a mode more suited to acute illness than chronic care. Information systems have not yet arisen in common practice to channel clinicians' attention to the problems associated with chronic care.

Table 2-3 reflects the changes in the common causes of death from 1900 to 2000. Many of those common at the turn of the twentieth century are no longer even listed. Today, the pattern of death in old age is generally similar to that of the population as a whole. The leading causes are basically the same, but there are some differences in the rankings. The leading causes of death are heart disease, cancer, stroke, chronic obstructive pulmonary disease (COPD), and influenza/pneumonia. Alzheimer disease features prominently.

Although the most dramatic reduction of mortality has occurred in infants and mothers, there has been a perceptible increase in survival even after age 65. Our stereotypes of what to expect from older people may therefore need reexamination. The average 65-year-old woman can expect to live another 19.2 years and a 65-year-old man another 16.3 years. Even at age 85, there is an expectation of more than 5 years.

However, this gain in survival includes both active and dependent years. Indeed, one of the great controversies of modern gerontological epidemiology is whether the gain in life expectancy brings with it equivalent gains in years free of

TABLE 2-3   CHANGES IN COMMONEST CAUSES OF DEATH, 1900-2000, ALL AGES AND THOSE 65 YEARS AND OLDER

| | RATE PER 100,000 | | | | | |
| | ALL AGES | | | | AGE 65+ | |
	1900	RANK	2000	RANK	2000	RANK
Diseases of heart	13.8	4	257.9	1	1712.2	1
Malignant neoplasms	6.4	8	200.5	2	1127.4	2
Cerebrovascular diseases	10.7	5	60.3	3	421.9	3
Chronic lower respiratory diseases	4.5	9	44.9	4	310.2	4
Influenza and pneumonia	22.9	1	24.3	7	173.3	5
Diabetes mellitus	1.1		24.9	6	149.8	6
Alzheimer disease			17.8	8	139.4	7
Senility	5.0	10				
Nephritis, nephritic syndrome, and nephrosis	8.9	6	13.7	9	90.8	8
Accidents	7.2	7	34.0	5	90.1	9
Septicemia			11.5	10	72.3	10
Tuberculosis	19.4	2				
Diarrhea and enteritis	14.3	3				

Data for 1900 from Linder and Grove, 1947; 2000 data from Minino, AM, Smith BL Deaths: Preliminary Data for 2000, National Vital Statistics Report, vol 49, No. 12, October 9, 2001, National Center for Health Statistics, Centers for Disease Control and Prevention.

dependency. The answer lies somewhere between. Although increased survival may be associated with more disability, the overall effect has been a pattern of decreasing disability (Cutler, 2001). Moreover, not all disability is permanent. Some older people experience transient episodes.

Some analysts have used disability as the basis for defining quality of life. They have then seized on the concept of active life expectancy to create a concept of quality-adjusted life years (QALYs). Under this formulation, which is especially popular with economists who are seeking a common denominator against which to weigh all interventions, the goal of health care is to maximize individuals' periods of disability-free time. However, such a formulation immediately raises concerns about the care of all those who are already frail; they would derive no benefit from any actions on their behalf unless they could convert them to a disability-free state.

DISABILITY

The World Health Organization distinguishes between impairments, disabilities, and handicaps. A disease may create impairment in organ function. That failure can eventually lead to a reduced ability to perform certain tasks. This inability to perform may become a handicap when those tasks are necessary to carry out social activities.

Hence, a handicap is the result of external demands and may be mitigated by environmental alterations. The distinction can provide a useful framework within which to consider the care of older persons.

There is a general pattern of increased impairment in the senses and in orthopedic problems with age. Because they tend to accumulate over time, the prevalence of chronic conditions increases with age. However, the nature of survivorship produces the occasional twist. The association between prevalence and age is not absolute. Those afflicted with diabetes and those with chronic lung disease, for example, do not survive as readily to age 85 and above. Despite having more chronic conditions and impairments, older people tend to report their health as generally good; 40% of those aged 65 and older rate their health as very good or excellent and another 32% rate it as good. This contrast highlights the coping abilities of elderly persons discussed in Chap. 1.

Because physicians tend to see the sick, they may form a distorted picture of the senior citizens. Most older persons are indeed self-sufficient and able to function on their own or with minimal assistance.

Those who need help are likely to be the very old. Functioning can be measured in a variety of ways. Commonly, we use the ability to perform specific tasks as a reflection of independence. These are grouped into two classes of measures. The term instrumental activities of daily living (IADLs) refers to tasks required to maintain an independent household. IADLs include such tasks as using the telephone, managing money, shopping, preparing meals, doing light housework, and getting around the community. They generally demand a combination of both physical and cognitive performance. Even among those at age 85 and above, more than half the population living in the community can still perform these tasks independently.

The ability to carry out basic self-care activities is reflected in the so-called activities of daily living (ADL). Dependencies in terms of ADL—which include

TABLE 2-4   PERCENT OF OLDER ADULTS HAVING ANY DIFFICULTY
PERFORMING SELECTED ACTIVITIES

	PERCENT		
	60-69 YEARS	70-79 YEARS	80+ YEARS
Managing money	6	10	24
Walking one-fourth mile	21	30	49
Lifting/Carrying 10 lb	22	28	46
Preparing own meals	8	12	27
Standing from armless chair	17	26	45
Getting in/out of bed	14	15	28
Dressing oneself	10	13	24
Going out for shopping, movies, etc	15	21	39

Ervin, RB Prevalence of Functional Limitations among Adults 60 Years of Age and Over:
United States, 1999-2002 Advance Data from Vital and Health Statistics No. 375, National
Center for Health Statistics, Centers for Disease Control and Prevention August, 2006.

such tasks as eating, using the toilet, dressing, transferring, walking, and bathing—
are less common than IADL losses. As shown in Table 2-4, even among the oldest groups, the prevalence of ADL dependency is quite low. Forty percent of
females aged 85 or more living in the community needed no assistance with any
IADL and more than 60% needed no help with ADL. Overall, among those aged
85 or more of both sexes living in the community, 16% needed help with one
ADL, 10% with two or three ADLs, and 9% with four or more ADLs.

SOCIAL SUPPORT

An important feature in determining an older person's ability to live in the
community is the extent of support available. The family is the heart of long-term
care (LTC). Family and friends provide the bulk of services in each category with,
or more often without, the help of formal caregivers. Informal care is largely provided by women.

Because women are both the major givers and receivers of LTC, a natural
coalition has formed between those advocating for improved LTC and women's
organizations. Even as women are entering the workforce in large numbers, they

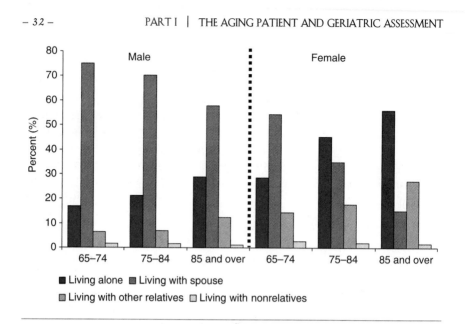

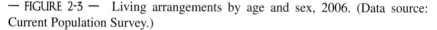

— FIGURE 2-3 — Living arrangements by age and sex, 2006. (Data source: Current Population Survey.)

continue to bear the majority of the caregiving load. Largely because they outlive men, over twice as many older women, as compared with men, live alone (Fig. 2-3), but the gap narrows by age 85. Wives and daughters are the most important source of family support for older persons.

Survey data suggest that more than 70% of persons aged 65 and older have surviving children. (Remember that the children of persons age 85 and older may themselves be aged 65 or older.) These "children" provide more than a third of the informal care.

The difference between needing and not needing a nursing home can depend on the availability of such support. Extrapolating from available data, we estimate that for every person older than age 65 in a nursing home, there are from one to three people equally disabled living in the community. The importance of social support must be kept continuously in mind. Formal community supports will continue to rely heavily on family and friends to see that adequate amounts of care are provided to maintain an elderly individual in the community. Efforts to reduce the burden of caregiving include encouraging respite care and providing direct assistance to the caregivers, both formal care to share the burden and pragmatic instruction about how to cope with the behavioral problems of demented patients. The physician must work diligently to maintain and bolster such support so as to avoid nursing home placement.

USE OF SERVICES

Chronic disease is more common with age. Figure 2-4 shows the prevalence of several common conditions in older persons. In general, the use of health-care services increases with age. The exception to the pattern of age-related increase is seen with dental care; it is not clear whether this reflects the lack of coverage under Medicare or a loss of teeth, but probably is at least greatly influenced by the former. Older people are more likely to see physicians because of chronic problems.

The introduction of a prospective payment system (PPS) for hospitals under Medicare in 1984 was associated with shorter lengths of stay and decreased admission rates. Table 2-5 shows the most common discharge diagnoses and surgical procedures in 2004. Heart disease, cancer, stroke, and pneumonia continue to dominate the scene. The growth of technology can be seen in the frequent use of procedures, especially catheterization and endoscopy.

The introduction of PPS greatly spurred the use of postacute care. Patients discharged earlier from hospitals often needed someplace to recuperate. As a result, Medicare began paying twice for hospital care. It paid a fixed amount for shorter stays and then often again for the posthospital care. Indeed, postacute care has been the fastest growing segment of Medicare. In reaction, the 1997 Balanced Budget Act imposed separate prospective payment methods on each of the predominate modes of postacute care (home health care, skilled nursing facilities, and inpatient rehabilitation). Table 2-6 shows the effects of the 1997 Balanced Budget Act on

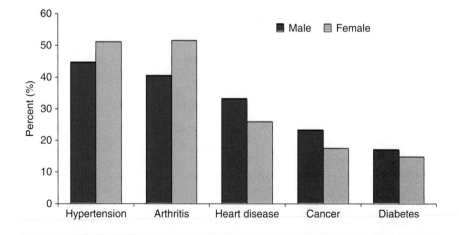

— FIGURE 2-4 — Percent of persons age 65 and over (age-adjusted) reporting selected chronic conditions by sex, 2004-2005. (Data source: National Health Interview Survey.)

TABLE 2-5   HOSPITAL DISCHARGE DIAGNOSES AND PROCEDURES
FOR PERSONS AGE 65 YEARS AND OLDER

DIAGNOSES	RATE PER 10,000 POPULATION
CONGESTIVE HEART FAILURE	225.0
Pneumonia	220.4
Cerebrovascular disease	175.6
Malignant neoplasms	172.2
Coronary atherosclerosis	158.6
Cardiac dysrhythmias	145.0
Acute myocardial infarction	126.6
Osteoarthritis	117.7
Chronic bronchitis	88.9
Fracture, neck of femur	79.6
Volume depletion	67.6
Psychoses	60.7
Diabetes mellitus	58.2
PROCEDURES	
Arteriography and angiography using contrast material	290.1
Cardiac catheterization	175.7
Endoscopy of small intestine	101.5
Balloon angioplasty of coronary artery	94.3
Insertion of coronary stent	87.2
Insertion, replacement, removal of cardiac pacemaker	84.3
Total knee replacement	80.3
Reduction of fracture	73.6
Coronary artery bypass graft	59.3
Cholecystectomy	40.9
Total hip replacement	37.3
Prostatectomy	29.1
Respiratory therapy	137.0
Diagnostic ultrasound	111.7
Computerized axial tomography	109.0
Hemodialysis	81.5
Insertion of endotracheal tube	71.9
Endoscopy of large intestine	64.3

DeFrances, CJ and Podgornik, 2004 National Hospital Discharge Survey. Advance Data from Vital and Health Statistics, Number 371, National Center for Health Statistics, Centers for Disease Control and Prevention, 2006.

TABLE 2-6   POSTACUTE CARE USED WITHIN 30 DAYS, 1996 AND 2000

	ANY PAC	SNF	REH	HHA	COMBINATION
Stroke, DRG 14					
1996	70%	37%	16%	33%	16%
2000	66%	37%	18%	26.7%	16%
Hip procedure, DRG 209					
1996	86%	43%	20%	57%	34%
2000	85%	43%	25%	51%	33%
Hip fracture, DRG 210 and 211					
1996	89%	68%	14%	33%	26%
2000	89%	70%	16%	29%	25%
COPD, DRG 88					
1996	42%	12%	NA	33%	4%
2000	36%	15%	NA	24%	5%
Pneumonia, DRG 89 and 90					
1996	46%	21%	NA	29%	5%
2000	42%	24%	NA	22%	5%
CHF, DRG 127					
1996	50%	15%	NA	39%	5%
2000	44%	18%	NA	29%	6%

CHF, chronic heart failure; COPD, chronic obstructive heart failure; DRG, diagnosis-related group; HHA, home health agency; NA, not applicable; PAC, postacute care; REH, inpatient rehabilitation unit; SNF, skilled nursing facility.

TABLE 2-7   PERCENT OF OFFICE VISITS BY SELECTED MEDICAL
CONDITIONS, 2005

	45-64 YEARS	65-74 YEARS	75+ YEARS
Arthritis	18.3	22.8	29.7
Ischemic heart disease	3.6	10.2	12.3
Congestive heart failure	1.3	2.9	6.5
Chronic obstructive pulmonary disease	4.0	9.1	8.4
Depression	12.4	7.2	7.8
Diabetes	13.6	20.0	16.7
Hypertension	29.9	43.8	46.4
Obesity	10.4	7.8	3.9

Cherry, DK, Woodwell, DA and Rechsteiner, EA National Ambulatory Medical Care
Survey: 2005 Summary. Advance Data from Vital and Health Statistics No. 387,
National Center for Health Statistics, Centers for Disease Control and Prevention,
2007.

postacute care use, for several conditions commonly associated with it. For those
often requiring active rehabilitation, the overall effects were minimal although there
was a shift away from home health-care use, but for the more medical conditions
there was a decrease in postacute care use, especially in home health care.

Table 2-7 describes the patterns for ambulatory visits at various ages. Despite
the general principle that bad things are more common with increasing age after
age 75, not all diagnoses increase with age.

NURSING HOME USE

The nursing home has traditionally been used as the touchstone for LTC, but
its role has changed with the changes in hospital payment under Medicare. The
fixed-payment approach and the consequent shortening of hospital stays have
spawned a new industry of posthospital care, sometimes called subacute care. In
effect, care that was formerly rendered in a hospital is now provided in other settings, including the nursing home and the home of the patient.

Some nursing homes have sought to increase their capacity to support such
care by upgrading their nursing staffs, but others have adopted the new title without

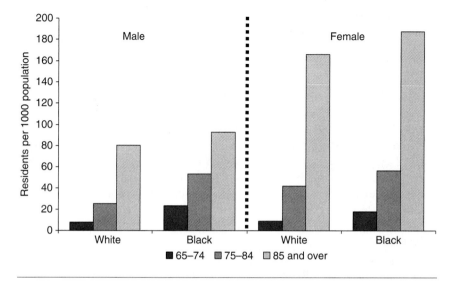

— FIGURE 2-5 — Nursing home residents per 1000 population by age, sex, and race/ethnicity, 2004. (Data source: The National Nursing Home Survey.)

changing their modus operandi. Thus, the distinction between long-stay and short-stay nursing home residents has become more exaggerated. Some residents are there for chronic care, whereas others are just visiting for a brief spell of recuperation and rehabilitation.

While nursing homes have increased their Medicare business dramatically, their long-stay business has been threatened by a growing disinclination to use such facilities. New forms of care, like assisted living, have provided other options, especially for those who can pay for such care.

We are prone to cite an estimated 5% for the proportion of those aged 65 years and older who are in nursing homes at any moment. Such a figure is a potentially misleading generalization in two respects. As Fig. 2-5 suggests, age is a very important factor. Among those age 65 to 74 years old, the rate is less than 2%. It rises to approximately 7% for those aged 75 to 84 and then jumps to 20% for those aged 85 and older. Moreover, what were formerly considered permanent stays have increasingly become transient visits. Thus, it is important to distinguish between these prevalence rates and the lifetime probability of entering a nursing home. Longitudinal studies suggest that persons age 65 have better than a 40% chance of spending some time in a nursing home before they die. Of those who enter a nursing home, 55% will spend at least 1 year there and 21% will spend 5 years or more (Kemper and Murtaugh, 1991). The proportion of persons spending at least some time in a nursing home is likely to increase if nursing homes continue to play a role in subacute care.

Nursing homes are needed not only because of the presence of diseases or even functional disabilities, but also as a result of a lack of social support. Often the family becomes exhausted after caring for an elderly patient for a long period. Family fatigue is especially a problem when the patient has symptoms that are very disruptive.

Among the most disturbing are incontinence and behavior problems that involve wandering or disruptive behavior. Table 2-8 summarizes the factors associated with increased likelihood of nursing home placement.

Approximately three-fourths of nursing home admissions come from hospitals. A 3-day hospital stay is a prerequisite for nursing home coverage available under Medicare (unless the patient is covered under a managed care plan). The hospitalization often represents the last step in a series of steps involving the deterioration of the patient and the patient's social supports. For others, the hospitalization results from an acute event, for example, a broken hip or a stroke, which then necessitates LTC.

In 2004, almost 20% of hospital patients aged 65 and older were discharged to nursing homes. As with those from the community, the rate of nursing home placement increases with age and is greater for females than for males. Table 2-8 summarizes some of the factors that can identify those older patients in hospitals at risk of nursing home placement. The most significant single factor predicting discharge to a nursing home is being admitted from one. Effectively all of the nursing home residents who survive their hospital stay will be returned to a nursing home. For those patients originating from the community, the most important factors are associated with dependency and cognitive status. Compared with those going home or to a rehabilitation unit, nursing home admissions are likely to have worse functional status and more confusion (Kane et al., 1996). Models have been developed to predict the time to nursing home admission for persons with Alzheimer disease (Stern et al., 1997).

Especially now that nursing home care includes both subacute and LTC, any analysis of nursing home residents must carefully distinguish between data based on a study of those who reside in a facility at a given time and those entering or leaving the facility. The conclusions reached about the nursing home population may be quite different depending on which groups are examined.

Short-stay and long-stay residents have distinct characteristics. The former tend to be younger, have more physical problems, and enter from the hospital. The long-term residents are more likely to be older, confused, and incontinent.

Nursing home data can be very confusing. Not only must one distinguish between admissions and residents but one must also look at the time course of former residents to appreciate the true nature of such LTC. On the one hand, the picture is much more dynamic than is usually suspected. The majority of persons admitted to a nursing home are discharged within 3 months. On the other hand, many of these people die in the nursing home, and many of the discharges are really transfers to hospitals. From there a majority of patients either return to the

TABLE 2-8   FACTORS AFFECTING THE NEED FOR NURSING HOME ADMISSION

Characteristics of the individual
   Age, sex, race
   Marital status
   Living arrangements
   Degree of mobility
   Activities of daily living
   Instrumental activities of daily living
   Clinical prognosis
   Level of function prior to hospitalization
   Urinary continence
   Behavior problems
   Mental status/Memory impairment
   Mood disturbance
   Ability to distinguish both sides of body
   Vertigo and falls
   Ability to manage medication
   Income
   Payment eligibility
   Need for special services
Characteristics of the support system
   Family capability
      For married respondents, age of spouse
      Presence of responsible relative (usually adult child)
      Family structure of responsible relative
      Employment status of responsible relative
   Physician availability
   Amount of care currently received from family and others
Community resources
   Formal community resources
   Informal support systems
   Presence of long-term care institutions
   Characteristics of long-term care institutions

nursing home or die in a hospital. It is more accurate to talk about LTC "careers" than to think in terms of discrete episodes.

As we enter an era of more aged persons with chronic disease, physicians will find themselves working increasingly in institutions such as nursing homes. They will be challenged to provide leadership in upgrading the care available in such settings. They will need to be familiar with the array of resources available to meet the needs of their patients and the factors determining access to these resources. A guide to long-term care resources is presented in Chap. 15.

References

Cutler DM. Declining disability among the elderly. *Health Aff (Millwood)*. 2001;20(6):11-27.

Kane RL, Finch M, Blewett L, et al. Use of post-hospital care by Medicare patients. *J Am Geriatr Soc*. 1996;44:242-250.

Kemper P, Murtaugh CM. Lifetime use of nursing home care. *N Engl J Med*. 1991;324:595-600.

Linder FE, Grove RD. *Vital Statistics Rates in the United States 1900–1940*. Washington, DC: US Government Printing Office; 1947.

Stern Y, Tang MX, Albert MS, et al. Predicting time to nursing home care and death in individuals with Alzheimer disease. *JAMA*. 1997;277(10):806-812.

Weingarten SR, Henning JM, Badamgarav E, et al. Interventions used in disease management programmes for patients with chronic illness—which ones work? Meta-analysis of published reports. *BMJ*. 2002;325:925-932.

Suggested Readings

Cutler DM, Rosen AB, Vijan S. The value of medical spending in the United States, 1960–2000. *New Engl J Med*. 2006;355(9):920-927.

Fries JF. Aging, natural death, and the compression of morbidity. *N Engl J Med*. 1980;303:130-136.

Gill TM, Williams CS, Tinetti ME. Assessing the risk for the onset of functional dependence among older adults: the role of physical performance. *J Am Geriatr Soc*. 1995;43:603-609.

Moon M. What Medicare has meant to older Americans. *Health Care Fin Rev*. 1996;18(2):49-59.

Vita AJ, Terry RB, Hubert HB, et al. Aging, health risks, and cumulative disability. *N Engl J Med*. 1998;338:1035-1041.

CHAPTER 3

EVALUATING THE GERIATRIC PATIENT

Comprehensive evaluation of an older individual's health status is one of the most challenging aspects of clinical geriatrics. It requires sensitivity to the concerns of people, awareness of the many unique aspects of their medical problems, ability to interact effectively with a variety of health professionals, and often a great deal of patience. Most importantly, it requires a perspective different from that used in the evaluation of younger individuals. Not only are the a priori probabilities of diagnoses different, but one must be attuned to more subtle findings. Progress may be measured on a finer scale. Special tools are needed to ascertain relatively small improvements in chronic conditions and overall function compared with the more dramatic cures of acute illnesses is often possible in younger patients. Creativity is essential in order to incorporate these tools efficiently in a busy clinical practice.

The purpose of the evaluation and the setting in which it takes place will determine its focus and extent. Considerations important in admitting a geriatric patient with a fractured hip and pneumonia to an acute care hospital during the middle of the night are obviously different from those in the evaluation of an older demented patient exhibiting disruptive behavior in a nursing home. Elements included in screening for treatable conditions in an ambulatory clinic are different from those in assessment of older individuals in their own homes or in long-term care facilities.

Despite the differences dictated by the purpose and setting of the evaluation, several essential aspects of evaluating older patients are common to all purposes and settings. Figure 3-1 depicts these aspects. Several comments on addressing them are in order:

1. Physical, psychological, and socioeconomic factors interact in complex ways to influence the health and functional status of the geriatric population.
2. Comprehensive evaluation of an older individual's health status requires an assessment of each of these domains. The coordinated efforts of several different health-care professionals functioning as an interdisciplinary team are needed.

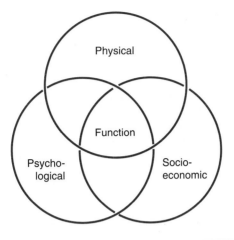

— FIGURE 3-1 —   Components of assessment of older patients.

3. Functional abilities should be a central focus of the comprehensive evaluation of geriatric patients. Other more traditional measures of health status (such as diagnoses and physical and laboratory findings) are useful in dealing with underlying etiologies and detecting treatable conditions, but in the geriatric population, measures of function are often essential in determining overall health, well-being, and the need for health and social services.

Just as function is the common language of geriatrics, assessment lies at the heart of its practice. Special techniques that address multiple problems and their functional consequences offer a way to structure the approach to complicated geriatric patients. The core of geriatric practice has been considered the comprehensive geriatric assessment, but its role has been actively debated. Geriatric assessment has been tested in a variety of forms. Table 3-1 summarizes the findings from a number of randomized controlled trials of different approaches to geriatric assessment. Annual in-home comprehensive geriatric assessment as a preventive strategy demonstrated the potential to delay the development of disability and reduce permanent nursing home stays (Stuck et al., 2002). Controlled trials of approaches to hospitalized geriatric patients suggest comprehensive geriatric assessment by a consultation team with limited follow-up does not improve health or survival of selected geriatric patients (Reuben et al., 1995), but that a special acute geriatric unit can improve function and reduce discharges to institutional care (Landefeld et al., 1995). A controlled multisite Veterans Affairs (VA) trial of inpatient geriatric evaluation and management demonstrated significant reductions in functional decline without increased costs

TABLE 3-1 EXAMPLES OF RANDOMIZED CONTROLLED TRIALS OF GERIATRIC ASSESSMENT

SETTING	EXAMPLES OF ASSESSMENT STRATEGIES	SELECTED OUTCOMES[*]
Community/Outpatients	Social worker assessment and referral Nursing assessment and referral Annual in-home assessment by nurse practitioner Multidisciplinary clinic assessment	Reduced mortality Reduced hospital use Reduced permanent nursing home use Delayed development of disability
Hospital inpatient (specialized units)	Interdisciplinary teams with focus on function, geriatric syndromes, rehabilitation	Reduced mortality Improved function Reduced acute hospital and nursing home use
Hospital inpatient consultation	Geriatric consultation teams	Mixed results Some studies improved function and lower short-term mortality Other studies show no effects

* Not all studies show improvements in all outcomes. See text and Rubenstein et al., 1991.

(Cohen et al., 2002). Results of outpatient geriatric assessment have been mixed and less compelling (Cohen et al., 2002). However, a randomized trial of outpatient geriatric assessment with an intervention to improve adherence to the recommendations prevented functional decline (Reuben et al., 1999).

There is considerable variation in approaches to the comprehensive assessment of geriatric patients. Various screening and targeting strategies have been used to identify appropriate patients for more comprehensive assessment. These strategies range from selection based on age to targeting patients with a certain number of impairments or specific conditions. Sites of assessment vary as well, and include the clinic, the home, the hospital, and different levels of long-term care. Geriatric assessment also varies in terms of which discipline carries out the different components of the assessment as well as in the specific assessment tools used. Despite the dramatic variation in approach to targeting, personnel used, and measures employed, a clear pattern of effectiveness has emerged. Taken together, these results are both heartening and cautioning. Systematic approaches to patient care are obviously desirable. The issue is more how formalized these assessments should be. Research suggests that the specifics of the assessment process seem to be less important than the very act of systematically approaching older people with the belief that improvement is possible.

A major concern about such assessments is efficiency. Because of the multi-dimensional nature of geriatric patients' problems and the frequent presence of multiple interacting medical conditions, comprehensive evaluation of the geriatric patient can be time consuming and thus costly. It is important to reduce duplication of effort. It is possible to have interprofessional collaboration in determining what data should be collected, but the actual data collection is best delegated to one or, at most, a few team members. Additional expertise can be brought to bear if the initial screening uncovers an area that requires it. Another crucial lesson is that assessment without follow-up is unlikely to make any difference. Thus, the term "geriatric assessment" has given way to the concept of geriatric evaluation and management. There must be strong commitment to act on the problems uncovered and to follow up long enough to be sure they have responded to the treatment prescribed.

Strategies that can make the evaluation process more efficient include the following:

1. The development of a close-knit interdisciplinary team with minimal redundancy in the assessments performed.
2. Use of carefully designed questionnaires that reliable patients and/or caregivers can complete before an appointment.
3. Incorporation of screening tools that target the need for further, more in-depth assessment.
4. Use of assessment forms that can be readily incorporated into a computerized relational database.
5. Integration of the evaluation process with case management activities that target services based on the results of the assessment.

This chapter focuses on the general aspects of assessing geriatric patients; sections on geriatric consultation, preoperative evaluation, and environmental assessments are included in the chapter.

Chapter 14 includes information on case management and other health services and Chap. 15 is devoted to the assessment and management of geriatric patients in the nursing home setting.

HISTORY

Sir William Osler's aphorism, "Listen to the patient, he'll give you the diagnosis," is as true in older patients as it is in younger patients. In the geriatric population, however, several factors make taking histories more challenging, difficult, and time consuming.

Table 3-2 lists difficulties commonly encountered in taking histories from geriatric patients, the factors involved, and some suggestions for overcoming these difficulties. Impaired hearing and vision (despite corrective devices) are common and can interfere with effective communication.

Techniques such as eliminating extraneous noises, speaking slowly and in deep tones while facing the patient, and providing adequate lighting can be helpful. The use of simple, inexpensive amplification devices with Walkman-style earphones can be especially effective, even among the severely hearing impaired. Patience is truly a virtue in obtaining a history; because thought and verbal processes are often slower in older than in younger individuals, patients should be allowed adequate time to answer in order not to miss potentially important information. At the same time, the cardinal rule of open-ended questions may need to be tempered to get the maximum amount of information in the time allocated.

Many older individuals underreport potentially important symptoms because of their cultural and educational backgrounds as well as their expectations of illness as a normal concomitant of aging. More aggressive probing may be necessary. Fear of illness and disability or depression accompanied by a lack of self-concern may also render the reporting of symptoms less frequent. Altered physical and physiologic responses to disease processes (see Chap. 1) can result in the absence of symptoms (such as painless myocardial infarction or ulcer and pneumonia without cough). Symptoms of many diseases can be vague and nonspecific because of these age-related changes. Impairments of memory and other cognitive functions can result in an imprecise or inadequate history and compound these difficulties. Asking specifically about potentially important symptoms (such as those listed in Table 3-3) and using other sources of information (such as relatives, friends, and other caregivers) can be very helpful in collecting more precise and useful information in these situations.

At the other end of the spectrum, geriatric patients with multiple complaints can frustrate the health-care professional who is trying to sort them all out. The multiplicity of complaints can relate to the prevalence of coexisting chronic and acute conditions in many geriatric patients. These complaints may, however, be deceiving. Somatic symptoms may be manifestations of underlying emotional distress rather than symptoms of a physical illness, and symptoms of physical conditions may be exaggerated by emotional distress (see Chap. 5). Getting to

TABLE 3-2   POTENTIAL DIFFICULTIES IN TAKING GERIATRIC HISTORIES

DIFFICULTY	FACTORS INVOLVED	SUGGESTIONS

Communication	Diminished vision
	Diminshed hearing
		Use well-lit room
		Eliminate extraneous noise
		Speak slowly in a deep tone
		Face patient, allowing
		  patient to see your lips
		Use simple amplification
		  device for severely
		  hearing impaired
		If necessary, write
		  questions in large print

	Slowed psychomotor performance	Leave enough time for the patient to answer

Underreporting of
symptoms
	Health beliefs
	Fear
	Depression
	Altered physical and
	  physiological responses
	  to disease process
	Cognitive impairment
		Ask specific questions
		  about potentially
		  important symptoms
		  (see Table 3-3)
		Use other sources of
		  information (relatives,
		  friends, other caregivers)
		  to complete the history

Vague or non
specific symptoms
	Altered physical and
	  physiological responses
	  to disease process
	Altered presentation of
	  specifc diseases
	Cognitive impairment
		Evaluate for treatable
		  diseases, even if the
		  symptoms (or signs) are
		  not typical or specific
		  when there has been a
		  rapid change in function
		Use other sources of infor-
		  mation to complete history

Multiple complaints	Prevalence of multiple
	  coexisting diseases
	Somatization of
	  emotions— "masked
	  depression"
	  (see Chap. 7)
		Attend to all somatic
		  symptoms, ruling out
		  treatable conditions
		Get to know the patient's
		  complaints; pay special
		  attention to new or
		  changing symptoms
		Interview the patient on
		  several occasions to
		  complete the history

TABLE 3-3   IMPORTANT ASPECTS OF THE GERIATRIC HISTORY

SOCIAL HISTORY

Living arrangements
Relationships with family and friends
Expectations of family or other caregivers
Economic status
Abilities to perform activities of daily living (see Table 3-8)
Social activities and hobbies
Mode of transportation
Advance directives (see Chap. 17)

PAST MEDICAL HISTORY

Previous surgical procedures
Major illnesses and hospitalizations
Previous transfusions

Immunization status
    Influenza, pneumococcus, tetanus

Preventive health measures
    Mammography
    Papanicolaou (Pap) smear
    Flexible sigmoidoscopy
    Antimicrobial prophylaxis
    Estrogen replacement

Tuberculosis history and testing

Medications (use the "brown bag" technique; see text)
    Previous allergies
    Knowledge of current medication regimen
    Compliance

Perceived beneficial or adverse drug effects

SYSTEMS REVIEW

Ask questions about general symptoms that may indicate treatable underlying disease such as fatigue, anorexia, weight loss, insomnia, recent change in functional status

TABLE 3-3　IMPORTANT ASPECTS OF THE GERIATRIC HISTORY
　　　　　　(*Continued*)

SYSTEMS REVIEW

Attempt to elicit key symptoms in each organ system, including the following:

SYSTEM	KEY SYMPTOMS
Respiratory	Increasing dyspnea Persistent cough
Cardiovascular	Orthopnea Edema Angina Claudication Palpitations Dizziness Syncope
Gastrointestinal	Difficulty chewing Dysphagia Abdominal pain Change in bowel habit
Genitourinary	Frequency Urgency Nocturia Hesitancy, intermittent stream, straining to void Incontinence Hematuria Vaginal bleeding
Musculoskeletal	Focal or diffuse pain Focal or diffuse weakness
Neurological	Visual disturbances (transient or progressive) Progressive hearing loss Unsteadiness and/or falls Transient focal symptoms
Psychological	Depression Anxiety and/or agitation Paranoia Forgetfulness and/or confusion

know patients and their complaints and paying particular attention to new or changing symptoms are helpful in detecting potentially treatable conditions.

Clinicians may become frustrated with older patients' slow pace and their tendency to wander from the subject at hand. In desperation, they shift their focus to the accompanying family members, who can provide a more lucid and linear history. But this tendency to bypass the older patient can have several serious effects. Not only does it diminish the self-image of the older patient and reinforce a message of dependency, it may miss important information that they patient knows but the family member does not.

Table 3-3 lists aspects of the history that are especially important in geriatric patients. It is often not feasible to gather all information in one session; shorter interviews in a few separate sessions may prove more effective in gathering these data from some geriatric patients.

Some topics that may be especially important to an older person's quality of life are often skipped over because they are embarrassing to the clinician or the patient. Issues like fecal and urinary incontinence and sexual dysfunction can be important areas to explore. Given its prevalence, its vulnerability to treatment and its ability to complicate the care of other conditions, it is important to screen for depression. Chapter 7 reviews the measures available for depression screening in older patients.

Often shortchanged in medical evaluations, the social history is a critical component. Understanding the patient's socioeconomic environment and ability to function within it is crucial in determining the potential impact of an illness on an individual's overall health and need for health services. Especially important is the assessment of the family's feelings and expectations. Many family caregivers of frail geriatric patients have feelings of both anger (at having to care for a dependent family member) and guilt (over not being able or willing to do enough) and have unrealistic expectations. Such unrealistic expectations are often based on a lack of information and can interfere with care if not discussed. Unlike younger patients, older patients often have had multiple prior illnesses. The past medical history is, therefore, important in putting the patient's current problems in perspective; this can also be diagnostically important. For example, vomiting in an elderly patient who has had previous intra-abdominal surgery should raise the suspicion of intestinal obstruction from adhesions; nonspecific constitutional symptoms (such as fatigue, anorexia, and weight loss) in a patient with a history of depression should prompt consideration of a relapse. Because older individuals are often treated with multiple medications, they are at increased risk of noncompliance and adverse effects (see Chap. 14). A detailed medication history (including both prescribed and over-the-counter drugs) is essential.

The brown bag technique is very helpful in this regard; have the patient or caregiver empty the patient's medicine cabinet (prescribed and over-the-counter drugs as well as nontraditional remedies) into a brown paper bag and bring it at each visit. More often than not, one or more of these medications can, at least in theory, contribute to geriatric patients' symptoms. Clinicians should not hesitate to turn to pharmacists for help in determining potential drug interactions.

A complete systems review, focusing on potentially important and prevalent symptoms in the elderly, can help overcome many of the difficulties described above. Although not intended to be all-inclusive, Table 3-3 lists several of these symptoms.

General symptoms can be especially difficult to interpret. Fatigue can result from a number of common conditions such as depression, congestive heart failure, anemia, and hypothyroidism. Anorexia and weight loss can be symptoms of an underlying malignancy, depression, or poorly fitting dentures and diminished taste sensation. Age-related changes in sleep patterns, anxiety, gastroesophageal reflux, congestive heart failure with orthopnea, or nocturia can underlie complaints of insomnia. Because many frail geriatric patients limit their activity, some important symptoms may be missed. For example, such patients may deny angina and dyspnea but restrict their activity to avoid the symptoms. Questions such as "How far do you walk in a typical day?" and "What is the most activity you carry out in a typical day?" can be helpful in patients suspected of limiting their activities to avoid certain symptoms.

PHYSICAL EXAMINATION

The common occurrence of multiple pathologic physical findings superimposed on age-related physical changes complicates interpretation of the physical examination. Table 3-4 lists common physical findings and their potential significance in the geriatric population.

An awareness of age-related physical changes is important to the interpretation of many physical findings and therefore subsequent decision making. For example, age-related changes in the skin and postural reflexes can influence the evaluation of hydration and volume status; age-related changes in the lung and lower-extremity edema secondary to venous insufficiency can complicate the evaluation of symptoms of heart failure.

Certain aspects of the physical examination are of particular importance in the geriatric population. Detection and further evaluation of impairments of vision and hearing can lead to improvements in quality of life. Evaluation of gait may uncover correctable causes of unsteadiness and thereby prevent potentially devastating falls (see Chap. 9). Careful palpation of the abdomen may reveal an aortic aneurysm, which, if large enough, might warrant consideration of surgical removal. The mental status examination is especially important; this aspect of the physical examination is discussed later and in Chap. 6.

TABLE 3-4   COMMON PHYSICAL FINDINGS AND THEIR POTENTIAL
              SIGNIFICANCE IN GERIATRICS

PHYSICAL FINDINGS	POTENTIAL SIGNIFICANCE
VITAL SIGNS	
Elevated blood pressure	Increased risk for cardiovascular morbidity; therapy should be considered if repeated measurements are high (see Chap. 11)
Postural changes in blood pressure	May be asymptomatic and occur in the absence of volume depletion. Aging changes, deconditioning, and drugs may play a role. Can be exaggerated after meals. Can be worsened and become symptomatic with antihypertensive, vasodilator, and tricyclic antidepressant therapy
Irregular pulse	Arrhythmias are relatively common in otherwise asymptomatic elderly; seldom need specific evaluation or treatment (see Chap. 11)
Tachypnea	Baseline rate should be accurately recorded to help assess future complaints (such as dyspnea) or conditions (such as pneumonia or heart failure)
Weight changes	Weight gain should prompt search for edema or ascites. Gradual loss of small amounts of weight common; losses in excess of 5% of usual body weight over 12 months or less should prompt search of underlying disease

TABLE 3-4   COMMON PHYSICAL FINDINGS AND THEIR POTENTIAL
SIGNIFICANCE IN GERIATRICS (*Continued*)

PHYSICAL FINDINGS	POTENTIAL SIGNIFICANCE
GENERAL APPEARANCE AND BEHAVIOR	
Poor personal grooming and hygiene (eg, poorly shaven, unkempt hair, soiled clothing)	Can be signs of poor overall function, caregiver's neglect, and/or depression; often indicates a need for intervention
Slow thought processes and speech	Usually represents an aging change; Parkinson disease and depression can also cause these signs
Ulcerations	Lower extremity vascular and neuropathic ulcers common Pressure ulcers common and easily overlooked in immobile patients
Diminished turgor	Often results from atrophy of subcutaneous tissues rather than volume depletion; when dehydration suspected, skin turgor over chest and abdomen most reliable
EARS (SEE CHAP. 13)	
Diminished hearing	High-frequency hearing loss common; patients with difficulty hearing normal conversation or a whispered phrase next to the ear should be evaluated further Portable audioscopes can be helpful in screening for impairment
EYES (SEE CHAP. 13)	
Decreased visual acuity (often despite corrective lenses)	May have multiple causes, all patients should have thorough optometric or ophthalmologic examination Hemianopsia is easily overlooked and can usually be ruled out by simple confrontation testing

TABLE 3-4   COMMON PHYSICAL FINDINGS AND THEIR POTENTIAL
             SIGNIFICANCE IN GERIATRICS (*Continued*)

PHYSICAL FINDINGS	POTENTIAL SIGNIFICANCE
EYES (SEE CHAP. 13)	
Cataracts and other abnormalities	Fundoscopic examination often difficult and limited; if retinal pathology suspected, thorough ophthalmologic examination necessary
MOUTH	
Missing teeth	Dentures often present; they should be removed to check for evidence of poor fit and other pathology in oral cavity Area under the tongue is a common site for early malignancies
SKIN	
Multiple lesions	Actinic keratoses and basal cell carcinomas common; most other lesions benign
CHEST	
Abnormal lung sounds	Crackles can be heard in the absence of pulmonary disease and heart failure; often indicate atelectasis
CARDIOVASCULAR (SEE CHAP. 11)	
Irregular rhythms	See Vital Signs at the beginning of the table
Systolic murmurs	Common and most often benign; clinical history and bedside maneuvers can help to differentiate those needing further evaluation Carotid bruits may need further evaluation

TABLE 3-4   COMMON PHYSICAL FINDINGS AND THEIR POTENTIAL
SIGNIFICANCE IN GERIATRICS (*Continued*)

PHYSICAL FINDINGS	POTENTIAL SIGNIFICANCE
CARDIOVASCULAR (SEE CHAP. 11)	
Vascular bruits	Femoral bruits often present in patients with symptomatic peripheral vascular disease
Diminished distal pulses	Presence or absence should be recorded as this information may be diagnostically useful at a later time (eg, if symptoms of claudication or an embolism develop)
ABDOMEN	
Prominent aortic pulsation	Suspected abdominal aneurysms should be evaluated by ultrasound
GENITOURINARY (SEE CHAP. 8)	
Atrophy	Testicular atrophy normal; atrophic vaginal tissue may cause symptoms (such as dyspareunia and dysuria) and treatment may be beneficial
GENITOURINARY (SEE CHAP. 8)	
Pelvic prolapse (cystocele, rectocele)	Common and may be unrelated to symptoms; gynecologic evaluation helpful if patient has bothersome, potentially related symptoms
EXTREMITIES	
Periarticular pain	Can result from a variety of causes and is not always the result of degenerative joint disease; each area of pain should be carefully evaluated and treated (see Chap. 10)

TABLE 3-4   COMMON PHYSICAL FINDINGS AND THEIR POTENTIAL
SIGNIFICANCE IN GERIATRICS (*Continued*)

PHYSICAL FINDINGS	POTENTIAL SIGNIFICANCE
	EXTREMITIES
Limited range of motion	Often caused by pain resulting from active inflammation, scarring from old injury, or neurologic disease; if limitations impair function, a rehabilitation therapist could be consulted
Edema	Can result from venous insufficiency and/or heart failure; mild edema often a cosmetic problem; treatment necessary if impairing ambulation, contributing to nocturia, predisposing to skin breakdown, or causing discomfort
	Unilateral edema should prompt search for a proximal obstructive process
	NEUROLOGIC
Abnormal mental status (ie, confusion, depressed affect)	See Chaps. 6 and 7
Weakness	Arm drift may be the only sign of residual weakness from a stroke Proximal muscle weakness (eg, inability to get out of chair) should be further evaluated; physical therapy may be appropriate

LABORATORY ASSESSMENT

Abnormal laboratory findings are often attributed to "old age." While it is true that abnormal findings are common in geriatric patients, few are true aging changes. Misinterpretation of an abnormal laboratory value as an aging change may result in underdiagnosis and undertreatment of conditions such as anemia.

Table 3-5 lists those laboratory parameters unchanged in the elderly and those commonly abnormal. Abnormalities in the former group should prompt further

TABLE 3-5 LABORATORY ASSESSMENT OF GERIATRIC PATIENTS

LABORATORY PARAMETERS UNCHANGED[*]
Hemoglobin and hematocrit
White blood cell count
Platelet count
Electrolytes (sodium, potassium, chloride, bicarbonate)
Blood urea nitrogen
Liver function tests (transaminases, bilirubin, prothrombin time)
Free thyroxine index
Thyroid-stimulating hormone
Calcium
Phosphorus

COMMON ABNORMAL LABORATORY PARAMETERS[†]	
PARAMETER	CLINICAL SIGNIFICANCE
Sedimentation rate	Mild elevations (10-20 mm) may be an age-related change
Glucose	Glucose tolerance decreases (see Chap. 12); elevations during acute illness are common
Creatinine	Because lean body mass and daily endogenous creatinine production decline, high-normal and minimally elevated values may indicate substantially reduced renal function
Albumin	Average values decline (< 0.5 g/mL) with age, especially in acutely ill, but generally indicate undernutrition
Alkaline phosphatase	Mild asymptomatic elevations common; liver and Paget disease should be considered if moderately elevated
Serum iron, iron-binding capacity, ferritin	Decreased values are not an aging change and usually indicate undernutrition and/or gastrointestinal blood loss

TABLE 3-5   LABORATORY ASSESSMENT OF GERIATRIC PATIENTS
(Continued)

COMMON ABNORMAL LABORATORY PARAMETERS[†]	
PARAMETER	CLINICAL SIGNIFICANCE
Prostate-specific antigen	May be elevated in patients with benign prostatic hyerplasia. Marked elevation or increasing values when followed over time should prompt consideration of further evaluation in patients for whom specific therapy for prostate cancer would be undertaken if cancer were diagnosed
Urinalysis	Asymptomatic pyuria and bacteriuria are common and rarely warrant treatment; hematuria is abnormal and needs further evaluation (see Chap. 8)
Chest radiographs	Interstitial changes are a common age-related finding; diffusely diminished bone density generally indicates advanced osteoporosis (see Chap. 12)
Electrocardiogram	ST-segment and T-wave changes, atrial and ventricular arrhythmias, and various blocks are common in asymptomatic elderly and may not need specific evaluation or treatment (see Chap. 11)

[*]Aging changes do not occur in these parameters; abnormal values should prompt further evaluation.
[†]Includes normal aging and other age-related changes.

evaluation; abnormalities in the latter group should be interpreted carefully. Table 3-5 also notes important considerations in interpreting commonly abnormal laboratory values.

FUNCTIONAL ASSESSMENT

General Concepts

Ability to function should be a central focus of the evaluation of geriatric patients (see Fig. 3-1). Medical history, physical examination, and laboratory findings are all of obvious importance in diagnosing and managing acute and chronic medical conditions in older people, as they are in all age groups. But once the dust settles, functional abilities are just as, if not more, important to the overall health, well-being, and potential need for services of older individuals. For example, in a patient with hemiparesis, the nature, location, and extent of the lesion may be important in the management, but whether the patient is continent and can climb the steps to an apartment makes the difference between going home to live or going to a nursing home.

The concern about function as a core component of geriatrics deserves special comment. Functioning is the end result of the various efforts of the geriatric approach to care. Optimizing function necessitates integrating efforts on several fronts. It is helpful to think of functioning as an equation:

$$\text{Function} = \frac{(\text{physical capabilities} \times \text{medical management} \times \text{motivation})}{(\text{social, psychological, and physical environment})}$$

This admitted oversimplification is meant as a reminder that function can be influenced on at least three levels. The clinician's first task is to remediate the remediable. Careful medical diagnosis and appropriate treatment are essential in good geriatric care. Adequate medical management, however, is necessary but not sufficient. Once those conditions amenable to treatment have been addressed, the next step is to develop the environment that will best support the patient's autonomous function.

Environmental barriers can be both physical and psychological. It is important to recognize how physical barriers may complicate functioning for persons with various conditions (eg, stairs for a person with dyspnea, inaccessible cabinets for the wheelchair bound, etc). Psychological barriers refer especially to the dangers of risk aversion. Those most concerned about the patient may restrict activity in the name of protecting the patient or the institution. For example, hospitals are notoriously averse to risk; older patients will be restricted to a wheelchair rather than risk them falling when walking.

This risk-averse behavior may be compounded by concerns about efficiency. Personal care is personnel intensive. It takes much more time and patience to work with patients to encourage them to do things for themselves than to step in and do the task. But that pseudoefficiency breeds dependence.

The third factor relates to the concept of motivation. If the care providers believe that the patient cannot improve, they will likely induce despair and discouragement in their charges. The tendency toward functional decline may become a self-fulfilling prophecy. Indeed, the opposite belief—that improvement is quite likely with appropriate intervention—may be the critical element in the success of geriatric evaluation units. Belief in the possibility of improvement can play another critical role in geriatric care. Psychologists have developed a useful paradigm referred to as "the innocent victim." The basic concept is that caregivers respond in a hostile manner to those they feel impotent to help. If given a sense of empowerment, perhaps by using assessment tools and intervention strategies such as the ones provided in this book, for approaching the complex problems of older persons, care providers are likely to feel more positive toward those individuals and be more willing to work with them rather than avoiding them. The more an information system can provide feedback on accomplishments and progress toward improved function, the more the provider will feel positively about the older patient.

Table 3-6 summarizes several other important concepts about comprehensive functional assessment in the geriatric population, which were identified in a Consensus Development Conference at the National Institutes of Health (NIH, 1988). To a large extent the purpose, setting, and timing of the assessment dictate the nature of the assessment process. Table 3-7 lists the different purposes and objectives of functional status measures. Generally, functional assessment begins with a case-finding or screening approach in order to identify individuals for whom more in-depth and interdisciplinary assessment might be of benefit. Assessment is often carried out at points of transition, such as a threatened or actual decline in health status or impending change in living situation. Without this type of targeting, the assessment of older people may be time consuming and not cost-effective. Numerous standardized instruments are available to assist in the assessment process.

Instruments designed for research use may not work in clinical practice, and vice versa. There are numerous potential pitfalls in the use of standardized assessment instruments (Kane and Kane, 2000; see Table 3-6). The critical concept in using standardized instruments is that they should fit the purposes and settings for which they are intended, and there must be a solid link between the assessment process and the follow-up provision of services. In addition, the assessment process should include a clear discussion of the patient's preferences and expectations, as well as the family's expectations and willingness to provide care. The importance of functional status assessment has been highlighted by data documenting the ability of functional status measures to predict mortality in older hospitalized patients (Inouye et al., 1998).

Assessment Tools for Functional Status

This chapter focuses on the assessment of physical and mental function. Mental function is also discussed in Chap. 6. Table 3-8 lists examples of measures of physical functioning. Physical functioning is measured along a spectrum. For disabled persons, one may focus on the ability to perform basic self-care tasks, often referred to as activities of daily living (ADLs). The patient is assessed on the ability to conduct each of a series of basic activities. Data usually come

TABLE 3-6   IMPORTANT CONCEPTS FOR GERIATRIC FUNCTIONAL
              ASSESSMENT

1. The nature of the assessment should be dictated by its purpose, setting,
    and timing (see Table 3-7)
2. Input from multiple disciplines is often helpful, but routine multidiscipli-
    nary assessment is not cost-effective
3. Assessments should be targeted
    a. Initial screening to identify disciplines needed
    b. Times of threatened or actual decline in status, impending change in
        living situation, and other stressful situations
4. Standard instruments are useful, but there are numerous potential pitfalls
    a. Instruments should be reliable, sensitive, and valid for the purposes
        and setting of the assessment
    b. How questions are asked can be critically important (eg, performance
        vs. capability)
    c. Discrepancies can arise between different informants (eg, self-report
        vs. caregiver's report).
    d. Self- or caregiver's report of performance, or direct observation of per-
        formance may not reflect what the individual does in everyday life.
    e. Many standard instruments have not been adequately tested for relia-
        bility and sensitivity to changes over time
5. Open-ended questions are helpful in complementing information from
    standardized instruments
6. The family's expectations, capabilities, and willingness to provide care
    must be explored
7. The patient's preferences and expectations should be elicited and consid-
    ered paramount in planning services
8. A strong link must exist between the assessment process and follow-up
    in the provision of services

from the patient or from a caregiver (eg, a nurse or family member) who has had
a sufficient opportunity to observe the patient. In some cases, it may be more useful to have the patient actually demonstrate the ability to perform key tasks.
Grading of performance is usually divided into three levels of dependency: (1)
ability to perform the task without human assistance (one may wish to distinguish
those persons who need mechanical aids like a walker but are still independent);

TABLE 3-7   PURPOSES AND OBJECTIVES OF FUNCTIONAL STATUS
             MEASURES

PURPOSE	OBJECTIVES
Description	Develop normative data Depict geriatric population along selected parameters Assess needs Describe outcomes associated with various interventions
Screening	Identify from among population at risk those individuals who should receive further assessment and by whom
Assessment	Make diagnosis Assign treatment
Monitoring	Observe changes in untreated conditions Review progress of those receiving treatment
Prediction	Permit scientifically based clinical interventions Make prognostic statements of expected outcomes on the basis of given conditions

(2) ability to perform the task with some human assistance; and (3) inability to perform, even with assistance. Distinguishing "independent without difficulty" from "independent with difficulty" may provide complementing prognostic information (Gill, Robison, and Tinetti, 1998).

It is helpful to appreciate that different disciplines approach functional measurement differently. A physician for example, may be content to ascertain whether a person can dress herself with or without assistance. By contrast, an occupational therapist might subdivide the act of getting dressed into a series of specific steps (eg, choosing appropriate clothes, getting them out of the closet or drawers, putting on different types of clothing, using various fasteners, etc). Likewise, performance can be further assessed in terms of the time required to complete the task and the skill with which it was done.

Commonly used tools for assessing physical function are included in the appendix. There may be discrepancies between patient's or caregiver's reports and what the individuals actually do in their everyday life. Moreover, there may be differences between reported physical functional status and actual measures of physical performance. Reuben's physical performance test is one example of a practical assessment that provides insights into actual performance and prognostic information (Reuben and Siu, 1990). (The physical performance test is

TABLE 3-8   EXAMPLES OF MEASURES OF PHYSICAL FUNCTIONING

Basic ADLs
Feeding
Dressing
Ambulation
Toileting
Bathing
Transfer (from bed and toilet)
Continence
Grooming
Communication

IADLs
Writing
Reading
Cooking
Cleaning
Shopping
Doing laundry
Climbing stairs
Using telephone
Managing medication
Managing money
Ability to perform paid employment duties or outside work (eg, gardening)
Ability to travel (use public transportation, go out of town)

ADL, activity of daily living; IADL, instrumental ADL.

included in the appendix.) In general, performance tests measure what occurs under standardized conditions, whereas reports address what is done under actual living conditions; hence, the latter may offer insights into the effects of the environment as well as the patient's abilities. Other performance-based assessments of gait and balance are discussed in Chap. 9.

In addition to these general geriatric measures of functional status, other functional assessment tools are commonly used in different settings. Examples include the following:

1. The Short Form 36—a global measure of function and well-being that is increasingly being used in outpatient settings. This measure has a disadvantage in the frail geriatric population because of a ceiling effect—that is, it does not distinguish well between sick and very sick older people.

2. The minimum data set (MDS)—a comprehensive assessment mandated on admission with quarterly updates in Medicare-/Medicaid-certified nursing facilities.
3. The functional independence measure (FIM, now part of the rehabilitation measure IRFPAI)—a detailed assessment tool commonly used to monitor functional status progress in rehabilitation settings.
4. The outcome and assessment information set (OASIS)—a comprehensive data collection system for use in home health care; it is mandatory for Medicare beneficiaries.

A new data system (CARE) is under development, which will replace MDS, OASIS, and IRFPAI, and introduce a common measurement system for all postacute care.

A structured assessment of cognitive function should be part of every complete geriatric functional assessment. Because of the high prevalence of cognitive impairment, the potential impact of such impairment on overall function and safety and the ability of patients with early impairments to mask their deficits, clinicians must specifically attend to this aspect of functional assessment. At a minimum, assessment should include a test for orientation and memory. A standardized geriatric mental status test is included in the appendix (the Folstein Mini-Mental State Examination). Although these tests do not probe the variety of intellectual functions appropriate for a more detailed assessment, they are quick, easy, scorable, and reliable. More detailed assessment of cognitive function is discussed in Chap. 6.

ENVIRONMENTAL ASSESSMENT

We emphasized earlier that patient function is the result of innate ability and environment. The clinician must, therefore, be particularly concerned with the older patient's environment. For many patients, the assessment should include an evaluation of the available and potential resources to maintain functioning. Just as physicians comfortably prescribe drugs, they should also be prepared to prescribe environmental interventions when necessary.

Rehabilitation therapists (ie, physical, occupational, speech) are especially skilled at functional assessment, developing and implementing rehabilitative plans of care targeted at potentially remediable functional impairments, and making specific recommendations about environmental modifications that can enhance safety and functional ability. An environmental prescription may include alterations in the physical environment (eg, ramps, grab bars, and elevated toilet seats), special services (eg, meals on wheels, homemaking, home nursing), increased social contact (eg, friendly visits, telephone reassurance, participation in recreational activities), or provision of critical elements (eg, food or money).

An environmental assessment by an occupational therapist for essentially asymptomatic older persons has been shown to significantly reduce subsequent hospital use (Clark et al., 1997).

The ability to identify the environmental interventions and function supports needed to maintain in the community may be the essential difference between enabling an older person to remain at home versus transferring the person to an institution. Although identifying the need is not tantamount to providing the resource, it is an important first step.

ASSESSMENT FOR PAIN

Guidelines published by the American Geriatrics Society recommend that on initial presentation or admission of an older person to any health-care service, the patient should be assessed for evidence of persistent pain (AGS Panel on Persistent Pain in Older Persons, 2002). Patients with persistent pain that may affect physical function, psychosocial function, or other aspects of quality of life should undergo a comprehensive pain assessment. Tables 3-9 and 3-10 list important aspects of the history and physical examination in assessment of pain, respectively. For patients who are cognitively intact, assessment of pain should be by direct questioning of the patient. Quantitative assessment of pain should be recorded by use of a standard pain scale, such as a visual analog scale, where a patient can indicate where along the continuum their pain lies. A verbal scale of 0 to 10, with 0 meaning no pain and 10 meaning the worst pain possible, is frequently used. Other scales, pain thermometer and faces, studied in older populations, are illustrated in Fig. 3-2. In cognitively impaired and nonverbal patients,

TABLE 3-9   IMPORTANT ASPECTS OF THE HISTORY IN ASSESSMENT
OF PAIN

1. Characteristics of the pain
2. Relation of pain to impairments in physical and social function
3. Analgesic history (present, previous, prescribed, over-the-counter, alternative remedies, alcohol use, side effects)
4. Patient's attitudes and beliefs about pain and its management
5. Effectiveness of treatments
6. Satisfaction with current pain management
7. Social support and health-care accessibility

TABLE 3-10   IMPORTANT ASPECTS OF THE PHYSICAL EXAMINATION IN ASSESSMENT OF PAIN

1. Careful examination of the site of pain and common sites for pain referral
2. Focus on the musculoskeletal system
3. Focus on the neurological system including weakness and dysesthesia
4. Observation of physical function
5. Psychological function
6. Cognitive function

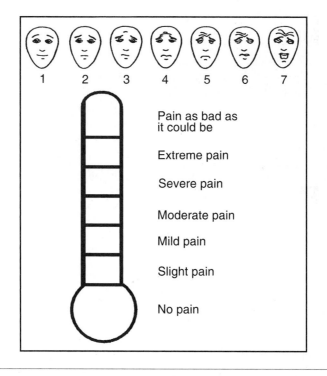

— FIGURE 3-2 —   Samples of two pain intensity scales that have been studied in older persons. Directions: Patients should view the figure without numbers. After the patient indicates the best representation of their pain, the appropriate numerical value can be assigned to facilitate clinical documentation and follow-up. Adapted with permission from Bieri D, et al. The faces pain scale for the self-assessment of the severity of pain experienced by children: Development, initial validation, and preliminary investigation for ration scale properties. *Pain.* May 1990; 41(2):139-150.

pain assessment should be by direct observation or history from caregivers. Patients should be observed for pain-related behaviors during movement. Unusual behavior in a patient with severe dementia should trigger assessment for pain as a potential cause.

NUTRITIONAL ASSESSMENT

Several parameters are used in assessing nutritional status in older adults. Some anthropometric variables are probably effective estimators of major aspects of body composition (Table 3-11). They cannot provide a complete description of the nutritional status of an individual and are not highly correlated with biochemical or hematologic indicators of nutritional status.

Although weight is a global measure, it can be obtained easily from adults and is useful in the absence of edema. Body mass index (BMI = kg/m^2) is best correlated with total body fat. Triceps and subscapular skin folds are highly correlated with the percentage of body fat in older adults. Waist to hip ratio is a parameter of central adiposity. Upper arm circumference is correlated with lean body mass and may be particularly helpful in edematous patients in whom weight is misleading. The effect of the aging process on lean body mass is so great that it remains a poor reflection of nutritional status in older adults.

Serum albumin is a practical indicator of malnutrition in older adults. However, liver disease, proteinuria, and protein-losing enteropathies must be excluded. A low serum albumin may be indicative of malnutrition, but a normal or increased serum albumin concentration does not necessarily indicate normality. Thyroxine-binding prealbumin and/or retinol-binding protein are more sensitive indices than are albumin and transferrin.

TABLE 3-11   ASSESSMENT OF BODY COMPOSITION

Assessment	Component
Weight	Global
Body mass index	Total fat
Skin fold	Percent fat
Waist:hip ratio	Central adiposity
Upper arm circumference	Lean body mass

TABLE 3-12   CRITICAL QUESTIONS IN ASSESSING A PATIENT FOR
MALNUTRITION

Is there any reason to suspect malnutrition?

If so, of which nutrient(s) and to what extent?

What are the pathophysiological mechanisms (eg, alteration in nutrient
intake, digestion and absorption, metabolism, excretion, or requirements)?

What etiology underlies the pathophysiological mechanism(s)?

In animals, dietary deprivation of protein results in anemia. Because anemia is one of the earliest manifestations of protein–calorie malnutrition, its presence should alert the physician to the possibility of malnutrition. Total lymphocyte count may be a very good marker for nutritional problems.

Some important factors need to be considered in evaluating a given patient. Table 3-12 presents some issues that should be considered in assessing older patients at risk for malnutrition. Individuals with such problems should have an evaluation of nutritional status. Some patients may have several concurrent diseases that impair nutritional status (Table 3-13). Protein–energy malnutrition may

TABLE 3-13   FACTORS THAT PLACE OLDER ADULTS AT RISK FOR
MALNUTRITION

Drugs (eg, reserpine, digoxin, antitumor agents)

Chronic disease (eg, congestive heart failure, renal insufficiency, chronic
gastrointestinal disease)

Depression

Dental and periodontal disease

Decreased taste and smell

Low socioeconomic level

Physical weakness

Isolation

Food fads

ensue and is associated with poor prognosis. The Mini Nutritional Assessment (MNA) and Subjective Global Assessment (SGA) predict mortality in geriatric patients (Persson et al., 2002), and are valuable tools for the assessment of nutritional status in older adults. The Short-Form Mini Nutritional Assessment (MNA-SF) can be used in a two-step screening process in which persons identified as at risk on the MNA-SF would receive additional assessment (Rubenstein et al., 2001; Table 3-14). The MNA (Guigoz, Vellas, and Garry, 1996) may be advantageous for the latter since it classified fewer patients than the SGA as well-nourished and those identified as well-nourished on the MNA had a better 3-year survival than those well-nourished by the SGA (Persson et al., 2002).

GERIATRIC CONSULTATION

Geriatric consultation may be requested to address specific clinical issues (eg, confusion, incontinence, recurrent falling), to perform a comprehensive geriatric assessment (often in the context of determining the need for placement in a difficult living setting), or to perform a preoperative evaluation of a high-risk geriatric patient. In this chapter, we discuss the latter two types of consultation.

Comprehensive Geriatric Consultation

A comprehensive geriatric consultation includes the following:

1. A geriatric-oriented history and physical examination attending to the issues reviewed earlier in this chapter.
2. Medication review; in addition, geriatric patients should be questioned about alcohol abuse.
3. Functional assessment.
4. Environmental and social assessment, focusing especially on caregiver's support and other resources available to meet the patient's needs.
5. Discussion of advance directives.
6. A complete list of the patient's medical, functional, and psychosocial problems.
7. Specific recommendations in each domain.

A systematic screening process to identify potentially remediable geriatric problems may be a useful tool for the comprehensive consultation.

One such screening strategy is illustrated in Table 3-15 (Moore and Siu, 1996). It may also be useful, especially in capitated systems, to use a tool that identifies risk for crises and expensive health-care utilization. The probability of repeated admissions (Pra) instrument is one such tool (Table 3-16; Pacala et al., 1997).

TABLE 3-14   MINI NUTRITION ASSESSMENT

A. Has food intake declined over the past 3 months due to loss of appetite, digestive problems, chewing or swallowing difficulties?
   0 = severe loss of appetite
   1 = moderate loss of appetite
   2 = no loss of appetite   ☐

B. Weight loss during last 3 months
   0 = weight loss > 3 kg (6.6 lb)
   1 = does not know
   2 = weight loss between 1 and 3 kg (2.2 and 6.6 lb)
   3 = no weight loss   ☐

C. Mobility
   0 = bed or chair bound
   1 = able to get out of bed/chair but does not go out
   2 = goes out   ☐

D. Has suffered psychological stress or acute disease in the past 3 months
   0 = yes
   2 = no   ☐

E. Neuropsychological problems
   0 = severe dementia or depression
   1 = mild dementia
   2 = no psychological problems   ☐

F. Body mass index (BMI) (weight in kg)/(height in m)^2
   0 = BMI less than 19
   1 = BMI 19 to less than 21
   2 = BMI 21 to less than 23
   3 = BMI 23 or greater   ☐

Screening score (subtotal max. 14 points)
   12 points or greater: Normal—no need for further assessment   ☐☐
   11 points or below: Possible malnutrition—continue assessment

Note: if greater specificity is desired consider 10 points or below as possible malnutrition.
Alternative height calculations using knee to heel measurements:
with knee at 90° angle (foot flexed or flat on floor or bed board), measure from bottom of heel to top of knee.
Men = (2.02 × knee height, cm) × (0.04 × age) + 64.19
Women = (1.83 × knee height, cm) × (0.24 × age) + 84.88
Body weight calculations in amputees:
For amputations, increase weight by the percentage below for contribution of individual body parts to obtain the weight to use to determine body mass index.
Single below knee 6.0% Single at knee 9.0%
Single above knee 15.0% Single arm 6.5%
Single arm below elbow 3.6%
Reproduced with permission from Rubenstein et al., 2001.

TABLE 3-15   EXAMPLE OF A SCREENING TOOL TO IDENTIFY POTENTIALLY
REMEDIABLE GERIATRIC PROBLEMS

Problem	Screening Measure	Positive Result
Poor vision	Ask, "Do you have difficulty driving, watching television, reading, or doing any of your daily activities because of your eyesight?" If yes, then test acuity with Snellen chart, with corrective lenses	Inability to read better than 20/40 on Snellen chart
Poor hearing	With audioscope set at 40 dB, test hearing at 1000 and 2000 Hz	Inability to hear 1000 or 2000 Hz in both ears or either frequency in one ear
Poor leg mobility	Time the patient after asking, "Rise from the chair. Walk 20 feet briskly, turn, walk back to the chair, and sit down."	Unable to complete task in 15 s
Urinary incontinence	Ask, "In the past year, have you ever lost your urine and gotten wet?" If yes, then ask, "Have you lost urine on at least 6 separate days?"	Yes to both questions
Malnutrition and weight loss	Ask, "Have you lost 10 pounds over the past 6 months without trying to do so?" and then weigh the patient	Yes to the question or weight < 100 lb
Memory loss	Three-item recall	Unable to remember all three items after 1 min
Depression	Ask, "Do you often feel sad or depressed?"	Yes to the question

TABLE 3-15   EXAMPLE OF A SCREENING TOOL TO IDENTIFY POTENTIALLY
REMEDIABLE GERIATRIC PROBLEMS (*Continued*)

PROBLEM	SCREENING MEASURE	POSITIVE RESULT
Physical disability	Ask six questions: "Are you able to: • Do strenuous activities such as fast walking or bicycling? • Do heavy work around the house like washing windows, walls, or floors? • Go shopping for groceries or clothes? • Get to places that are out of walking distance? • Bathe: either a sponge bath, tub bath, or shower? • Dress, including putting on a shirt, buttoning and zipping, and putting on shoes?"	No to any question

Reproduced with permission from Moore and Siu, 1996.

Among frail, dependent geriatric patients, screening for risk factors and elder abuse is important. Elder abuse is more common among older people who are in poor health and who are physically and cognitively impaired. Additional risk factors include shared living arrangements with a relative or friend suspected of alcohol or substance abuse, mental illness, or a history of violence.

Frequent emergency room visits for injury or exacerbations of chronic illness should also raise suspicion for abuse. Table 3-17 illustrates an example of an effective format for documenting the results of the consultation, listing the problems and recommendations first.

PREOPERATIVE EVALUATION

Geriatricians are often called upon by surgeons and anesthesiologists to assess elderly patients before surgical procedures. Table 3-18 lists several of the

TABLE 3-16   QUESTIONS ON THE PRA INSTRUMENT FOR IDENTIFYING
GERIATRIC PATIENTS AT RISK FOR HEALTH SERVICE USE

1. In general, would you say your health is:
   (excellent, very good, good, fair, poor)

2. In the previous 12 months, have you stayed overnight as a patient in a hospital?
   (not at all, one time, two or three times, more than three times)

3. In the previous 12 months, how many times did you visit a physician or clinic?
   (not at all, one time, two or three times, four to six times, more than six times)

4. In the previous 12 months, did you have diabetes?
   (yes, no)

5. Have you ever had: Coronary heart disease? (yes, no)
   Angina pectoris? (yes, no)
   A myocardial infarction? (yes, no)
   Any other heart attack? (yes, no)

6. Your sex?
   (male, female)

7. Is there a friend, relative, or neighbor who would take care of you for a few days if necessary?
   (yes, no)

8. Your date of birth?
   (month   , day   , year   )

key factors involved in the preoperative evaluation of geriatric patients. Although older patients (age > 70 years) have higher rates of major perioperative complications and mortality after nonemergent major noncardiac surgical procedures than do younger patients, mortality is low, even in patients 80 years of age or older (Polanczyk et al., 2001). Morbidity and mortality, however, are influenced to a greater extent by the presence and severity of systemic illnesses and whether the procedure is elective versus emergent. Thus, evaluating a geriatric patient's preoperative status and risk for surgery necessitates a thorough assessment of cardiopulmonary and renal function as well as nutritional and hydration status.

TABLE 3-17   SUGGESTED FORMAT FOR SUMMARIZING THE RESULTS OF
A COMPREHENSIVE GERIATRIC CONSULTATION

1. Identifying data, including referring physician
2. Reason(s) for consultation
3. Problems
   a. Medical problem list
   b. Functional problem list
   c. Psychosocial problem list
4. Recommendations
5. Standard documentation
   a. History, including medications, significant past medical
      and surgical history, system review
   b. Social and environmental information
   c. Functional assessment
   d. Advance directive status
   e. Physical examination
   f. Laboratory and other test data

Factors that increase the risk of perioperative cardiac complications in patients undergoing noncardiac surgery include ischemic heart disease, congestive heart failure, diabetes mellitus, and renal insufficiency (Lee et al., 1999). Patients with a recent history of myocardial infarction, active angina, pulmonary edema, and severe aortic stenosis are at especially high risk (Mangano and Goldman, 1995). Preoperative pulmonary function tests and arterial blood gases are rarely of prognostic value. Assessment of exercise tolerance may be helpful, for example, the ability to climb one flight of stairs. In patients at low risk for cardiac complications, no beta-blockade is necessary. In patients at increased risk for cardiac complications, modified exercise testing, dipyridamole thallium scanning, or dobutamine echocardiography may be indicated (Palda and Detsky, 1997). Coronary artery bypass grafting or percutaneous coronary revascularization should be limited to patients who have a clearly defined need for the procedure that is independent of the need for noncardiac surgery (Fleisher and Eagle, 2001).

Underlying conditions that are prevalent in the geriatric population, such as hypertension, congestive heart failure, chronic obstructive lung disease, diabetes mellitus, anemia, and undernutrition, need particularly careful management in the preoperative period (Thomas and Ritchie, 1995; Schiff and Emanuele, 1995). Medication regimens should be scrutinized in order to determine whether specific

TABLE 3-18   KEY FACTORS IN THE PREOPERATIVE EVALUATION OF THE GERIATRIC PATIENT

1. Age > 70 is associated with an increased risk of complications and death
   a. Risk varies with the type of procedure and local complication rates
   b. Emergency procedures are associated with much higher risk
   c. Comorbid conditions, especially cardiovascular, are more important risk factors than age per se
2. The appropriateness and risk-benefit ratio of the proposed surgery must be carefully considered
3. Underlying conditions must be evaluated and optimally managed before nonemergency surgery, eg:
   a. Cardiovascular disease, especially heart failure
   b. Pulmonary status
   c. Renal function
   d. Diabetes mellitus
   e. Thyroid disease (which is often occult)
   f. Anemia
   g. Nutrition
   h. Hydration and volume status, especially in patients on diuretics
4. Medication regimens should be carefully planned; some drugs should be continued, others should be withheld, and some necessitate dosage adjustments
5. Several cardiovascular conditions substantially increase risk, including:
   a. Myocardial infarction within 6 months
   b. Pulmonary edema
   c. Angina (especially if unstable)
   d. Severe aortic stenosis
6. Specific laboratory evaluations may be helpful in some situations, eg:
   a. Pulmonary function tests and arterial blood gas with respiratory symptoms, obesity, chest deformity (eg, kyphoscoliosis), abnormal chest radiographs, planned thoracic or upper abdominal procedure
   b. Noninvasive cardiac testing in high and intermediate risk for cardiac event patients
   c. Creatinine clearance with unstable or borderline renal function, or the use of nephrotoxic or renally excreted drugs
7. The documented effectiveness, risks, and benefits of perioperative prophylactic measures should be considered:
   a. Beta-blocker administration[*]
   b. Antithrombotic prophylaxis[†]
   c. Antimicrobial prophylaxis [‡]

---

[*] See Fleisher and Eagle, 2001.
[†] See Geerts et al., 2001.
[‡] See Medical Letter on Drugs and therapeutics, 1999.

drugs should be continued or withheld. Results from several well-designed clinical trials suggest that use of β-blockers perioperatively is associated with significant reductions in cardiac morbidity and mortality (Auerbach and Goldman, 2002). High and intermediate cardiac event risk patients with negative noninvasive test results should begin beta-blockade therapy. Those with positive noninvasive test results should have consideration of additional therapies to reduce risk, for example, coronary revascularization. Careful consideration should also be given to perioperative prophylactic measures for the prevention of thromboembolism and infection, many of which have documented efficacy in specific situations (Medical Letter on Drugs and Therapeutics, 1999; Geerts et al., 2001).

Many surgeons and anesthesiologists tend to favor regional over general anesthesia for geriatric patients. Regional anesthesia (eg, epidural), however, may have several potential disadvantages. Patients may require added intravenous sedation and/or analgesia, thus increasing the risks of perioperative cardiovascular and mental status changes. Significant cardiovascular changes can, in fact, occur during regional anesthesia; thus invasive monitoring may be required in some patients. Neither the incidence of deep vein thrombosis nor the amount of blood loss seems to be substantially decreased compared to general anesthesia. Thus, decisions about the type of anesthesia should be carefully individualized on the basis of patient factors, the nature of the procedure, and the preferences of the surgical team.

References

AGS Panel on Persistent Pain in Older Persons. The management of persistent pain in older persons. *J Am Geriatr Soc.* 2002;50:S205-S224.

American College of Physicians. Guidelines for assessing and managing the perioperative risk from coronary artery disease associated with major noncardiac surgery. *Ann Intern Med.* 1997;127:309-312.

Auerbach AD, Goldman L. β-Blockers and reduction of cardiac events in noncardiac surgery: scientific review. *JAMA.* 2002;287:1435-1444.

Bula CJ, Berod AC, Stuck AE, et al. Effectiveness of preventive in-home geriatric assessment in well-functioning, community-dwelling older people: secondary analysis of a randomized trial. *J Am Geriatr Soc.* 1999;47:389-395.

Clark F, Azen SP, Zemke R, et al. Occupational therapy for independent-living older adults: a randomized controlled trial. *JAMA.* 1997;278(16):1321-1326.

Cohen HJ, Feussner JR, Weinberger M, et al. A controlled trial of inpatient and outpatient geriatric evaluation and management. *N Engl J Med.* 2002;346:905-912.

Fleisher LA, Eagle KA. Lowering cardiac risk in noncardiac surgery. *N Engl J Med.* 2001;345:1677-1682.

Geerts WH, Heit JA, Clagett GP, et al. Prevention of venous thromboembolism. *Chest.* 2001;119:132S-175S.

Gill TM, Robison JT, Tinetti ME. Difficulty and dependence: two components of the disability continuum among community-living older persons. *Ann Intern Med.* 1998;128:96-101.

Guigoz Y, Vellas B, Garry PJ. Assessing the nutritional status of the elderly: the Mini Nutritional Assessment as part of the geriatric evaluation. *Nutr Rev.* 1996;54:559-565.

Inouye SK, Peduzzi PN, Robison JT, et al. Importance of functional measures in predicting mortality among older hospitalized patients. *JAMA.* 1998;279:1187-1993.

Kane RL, Kane RA. *Assessing Older Persons: Measures, Meaning, and Practical Applications.* New York, NY: Oxford University Press; 2000.

Katz S, Ford A, Moskowitz R, et al. The index of ADL: a standardized measure of biological and psychosocial function. *JAMA.* 1963;185:914-919.

Landefeld CS, Palmer RM, Kresevic DM, et al. A randomized trial of care in hospital medical unit especially designed to improve the functional outcomes of acutely ill older patients. *N Engl J Med.* 1995;332:1338-1344.

Lee TH, Marcantonio ER, Mangione CM, et al. Derivation and prospective validation of a simple index for prediction of cardiac risk of major noncardiac surgery. *Circulation.* 1999;100:1043-1049.

Mangano DT, Goldman L. Preoperative assessment of patients with known or suspected coronary disease. *N Engl J Med.* 1995;333:1750-1756.

Medical Letter on Drugs and Therapeutics. Antimicrobial prophylaxis in surgery. *Med Lett.* 1999;41(1060):75-80.

Moore AA, Siu AL. Screening for common problems in ambulatory elderly: clinical confirmation of a screening instrument. *Am J Med.* 1996;100:438-443.

NIH Consensus Development Conference Statement. Geriatric assessment methods for clinical decision making. *J Am Geriatr Soc.* 1988;36:342-347.

Pacala JT, Boult C, Reed RL, et al. Predictive validity of the Pra instrument among older recipients of managed care. *J Am Geriatr Soc.* 1997;45:614-617.

Palda VA, Detsky AS. Perioperative assessment and management of risk from coronary artery disease. *Ann Intern Med.* 1997;127:313-328.

Persson MD, Brismar KE, Katzarski KS, et al. Nutritional status using Mini Nutritional Assessment and Subjective Global Assessment predict mortality in geriatric patients. *J Am Geriatr Soc.* 2002;50:1996-2002.

Polanczyk CA, Marcantonio E, Goldman L, et al. Impact of age on perioperative complications and length of stay in patients undergoing noncardiac surgery. *Ann Intern Med.* 2001;134:637-643.

Reuben DB, Siu A, Kimpau S. The predictive validity of self-report and performance-based measures of function and health. *J Gerontol Med Sci.* 1992;47:106-110.

Reuben DB, Borok GM, Wolde-Tsadik G, et al. A randomized trial of comprehensive geriatric assessment in the care of hospitalized patients. *N Engl J Med.* 1995;332:1345-1350.

Reuben DB, Frank JC, Hirsch SH, et al. A randomized clinical trial of outpatient comprehensive geriatric assessment coupled with an intervention to increase adherence to recommendations. *J Am Geriatr Soc.* 1999;47:371-372.

Rubenstein LZ, Stuck AE, Sill AL, et al. Impacts of geriatric evaluation and management programs on defined outcomes: overview of the evidence. *J Am Geriatr Soc.* 1991;39(suppl):85-165.

Rubenstein LZ, Harker JO, Salva A, et al. Screening for undernutrition in geriatric practice: developing the Short-Form Mini-Nutritional Assessment (MNA-SF). *J Gerontol A Biol Sci Med Sci.* 2001;56A:M366-M372.

Schiff RL, Emanuele MA. The surgical patient with diabetes mellitus: guidelines for management. *J Gen Intern Med.* 1995;10:154-161.

Stuck AE, Aronow HU, Steiner A, et al. A trial of annual in-home comprehensive geriatric assessments for elderly people living in the community. *N Engl J Med.* 1995;333: 1184-1189.

Stuck AE, Egger M, Hammer A, et al. Home visits to prevent nursing home admission and functional decline in elderly people: systematic review and meta-regression analysis. *JAMA.* 2002;287(8):1022-1028.

Thomas DR, Ritchie CS. Preoperative assessment of older adults. *J Am Geriatr Soc.* 1995;43:811-821.

Suggested Readings

Applegate WB, Blass JP, Williams TF. Instruments for functional assessment of older patients. *N Engl J Med.* 1990;322:1207-1214.

Crum RM, Anthony SC, Bassett SS, et al. Population-based norms for the Mini-Mental State Examination by age and educational level. *JAMA.* 1993;269:2386-2391.

Feinstein AR, Josephy BR, Wells CK. Scientific and clinical problems in indexes of functional disability. *Ann Intern Med.* 1986;105:413-420.

Finch M, Kane RL, Philp I. Developing a new metric for ADLs. *J Am Geriatr Soc.* 1995;43:877-884.

Fleming KC, Evans JM, Weber DC, et al. Practical functional assessment of elderly persons: a primary-care approach. *Mayo Clin Proc.* 1995;70:890-910.

Folstein MF, Folstein S, McHuth PR. Mini-Mental State: a practical method for grading the cognitive state of patients for the clinician. *J Psychiatr Res.* 1975;12:189-198.

Gill TM, Feinstein AR. A critical appraisal of the quality of quality-of-life measurements. *JAMA.* 1994;272:619-626.

Reuben DB, Siu AL. An objective measure of physical function of elderly persons: the physical performance test. *J Am Geriatr Soc.* 1990;38:1105-1112.

Scheitel SM, Fleming KC, Chutka DS, et al. Geriatric health maintenance. *Mayo Clin Proc.* 1996;71:289-302.

Siu A. Screening for dementia and its causes. *Ann Intern Med.* 1991;115:122-132.

Williams ME, Hadler N, Earp JA. Manual ability as a mark of dependency in geriatric women. *J Chronic Dis.* 1987;40:481-489.

CHAPTER 4

CHRONIC DISEASE MANAGEMENT

Geriatrics can be thought of as the intersection of gerontology and chronic disease management. At a time when medical care in general is awakening to the importance of good chronic disease care, geriatrics has been at it for years. Many of the principles of geriatrics are basically those of good chronic care. The basic tenets of good chronic care are summarized in Table 4-1.

Professional roles need to be reexamined to look for opportunities to delegate to less expensive personnel many tasks formerly performed by more trained professionals. For example, nurse practitioners have been shown capable of proving a good deal of primary care that was formerly the exclusive purview of physicians (Horrocks, Anderson, and Salisbury, 2002; Mundinger et al., 2000).

Expectations must be recalibrated. The familiar dichotomy of care versus cure must be expanded to recognize the role of disease management. Because the natural course of chronic illness is deterioration, successful care must be defined as doing better than would be expected otherwise. This phenomenon is illustrated in Fig. 4-1. The bold line represents the effects of good care. The dotted line represents the effects of the absence of such care. Both lines show decline over time. The difference between them represents the effects of good care. Most of the time this contrast is invisible. All that is seen is decline despite the best efforts. Improving care will require developing information systems that can contrast actual and expect clinical courses.

Appreciating this contrast is critical to both policy and morale. The importance of measuring success by comparing the actual clinical course to a generated expected course is central to concepts of quality in chronic disease. It is also important in maintaining the morale of workers in this field. People who see only decline despite their best efforts become discouraged (Lerner and Simmons, 1966). They need to appreciate the value of their care if they are to continue to give it in the face of so much frailty and disability. Slowing the rate of decline must be seen as positive achievement.

Likewise policy makers, and indeed the general public, are unlikely to support needed efforts to improve chronic care if they do not believe that such care

TABLE 4-1 CHRONIC CARE TENETS

Aggressive primary care

Proactive monitoring

Early intervention to avoid catastrophes

Patient-centeredness, meaningful patient involvement in the care process

Use of information technology

Teamwork, delegation

Use of time

Assessing benefit in terms of slowing decline

can make a difference. They must be educated to appreciate these differences and they must be given the information to demonstrate these differences.

Chronic care requires better data systems. Information technology is probably the most important technological breakthrough for chronic care. Structured protocols, based on strong empirical data, become the basis for planning, monitoring, and

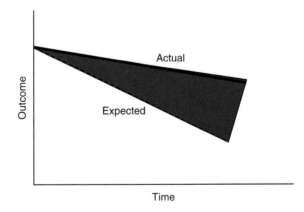

— FIGURE 4-1 — A conceptual model of the difference between expected and actual care. The heavier line represents what is usually observed in clinical chronic care. Despite good care, the patient's course deteriorates. The true benefit, represented by the area between the dark line and the dotted line, is invisible unless some means is found to display the expected course in the absence of good care. Such data could be developed on the basis of clinical prognosis or it could be derived from accumulated data once such a system is in place.

implementing care. These protocols need not always be clinical guidelines, which should be based on strong scientific evidence.

Structuring data helps to focus the clinician's attention on what is most relevant. The goal of a good information system should be to present clinicians with pertinent information at the right time in the form that will capture their attention. Identifying what is salient at the moment is critical, especially in view of the brief contact times allowed. Too much information can be as dysfunctional as too little, because the pertinent facts get lost in a sea of data.

Elderly patients are in danger of being dismissed as hopeless or not worth the effort on the basis of their age. Physicians faced with the question of how much time and resources to spend in searching for a diagnosis will want to consider the probability of benefit for the investment. In some cases, older patients are better investments than younger ones. This apparent paradox occurs in the case of some preventive strategies when the high risk of susceptibility and the discounted benefits of future health favor older persons. But it also arises in situations where small increments of change can yield dramatic differences.

Perhaps the most striking example of the latter is found in the case of nursing home patients. Ironically, very modest changes in their routine, such as introducing a pet, giving them a plant to tend, or increasing their sense of control over their environment, can produce dramatic improvements in mood and morale.

At the same time, the risk-benefit ratio is different with older patients. Treatments that might be easily tolerated in younger patients may pose a much greater risk of producing harmful effects in older patients. As shown in Fig. 4-2,

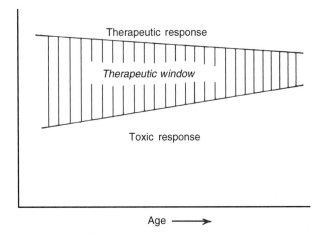

— FIGURE 4-2 — Narrowing of the therapeutic window.
This diagram portrays in a conceptual manner how the space between a therapeutic dose and a toxic dose narrows with age.

the therapeutic window that separates benefit from harm is narrower. In effect, the dosage that will produce a positive effect more closely approaches one that can lead to a toxic effect. As noted earlier, one of the hallmarks of aging is a loss of responsiveness to stress. In this context, treatment may be viewed as a stress.

Those who treat older patients must also consider the theory of competitive risks. Because older persons often suffer from multiple problems, treating one problem may provide an opportunity for more adverse effects from another. In essence, eliminating one cause of death increases the likelihood of death from other causes.

A useful tool for creating a more proactive and focused attitude among those who care for older persons is the flowchart. Focusing on a few clinical parameters that are both significant and most likely to be affected by treatment helps the clinicians focus their attention and recognize changes early. Because the changes are likely to be subtle, it is often helpful to establish treatment goals with time frames for achieving them. Both the health-care team and the patient can then agree on expectations and follow progress toward the goal.

The goals should be achievable. Small successes are very important and reinforcing. Thus the units of measurement should be capable of detecting small but meaningful changes. In many instances, small gains can, in fact, make an enormous difference. The stroke patient, for example, who regains the use of hand muscles has a greatly improved ability to function. Being able to change position in bed may mean the difference between getting pressure sores and not. Regaining a method of communication, whether by speech or some other means, can restore social contact.

By introducing gradual, small steps, a functional task may appear more achievable. We have all had some experience in getting a bedridden patient to resume a more active role. For an older person who has been on bed rest for a long period, this task requires overcoming both physiological and psychological problems. Small steps will often ease the transition and provide an opportunity to monitor the effects at each stage to minimize risk.

SPECIFIC AREAS OF GERIATRIC DISEASE MANAGEMENT

Cancer Care

Cancer is a frequent event in older persons. Its diagnosis and treatment poses special challenges. Physicians may become less enthusiastic about screening from cancer in elderly patients because they anticipate that these patients already have limited life expectancy and hence are unlikely to benefit from aggressive detection and treatment. These attitudes need careful reconsideration. Some cancers, like breast cancer, may indeed have a more indolent course in elderly patients. Some elderly patients may not be able to stand the stress imposed by aggressive cancer treatment; the therapeutic window concept discussed earlier in this chapter applies strongly here.

Nonetheless, cancer represents a substantial risk for older patients and should be approached carefully and deliberately. Figure 4-3 shows that many cancers have their peak incidence in old age. As seen in Fig. 4-4, older people do not survive long with cancer. Indeed, cancer is an important cause of death; about 50% of persons 85+ (75% of 75-84, 90% of 65-74) survive 5 years if they don't die from cancer. For older people, the effects of cancer on death are seen in the first 30 months. Age matters; cancer effects are greater for the oldest patients. Some cancers are more important in older people than is commonly believed. For example, cervical cancer is deadly in older people. Breast cancer affects the age group 85+ harder than those younger. Leukemia hits the elderly hardest. Therefore, physicians should consider active treatment option in older patients and weigh the risk-benefit ratio carefully and individually.

Older cancer patients deserve special consideration. Table 4-2 outlines some specific issues related to age in connection with treating selected cancers. Overall, cancer treatment in older patients requires individualized consideration based on risk–benefit analysis and a careful consideration of the older person's preferences (Downey, Livingston, and Stopeck, 2007).

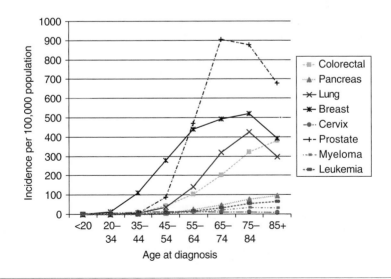

— FIGURE 4-3 — Age-specific incidence of selected cancers.

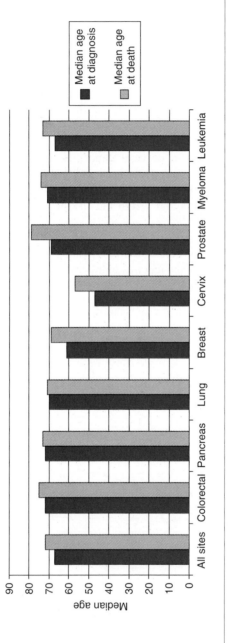

— FIGURE 4-4 — Mean age of diagnosis and death for selected cancers.

TABLE 4-2   CANCER TREATMENT ISSUES RELATED TO AGE

Disease	Age-Related Changes	Unresolved Issues
AML	• Decreased sensitivity tochemotherapy secondary to increased prevalence of *MDR1* • Unfavorable cytogenetic profiles	• Reversal of MDR1 • Role of low-dose cytarabine • Supportive care
Non-Hodgkin lymphoma, large cells	• Decreased duration of complete response, possibly secondary to increased circulating levels of interleukin-6	• Use of chemotherapy in higher doses • Biological treatment • Alternative regimens
Breast cancer	• More indolent course, secondary to higher prevalence of a well-differentiated hormone-receptor rich, slowly proliferating tumor(s) and to a hormonal and immunologic milieu that is unfavorable to tumor(s)	• Value of radiotherapy after lumpectomy • Primary hormonal treatment • Value of adjuvant chemotherapy • Value of lymph node dissection • Use of epirubicin or liposomal doxorubicin in lieu of doxorubicin
Colorectal cancer	• Decreased tolerance of fluorinated pyrimidines	• Alternative forms of adjuvant therapy
Lung cancer (non–small cell)	• Reduced tolerance of combined-modality treatment in stage III	• Alternative approaches
Ovarian cancer	• Decreased response to cytotoxic chemotherapy	• Alternative forms of treatment

AML, acute myelogenous leukemia; *MDR1*, multiple drug resistance gene.
Reproduced with permission from the NCCN v.2.2007 Senior Adult Oncology Guideline Clinical Practice Guidelines in Oncology. Copyright © National Comprehensive Cancer Network, 2007. Available at http://www.nccn.org. Accessed November 7, 2007. To view the most recent and complete version of the guideline, go to http://www.nccn.org.

End-of-Life Care

The physician's concern with the patient's functioning continues throughout the course of the chronic disease. Elderly patients will die. In many cases, death is not a reflection of medical failure. The approach to the dying patient will often raise difficult dilemmas. No simple answers suffice. Perhaps the best advice is not to take on the whole burden. Too often the dying patient is treated as an object. Ignored and isolated, the patient may be discussed in the third person.

Physicians must come to terms with death if they are to treat elderly patients. Often the patients are more comfortable with the subject than are their physicians. Fleeing from the dying patient is inexcusable. Dying patients need their doctors. At a very basic level, everything should be done to keep the patient as comfortable as possible. One simple step is to identify the pattern of discomforting symptoms and arrange the dosage schedule of palliatives to prevent rather than respond to the symptoms.

Patients need an opportunity to talk about their death. Not everyone will take advantage of that chance, but a surprising number will respond to a genuine offer made without time pressure. Such discussions are not conducted on the run. Often several invitations accompanied by appropriate behavior (eg, sitting down at the bedside) are necessary.

Some physicians are unable to confront this aspect of practice. For them, the challenge is to recognize their own behavior and get appropriate help. Such help is available at various levels: help for the physician and for the patient. Groups and therapy are readily available to assist doctors to deal with their feelings. Patients of doctors who fear death need the help of other caregivers. Often other professionals (nurses, social workers) who are working with these patients already can play the lead role in helping them work through their feelings. But the active intervention of another caregiver is not justification to ignore the patient.

The rise of the hospice movement has created a growing cadre of persons and settings to help with the dying patient. The lessons coming from this experience suggest that much can be done to facilitate this stage of life, although the formal studies done to evaluate hospice care do not show dramatic benefits.

Patients should be encouraged to be as active as possible and as interactive as they wish. Even more than in other aspects of care, the unique condition of the dying patient necessitates that the physician be prepared to listen carefully to the patient and to share in decision making about how and when to do things.

Medical care has evolved in such a way that special exemptions are made for the period at the end of life. Hospice care was created to reverse the overuse of technology and denial of dying (see Chap. 15). It can be viewed as both a success and a failure. On the one hand, it is still probably used too little and too late, only after more drastic measures have been tried. At the same time, it has led to serious reconsideration of how medicine handles the process of dying. It has spawned the concept of palliative care, an idea that many aspects of support and comfort can be applied coincident with active treatment (Morrison, 2004). It has forced a reassessment of how pain is managed, with more attention to proactive treatment in adequate doses.

SPECIAL ISSUES IN CHRONIC DISEASE MANAGEMENT

Clinical Glide Paths

Providing effective chronic care relies on a longitudinally oriented information system that is sensitive to change. Each clinical encounter with a chronically ill patient is essentially a part of a continuing episode of care; it has a history and a future. Caring for a chronically ill patient, especially one with multiple problems, demands an enormous feat of memory as the patient's list of problems is unearthed and the history, treatments, and expectations associated with each are reviewed. Clinicians caring for such patients (often under enormous time pressures) may find themselves either overwhelmed with large volumes of data from which they must quickly extract the most salient facts or, alternatively, relying on inadequate data from which to reconstruct the patient's clinical course. Moreover, because patients live with their disease 24 hours a day, 7 days a week, they are best positioned to make regular observations about its progress. Such patient-constructive involvement responds to another principle of chronic care. These goals can be achieved using a simple information system that can focus the clinician's attention on salient parameters.

One approach to organizing clinical information and actively involving patients in their own care is the clinical glide path. The underlying concept is based on landing an airplane. Basically, the goal is to keep the patient within the expected trajectory to avoid the need for dramatic midcourse corrections. An expected clinical course (with provision for confidence intervals) is created. Ideally this clinical trajectory would be derived from a large statistical database that shows how similar patients have done previously. However, in the absence of such a database, the expected clinical path can be based on the clinician's experience and intuition. A separate glide path is used for each chronic problem. For each condition, the clinician selects one (or at the most two) clinical parameters to track. Ideally these should reflect how the problem manifests in that patient. The parameter can be a sign or a symptom, or even a laboratory value. The data on this parameter are collected regularly, several times a week or even daily. In most cases, the patients can provide the information, having been taught to make careful, consistent observations. These are recorded on the equivalent of flow sheets, which can be entered into a computer program that produces a graphic display. The key to this monitoring is the early warning. Observations falling outside the confidence intervals prompt strong exception messages. Any pattern of deviation is the cue for action and early intervention to assess the patient's condition and to take appropriate action. These cases should be seen quickly and with enough time to evaluate the reasons for the changes in status. Figure 4-5 shows a hypothetical example of such a clinical glide path. The patient's progress (marked with dia-monds) is within the confidence interval (which indicates a path of gradual

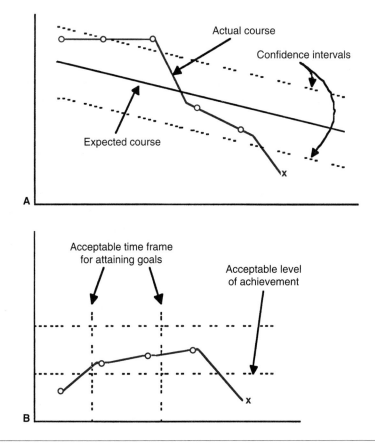

— FIGURE 4-5 —   Clinical glide path models. In this model (A), the expected course (solid line) calls for gradual decline. The confidence intervals are shown as dotted lines. Actual measures that are within or better than the glide path are shown as o. When the patient's course is worse than expected, the o changes to an x. The design shown uses confidence intervals with upper and lower bounds, but actually only the lower bound is pertinent. Any performance above the upper confidence interval boundary is very acceptable. The design of the glide path can also take another form, (B). It may be preferable to think in terms of reaching a threshold level within a given time window (eg, in recuperating from an illness) and then maintaining that level.

decline) until the last observation (noted with a star), which falls outside the confidence interval and hence should trigger a warning.

Patients (or their caregivers) can be trained to make systematic observations about salient clinical parameters and to report meaningful changes (determined by established protocols) to their clinicians. Even better, they can enter such observations into a simple computerized data system that has been programmed to notify clinicians when the patterns exceed predetermined algorithms. Routine data are not actionable, only meaningful changes.

The clinician's task is then to evaluate the meaning of such a change. The patient should be seen quickly (either by a physician or another clinician) to have the findings analyzed. The basic approach addresses three questions:

Is the data accurate? Has there been a real change?
Has the patient adhered to his/her prescribed regimen?
Has there been an intervening event (eg, infection, change in diet)?

If the answers to all three questions are negative, then a full assessment is warranted to determine the reason for the deviation.

The glide path approach meets several needs for chronic care. (1) It helps to focus physicians' attention on salient parameters. It provides an indication of early problems in time to make midcourse corrections. (2) It provides a means to involve patients more actively in their care. They learn about what is important and assume greater responsibility. (3) It is a basis for reapportioning time and effort to focus attention where an intervention is likely to produce a greater impact.

It is important to distinguish the clinical glide path approach from clinical pathways. The latter specify an expected course with specific milestones and dictates what care should be provided at specific junctures. This approach works well in very predictable situations such as postoperative recovery and even some instances of rehabilitation, but most of chronic care management is not as predictable. The glide path method specifies what data should be collected, not what actions should be taken. Its underlying premise holds that when clinicians can be aided in focusing their attention on a patient's salient parameters, they will be able to manage the chronic problems better.

Nursing home care has never attracted a great deal of physician enthusiasm, but this need not continue to be the case. If we can implement a new form of record keeping that provides better information to staff and demands better performance from them, we would see an improvement in morale and hence a more attractive atmosphere in which to practice.

Targeting and Tracking

Case management has received a lot of attention, although its efficacy has yet to be established. One of the problems in assessing the benefits of case management has been the multiple ways the term has been used. (For a discussion of case management, see Chap. 15.)

Focusing attention on the management of specific problems has become a consistent theme in the effort to improve the management of chronic illness. Disease management is most commonly used by health plans, which use the available administrative data from encounters, drug records, and laboratory tests to identify all enrollees with a given condition. Protocols can then be applied to look for errors of both omission and commission. In some cases, potential complications can be flagged and checks built in to try to avoid untoward events such as drug interactions.

A more active approach to disease management uses case managers for patients who are determined to need special attention, either because they have a diagnosis that suggests high risk of subsequent use or their history indicates problems in controlling their disease(s). These case managers work with the patients to be sure that they understand their regimens. They encourage the patients to raise any questions early. They telephonically monitor the course of the illness using parameters like those described above. They may make home visits to ascertain how the patients are doing and to ensure that they can function effectively in their natural habitats. The positive reports from trials of this approach have encouraged many replications.

Another variation on disease management being practiced in a few managed care organizations is group care. Here patients with a given disease (sometimes a more heterogeneous cluster of patients is assembled) are brought together for periodic sessions that include health education and group support, as well as individual clinical attention. It has proven more efficient to use groups in this way. The same sessions can draw upon specialists to see problematic cases more efficiently.

Particularly in the context of managed care, there is a strong incentive to try to identify high-risk patients in order to attend to them before they develop into high-cost cases. Various predictive models have been developed to identify such cases. One widely used model is the probability of repeat admissions (Pra). (See Chap. 3.)

This tool uses an eight-item questionnaire to flag older patients who are most likely to have two or more hospital admissions in the next several years (Boult et al., 1993; Pacala, Boult, and Boult, 1995). A modification of this method has been developed to use administrative databases as well. A similar approach is being developed to identify those at high risk for needing long-term care. Once these patients have been targeted, an intervention is needed to change the predicted course. The Pra model does not specify what actions should be taken; it was initially developed as a method for identifying those in need of a comprehensive geriatric examination.

Other efforts have sought to target high-risk groups. An analysis of the Medicare Current Beneficiary Survey identified a model that could identify older persons at risk of death or functional decline (Saliba et al., 2001). Another index can identify older adults who have an increased risk of death 1 year after hospitalization (Walter et al., 2001).

Interventions have also been developed to address those at highest risk. A meta-analysis of geriatric assessment declared it a substantial boon to care, because it was associated with reduced mortality and improved function (Stuck et al., 1993). Another meta-analysis suggests that home visits to basically well older persons can prevent nursing home admissions and functional decline (Stuck et al., 2002).

Function has proven to be an important predictive risk factor for both subsequent use of expensive services and or outcomes in general. Poor functional status in hospital patients predicts later mortality over and above the effects of burden-of-illness measures.

Minimum Data Set for Nursing Homes

The field of postacute care has evolved into at least three separate silos: inpatient rehabilitation, skilled nursing facilities, and home health care. Each has developed its own set of measures, which have subsequently been used for prospective payment. Nursing homes use the minimum data set (MDS). Rehabilitation uses a variant of the function improvement measure (FIM). Home health uses the outcome and assessment information set (OASIS). This inefficient parallelism has precluded good comparisons of the relative effectiveness of these different approaches. A new universal assessment tool for postacute care, CARE, is being tested.

The Omnibus Budget Reconciliation Act of 1987 (OBRA 1987) produced many changes in the way nursing homes were regulated. Perhaps none was as influential as the requirement that all nursing home residents covered by federal funds be assessed regularly using a standardized form, the MDS, for nursing home resident assessment and care screening. This information is designed to be completed by a nurse, but it draws on data from a number of disciplines.

The MDS summarizes a number of facets about each resident, including functional levels, cognitive and behavioral problems, special care needs, skin condition, nutritional status, and psychosocial well-being (the last not very well).

In addition to serving as a basic data set, problems identified trigger more detailed required documentation, called resident assessment protocols (RAPs), in 18 areas. Table 4-3 lists the RAPs.

The MDS is intended to provide a basis for developing better plans of care and for assessing the changes in functional levels over time. It can also prove a useful tool for physicians. It is a compact source of information about various aspects of each nursing home resident. If the pertinent parameters for goals determined to be achieved in the care plan were systematically charted in a flow sheet, it would be possible to see progress at a glance or to recognize the need for a change in the plan of care. Physicians can play a key role in helping nursing home staff to see how such information can be used to improve care, not just to meet external mandates for better documentation.

TABLE 4-3   RESIDENT ASSESSMENT PROTOCOL (RAP) TOPICS

Delirium	Cognitive loss/Dementia
Visual function	Communication
ADL functional/Rehabilitation potential	Urinary incontinence
Psychosocial well-being	Mood state
Behavior problem	Activities
Falls	Nutritional status
Feeding tubes	Dehydration/Fluid maintenance
Dental care	Pressure ulcers
Psychotropic drug use	Physical restraints

ADL, activity of daily living.

However, several important shortcomings of the MDS must be acknowledged. The MDS was designed to be a means of recording judgments. These judgments inevitably pass through several hands. The persons with the most direct opportunity to observe behavior are the nurses' aides, who then communicate their observations to the nurses completing the forms. The overall reliance on observations means that, in effect, all nursing home residents are being assessed as though they were cognitively impaired. This limitation is especially severe, because the MDS purports to measure critical elements of quality of life. Assuming that one can truly infer another person's emotional state, the degree to which they are engaged in meaningful activities or whether they have real social relationships seems like an act of hubris. Even using observations to determine a person's cognitive capacity seems to require heroic assumptions. It may be possible to detect extremes of behavior, but no one would want to argue that such an approach is the best way to assess many of these critical domains. Nonetheless, the MDS does not use specific questions put to those patients who can respond. Work is currently underway to test methods to assess quality of life among nursing home residents. Many, including those who are cognitively impaired can be interviewed directly. The challenge comes in how to gather information on those who cannot respond reliably. Proxy use works poorly at the individual level, although the mean values correspond well with those obtained from residents and thus can be used to assess the performance of nursing home as a whole. The new version of the MDS contains specific questions to pose to nursing home residents.

The MDS has also been used as the basis for assessing the quality of nursing home care. A set of quality indicators has been developed on the basis of MDS information. These are now being nationally normed, although more work is needed on risk adjustment to allow for valid comparisons among nursing homes that may have quite different case mixes.

Outcome and Assessment Information Set (OASIS)

The federal government has also prescribed a data system for home health care. OASIS is intended to play much the same role in this venue that MDS does in the nursing home, providing both a consistent information base for quality assessment and serving as the basis for better care planning.

ROLE OF OUTCOMES IN ASSURING QUALITY OF LONG-TERM CARE

Quality of care remains a critical, if elusive, goal for long-term care. As we consider steps for resource allocation, we might first address the question of whether we are spending our current funds most wisely. There is at once a growing demand for more creativity and more accountability in long-term care. It may be possible to reduce the regulatory burden, increase the meaningful accountability, and make the incentives within the system more rational. Progress in long-term care and chronic care will require not only more innovation and creativity, but also accountability. Outcome monitoring (and ultimately outcome-based rewards) allow both to coexist.

Before we can talk about how to package care or how to buy it cheaper, we need a better understanding of what we are really buying. One hears more and more about the value of shifting attention from the process of care to the actual outcomes achieved in acute care. These arguments apply at least as strongly to long-term care.

Two basic concepts must be kept in mind when discussing outcomes.

1. The term outcomes is used to mean the relationship between achieved and expected.
2. Because outcomes rely on probabilities, it is inappropriate to base assessments of outcomes on an individual case. Outcomes are averages and are always judged on the basis of group data.

Table 4-4 summarizes the reasons for looking toward outcomes as the way to assess and assure quality.

Nonetheless, clinicians frequently balk at being judged on the basis of outcomes. This discomfort can be traced to several issues.

1. Virtually all of clinical training addresses the process of care. Clinicians are schooled in what to do for whom. They reasonably believe, therefore, that if they do the right thing well, they have provided a quality service. They do not like to discuss clusters of patients, preferring to review their care one patient at a time.
2. Many factors can affect the outcomes of care that are out of the clinicians' control. They have difficulty with the concept of probability and prefer to either be responsible or not.

TABLE 4-4   RATIONALE FOR USING OUTCOMES

1. Outcomes encourage creativity by avoiding domination by current professional orthodoxies or powerful constituencies

2. Outcomes permit flexibility in the modality of care

3. Outcomes permit comparisons of efficacy across modalities of care

4. Outcomes permit more flexible responses to different levels of performance, and thus avoid the "all-or-none" difficulties of many sanctions. At the same time, outcomes have some limitations

5. Outcomes necessitate a single point of accountability; all the actors— facility operators, agencies, staff, physicians, patients, and family— contribute to them. Under this approach the role of the provider includes motivating others

6. Outcomes are largely influenced by the patient's status at the beginning of treatment. The easiest and most direct way to address this issue is to think of the relationship between achieved and expected outcomes as the measure of success

7. Outcomes must also take cognizance of case mix. Predicting outcomes necessitates information about disease characteristics (eg, diagnosis, severity, and comorbidity) and patient's characteristics (eg, demographic factors, prior history, and social support)

3. Outcomes are by their nature post hoc. Often, a long period can elapse between the time of an action and the report of its success. It is thus too late to intervene in that case.

4. Outcomes indicate a problem but offer no solution. Outcomes do not often point to specific actions that must be taken to correct the problems.

Hence, introducing outcomes, however rational, has not been easy. Making clinicians comfortable with an outcomes' philosophy will require substantial training and new incentives. Physicians need to be trained to think in terms of both condition-specific and generic outcomes. They need access to data systems that can display the outcomes of their care for clinically relevant groups of patients under their care and compare them with what are reasonable outcomes for comparable patients receiving good care. Table 4-5 summarizes the key issues in outcomes measurement and its applications.

Outcomes should be used as the basis for quality assurance in long-term care. The outcome approach can be used in several ways.

TABLE 4-5   OUTCOMES MEASUREMENT ISSUES

ISSUE	COMMENTS
Need outcome measures that are both clinically meaningful and psychometrically sound	Use combination of condition-specific and generic measures Usually better to adapt extant measures than to develop measures de novo
Outcomes are always post hoc	Expand outcomes information systems to include data on risk factors. These data should be useful in guiding clinicians to collect information that will identify potential problems. Use these data to create risk warnings to flag high-risk cases
Every physician has all the tough cases	Need to include a wide variety of case-mix adjusters for severity and comorbidity Ask clinicians in advance to identify potential risk adjusters Collect almost any item that a clinician might want to see Test the ability of the potential risk factor to predict outcomes and discard if it has little predictive power
Because no two clinicians see the same cases, comparisons are unfair	Use risk adjustment Create clinically homogeneous subgroups; use risk propensities groups of patients with same a priori likelihood of developing the outcome
Cannot control for selection bias; patients may receive different treatments because of subtle differences	Adjust for all clinically identifiable differences Use statistical methods (eg, instrumental variables) to adjust for unmeasured differences

TABLE 4-6 EVIDENCE-BASED RECOMMENDATIONS DERIVED FROM ASSESSING CARE OF VULNERABLE
ELDERS (ACOVE)

TOPIC	RECOMMENDATION	LEVEL OF EVIDENCE
Venous thrombosis prophylaxis	Hospitalized patients at high risk for venous thrombosis should receive DVT prophylaxis (pharmacological or sequential or intermittent compression)	Strong
Endocarditis prophylaxis	Patients at moderate to high risk should receive antibiotic prophylaxis	Weak
Central venous catheter infection precautions	Patients with new temporary central venous catheter should receive maximum barrier precautions	Moderate
Indwelling bladder catheter	Catheters should be avoided whenever possible and removed as soon as possible	Weak
Delirium evaluation	Suspected delirium should be evaluated	Moderate
Mobilization	Patients should be ambulated within 48 h of admission unless they are receiving intensive or palliative care	Moderate
Falls	Falls should be investigated to ascertain prodromal symposiums and evaluate medications	Weak
Aspiration pneumonia	Patients who are tube fed should have a plan to reduce the risk of aspiration pneumonia, including elevating the head of the bed	Moderate
Preventing ventilator-associated pneumonia	Patients who are mechanically ventilated should have a plan to reduce the risk of pneumonia, including avoiding supine position and using the semirecumbent position	Moderate

Time for antibiotic therapy	Antibiotics should be administered to patients admitted with pneumonia within 4 h of admission	Moderate
Oxygen therapy	Patients with CAP with hypoxia (O_2 saturation < 90%) should receive oxygen	Weak
Changing parenteral to oral antibiotics	Patients with CAP should be switched to equivalently bioavailable oral antibiotics as soon as possible; evidence of a successful switch should include documentation of clinical improvement, toleration of the drugs, and hemodynamic stability	Strong
Discharge assessment	Hospital discharge assessment should include level of independence, need for home health services, and patient and caregiver readiness for discharge	Weak
Preoperative care	Preoperative evaluation for elective major surgery should include a pulmonary review of symptoms and chest auscultation, test for diabetes mellitus, assessment for risk factors for delirium	Weak
Preoperative antibiotics	Patients undergoing major elective surgery should receive prophylactic antibiotics 1 h before incision that are discontinued within 24 h after surgery	Strong
Anticoagulation	Patients who have a hip fracture or have undergone total hip replacement should be started on anticoagulation preoperatively on the evening after surgery	Strong
Postoperative mobilization	Patients who were ambulatory prior to major surgery and are not in intensive care should be ambulated by postoperative day 2	Moderate
Perioperative diabetes control	Diabetic patients undergoing major surgery should have their blood sugar below 200 on the day of surgery and the first two postoperative days	Moderate

TABLE 4-6   EVIDENCE-BASED RECOMMENDATIONS DERIVED FROM ASSESSING CARE OF VULNERABLE
ELDERS (ACOVE) (*Continued*)

TOPIC	RECOMMENDATION	LEVEL OF EVIDENCE
Comprehensive palliative care plan	Vulnerable elders with metastatic cancer, oxygen-dependent pulmonary disease, NYHA class II or IV congestive heart failure, end-stage liver disease, end-stage renal disease, or dementia should have a documented plan for managing pain and other symptoms, spiritual and existential concerns, caregiver burdens and needs for practical assistance, and advance care planning	Weak
Gastrostomy tube placement	Careful discussion is needed	Weak
Advance care plan documentation	All vulnerable elders should have a plan for a surrogate decision maker in their outpatient charts	Weak
COPD and smoking	Patients with COPD should be actively urged and assisted to stop smoking	Strong
COPD and passive smoking	Patients with COPD should not be in environments where people smoke	Moderate
Screening for hypoxemia	Patients with COPD who do not use supplemental oxygen and have postbronchodilator $FEV_1 < 50\%$ should be assessed annually for oxygenation status	Strong
Rapid-acting bronchodilator	COPD patients (GOLD > I) should be prescribed a short-acting bronchodilator and taught how to use it properly	Weak
Long-acting bronchodilator	Patients with moderate to severe (GOLD stage II-IV) COPD with symptoms not controlled by as-needed bronchodilator or who have two or more exacerbations in the prior year should be prescribed long-acting bronchodilators	Moderate

Inhaled corticosteroids	Patients with severe to very severe (GOLD stage III-IV) COPD who had two or more exacerbations requiring antibiotics or oral corticosteroids in the past year should be prescribed inhaled steroids (in addition to long-acting bronchodilators), if not taking oral steroids	Strong
Performance scores in breast cancer	Physical and psychosocial status should be evaluated in women with breast cancer	Moderate
Comorbidities in breast cancer	Comorbidities should be evaluated	Moderate
Evaluation of estrogen and progesterone receptors	Estrogen and progesterone receptor status should be evaluated in locally invasive breast tumors	Strong
HER2/neu receptor status	HER2/neu receptor status should be evaluated in locally invasive breast cancer when chemotherapy is contemplated	Strong
Staging bone scan for locally invasive early breast cancer	In the presence of bone pain, elevated alkaline phosphatase, tumor size > 5 cm, or positive lymph nodes, radiographic bone imaging should be done	Weak
Lobular carcinoma in situ	If there is only lobular carcinoma in situ, no further surgical resection is indicated	Weak
Locally invasive cancer	Patients with early-stage breast cancer (I, IIA/B, T3N1M0) who undergo lumpectomy should discuss radiation therapy	Strong
Adjuvant chemotherapy	In a patient with locally invasive breast cancer and 4+ positive nodes and a life expectancy of 5+ years, adjuvant chemotherapy should be offered	Strong
Adjuvant chemotherapy for HER2/neu positive breast cancer	Patients with normal cardiac function and a life expectancy of 5+ years with locally invasive cancer and positive nodes, or who have metastatic cancer, who have HER2/neu receptor overexpression should be offered trastuzumab	Strong

TABLE 4-6   EVIDENCE-BASED RECOMMENDATIONS DERIVED FROM ASSESSING CARE OF VULNERABLE
ELDERS (ACOVE) (*Continued*)

TOPIC	RECOMMENDATION	LEVEL OF EVIDENCE
Aromatase inhibitors	Patients with advanced ER-positive breast cancer with bone metastasis and without extensive visceral involvement should be offered endocrine therapy	Strong
Performance score for patients with colorectal cancer	Physical and psychosocial status should be evaluated in women with colorectal cancer	Moderate
Pretreatment carcinoembryonic antigen level	Patients with a newly diagnosed colorectal cancer should have a pretreatment CEA level to assess prognosis	Moderate
Pretreatment CT scan	Patients with newly diagnosed colon or rectal cancer who are candidates for elective primary tumor resection and have an elevated or unknown CEA should have a CT scan of the abdomen and pelvis to guide treatment plans for surgery and adjuvant treatment	Weak
Preoperative ultrasound or MRI for rectal cancer	Newly diagnosed rectal cancer patients with normal CEA and candidates for elective resection of the primary tumor should have pelvic imaging by ultrasound, MRI, or CT to improve staging	Moderate
Preoperative total colonic examination	Patients who have new colorectal cancer and are candidates for potential cure should have a preoperative total colonic examination to look for synchronous carcinomas and polyps	Weak

Adjuvant therapy for stage III colon cancer	Patients with stage III colon cancer should receive adjuvant chemotherapy within 4 months of surgery	Strong
Preoperative neoadjuvant therapy for stage II and II rectal cancer	Patients with stage II or II mid-low rectal cancers who are candidates for surgery should receive preoperative neoadjuvant chemotherapy and radiation	Strong
Postoperative adjuvant therapy for stage II and II rectal cancer	Patients who undergo surgical resection for stage II or III rectal cancer and did not receive neoadjuvant therapy should receive postoperative adjuvant chemotherapy, radiation therapy, or both	Strong
Postoperative surveillance	Patients with greater than stage I undergo surgical resection for a cure should be followed every 6 months with a history and physical and CEA levels for the first 2 years and annually for years 3 through 5	Strong
Colonoscopy after surgery	Patients who undergo colorectal cancer resection for cure should have a colonoscopy within 3 years after surgery	Weak

Wenger and Shekelle, 2007
CAP, community-acquired pneumonia; CEA, carcinoembryonic antigen; COPD, chronic obstructive pulmonary disease; CT, computed tomography; DVT, deep vein thrombosis; GOLD, Global Initiative for Chronic Obstruction Disease; MRI, magnetic resonance imaging; NYHA, New York Heart Association.
Data compiled from Wenger NS, Roth CP, Shekelle P, ACOVE Investigators: Introduction to the assessing care of vulnerable elders-3 quality indicator measurement set. Journal of the American Geriatrics Society. Oct; 55 Suppl 2:S247-S52, 2007.

1. As reflected in the OBRA 1987 regulations (which, in turn, were stimulated by the Institute of Medicine's 1986 report), there is already growing national interest in increasing the emphasis on outcomes in regulatory activities. Outcome measures can be substituted for most of the current structure and process measures. It is appropriate to continue regulation in areas such as life safety. Concomitant with an outcomes' emphasis would be the reduction of regulatory burden. It is important to recognize, however, that it is not appropriate to dictate structure, process, and outcome at the same time. Such a policy removes all degrees of freedom and stifles creativity at the point when we want to encourage it. Under an outcome-regulated approach, providers whose patients do better than expected are rewarded and are less worried about their style of caregiving, whereas those whose patients do relatively poorly are investigated more closely.

2. Outcomes can be incorporated into the payment structure to link payment with effects of care. Payments, either in the form of bonuses and penalties or as a more fundamental part of the payment structure, can be used to reward and penalize good and bad outcomes, respectively. (eg, an outcome approach might use a factor reflecting the overall achieved/expected ratio for a patient as a multiplier against the costs of care to develop a total price paid for that period of time; or one might use a similar ratio to weigh the amount of money going to a given provider from a fixed pool of dollars committed to such care.) Such an approach must be viewed carefully within the context of our present case-mix reimbursement scheme for nursing homes, because the latter indirectly rewards deterioration in function. An outcome approach to payment is compatible with a case-mix approach that is used on admission only.

3. An outcomes approach can be incorporated into the basic caring process. Where the information base used in assessing patients and developing care plans is structured, the emphasis on outcomes can become a proactive force to guide care. Optimally, the information used to assess outcomes will come from the clinical records and will be the same information used to guide care. Using available computer technology, it is now feasible to collect such data, translate them into care plans, and aggregate these data for quality assurance at minimal additional cost. The great advantage of such a scheme is its potential both to provide a better information base with which to plan care and to reinforce the creative use of such information to achieve improvements in function. Much of the current efforts going into more traditional regulatory activities might be redirected to this effort, with assessors used to validate the assessment and to focus more intense efforts on the miscreants.

We have generally good consensus on the components of outcomes, which include elements of both quality of care and quality of life; but we are less clear

about how to sum them to produce composite scores. The gerontological literature consistently cites the following categories of outcomes:

- Physiologic function (eg, blood pressure control, lack of decubitus)
- Functional status (usually a measure of activities of daily living [ADLs])
- Pain and discomfort
- Cognition (intellectual activity)
- Affect (emotional activity)
- Social participation (based on preferences)
- Social relations (at least one person who can act as a confidant)
- Satisfaction (with care and living environment)

To these must be added more global outcomes, such as death and admission
to hospital.

Work is already available with nursing home residents to show that these
factors can be predicted with sufficient accuracy to be used in a regulatory
model. There is similar work to show that there is reasonable consensus across
a variety of constituencies about the relative weights to be placed on them for
different kinds of patients (eg, different levels of physical and cognitive function at baseline).

The outcomes approach offers significant assistance with a recurrent problem
in regulation—the development of standards. This approach may avoid many of
these difficulties by relying on empirical standards. Rather than arguing about
what is a reasonable expectation, the standard can be empirically determined.
Expectations can be derived from the actual outcomes associated with real care
given by those felt to represent a reasonable level of practice. This could include
the entire field or a designated subset. Under this arrangement, providers would
be comparing their achievements to each other's past records, with the possibility that everyone can do better.

TECHNOLOGY FOR QUALITY IMPROVEMENT

Ideally, one would like to see a measurement approach that

- Can cover the spectrum of performance
- Is easy and rapid to administer
- Is sensitive to meaningful change in performance
- Is stable within the same patient over time
- Performs consistently in different hands
- Cannot be manipulated to meet the needs of either the provider or the
  patient

The solution to this challenge is to create an assessment approach that incorporates the features designed to maximize these elements.

To cover the broad spectrum sought and still be relatively quickly adminis-tered, an instrument should have multiple branch points. These permit the user to focus on the area along the continuum where the patient is most likely to function and to expand that part of the scale to measure meaningful levels of performance. Branching can also ensure that the assessment is comprehensive but not burdensome.

By using key questions to screen an area, interviewers can ascertain whether to obtain more detailed information in each relevant domain. Where the initial response is negative, they can go on to the next branch point. Reliability is more likely to be achieved when the items are expressed in a standardized fashion tied closely to explicit behaviors. Whenever possible, performance is preferred over reports of behavior.

One cannot expect to totally avoid the gaming of an assessment. If the patient knows that poor performance is needed to ensure eligibility, they may be moti-vated to achieve the requisite low level. One can use some test of ripeness bias, such as measures of social desirability, but they will not prevent gaming the sys-tem or detect all cheating.

Computer Technology

Clinical medicine seems headed inevitably toward electronic medical records. This step could represent a major advance in the care of older people, if the opportunity is properly harnessed. Simply reproducing the current unstructured information set in a more legible and transmissible format will not suffice. Structured information provides the vehicle for assuring a more sys-tematic evaluation and follow-up of cases. By distinguishing between missing and normal values, it can provide the structure to focus clinicians' attention on salient items.

Computer technology can dramatically reduce redundancy. Properly mobi-lized, computers can provide the structure needed to assure a comprehensive assessment with no duplication of effort. Because they are interactive, they can carry out much of the desired branching and can even use simple algorithms to clarify areas of ambiguity and retest areas where some unreliability is suspected. Similar algorithms can look for inconsistency to screen for cheating.

Data stored on computers can be aggregated to display performance across patients by provider (eg, physician, nursing home, or agency). Data on a patient can be traced across time to look at changes in function and, in turn, can be aggregated.

The next important step in the progression is to move the focus from a single point of care to the linking of related elements of care. In an ideal system, patient information would be linked to permit tracing changes in status for that individ-ual as they move from one treatment modality to another. Thus, hospital admis-sion and discharge information, long-term care information, and primary care information would be merged into a common computer-linked record, which allows one to trace the patient's movements and status.

Finally, it would be desirable to have data on the process of care as well as the outcomes. This combination would permit analyses of what elements of care made a difference for which patients.

Such an approach to assuring quality is within our grasp if we are prepared to invest in data systems and to commit ourselves to collecting standardized information. It necessitates a shift in some of our fundamental paradigms from thinking about whether we did the right thing to deciding if it made any difference after all.

Two basic changes in thinking are necessary in order to establish an outcome-based philosophy, both of which are difficult for clinicians.

1. Thinking in the aggregate, using averages instead of examining each case; outcomes do not work well for individual cases because there is always a chance that something will go wrong, and life does not provide a control group.
2. Attributing responsibility to the whole enterprise rather than placing blame on an individual; a pattern of poor outcomes will mandate closer inspection of the process of care, but outcomes per se are a collective responsibility.

Computerized records greatly facilitate the task of monitoring the outcomes of care. Ideally, such a record system should be proactive, directing the collection of clinical information to encourage adequate coverage of relevant material. Long-term care is actually ahead of acute care in this regard, with the federal requirement for computerized versions of the MDS. Unfortunately, most of the systems in use are simply inputting mechanisms. They do not begin to tap the real potential of a computerized information system. Because long-term care depends heavily on poorly educated personnel for so much of its core services, the availability of an information support system, which can provide feedback and direction, is especially appropriate.

Computerization can provide both the flexibility and the brevity sought by using branching logic to expand a category when there is reason to explore it more thoroughly. It can avoid duplication by displaying data already collected by others while still permitting the second observer to correct and challenge earlier entries. More important, it can display information to show change over time, thus permitting both the regulators and the caregivers to look at the effects of care.

Once the data are in electronic form, they are easily transmitted and manipulated. It is not hard to envision a large set of data derived from these systematic observations that would permit calculations of expected courses for different types of long-term care patients. These could then be compared to individual patients' courses to assess the potential impact of care on outcomes.

The computer's ability to compare observed and expected outcomes extends beyond its role as a regulatory device. It could be a major source of assistance to caregivers. One of the great frustrations in long-term care, especially in the trenches, is the difficulty in sensing whether the caregiver is making a difference. Because so many patients enter care when they are already declining, the benefits of care are often best expressed as a slowing of that decline curve. Without some measure of expected course in the absence of good care, those who render care daily may not appreciate how much they are accomplishing and thereby may forgo one of the important rewards of their labors.

To display information about the change in patient's condition over time, a simple task for a computer, will assist the long-term caregiver to think more in terms of the overall picture, rather than a series of separate snapshots in time. Given the computer's ability to translate data into graphics, it is a simple procedure to develop pictorial representations of the changes occurring for a given patient or group of patients and to contrast those with what might be reasonably expected.

Again the effort is directed toward changing perceptions about older persons, especially those in long-term care. For too long, long-term care has worked in a negative spiral—a self-fulfilling prophecy that expected patients to deteriorate— served to discourage both care providers and patients. Such an attitude is hardly likely to attract the best and the brightest in any of the health professions. As noted earlier in this chapter, nursing home patients are among the most responsive to almost any form of intervention. Any information system that can reinforce a prospective view of long-term care, especially one that can display patient progress, represents an important adjunct to such care.

Assessing care of vulnerable elders (ACOVE) has also made a number of recommendations about steps in providing better care, but none are supported by strong evidence (Wenger and Shekelle, 2007). These recommendations include

- All patients should be able to identify a physician or clinic to call for medical care and know how to reach them.
- After a new medication is prescribed for a chronic illness the following should be noted at follow-up:
    - Medication is being taken as prescribed.
    - Patient was asked about the medication (eg, side effects, adherence, availability).
    - Medication was not started because it was not needed or changed.
    - If a patient is seen by two or more physicians and new medication is prescribed by one, the other(s) should be aware of the change.
    - If a patient is referred to a consultant, the referring physician should show evidence of the consultant's findings and recommendations.
- If a diagnostic test is ordered, the following should be documented at the next visit:
    - Result of test specifically acknowledged.
    - Note that test was not needed or not performed and why.
    - Note that test is pending.

- If a patient misses a scheduled preventive visit there should be a reminder.
- When patients are seen in an emergency department (ED) or admitted to hospital, the continuity physician should be notified within 2 days.
- Patients discharged from hospital and who survive 6 weeks should have some contact with their continuity physician who should be aware of the hospitalization.
- When patient is discharged to home from hospital and receives new chronic disease medication, the continuity physician should document the change in medication within 6 weeks.
- When patient is discharged to home or to a nursing home from hospital and tests are pending, the results should be available within 6 weeks.
- When patient is discharged to home or to a nursing home from hospital, there should be a discharge summary in the continuity physician's records.
- If a patient does not speak English, the interpreter or translated materials should be used.

SUMMARY

In many respects, geriatrics is the epitome of chronic disease care. New paradigms are needed, which recognize the changing role of patients their own care, the need to think differently about the payoff horizons for investments in care, and the tracking of the course of disease to identify when intervention is needed. With geriatrics and chronic disease in general, the benefits of good care may be hard to discern, because they represent a slowing of decline. This effect is invisible unless there is some basis for forming an expected clinical course against which to compare the actual course.

Physicians caring for older patients need to think in prospective terms. They will enjoy their practices more if they can learn to set reasonable goals for patients, to record progress toward these goals, and to use the failure to achieve progress as an important clinical sign of the need for reevaluation.

References

Beck A, Scott J, Williams P, et al. A randomized trial of group outpatient visits for chronically ill older HMO members: the cooperative health care clinic. *J Am Geriatr Soc.* 1997;45:543-549.

Boult C, Dowd B, McCaffrey D, et al. Screening elders for risk of hospital admission. *J Am Geriatr Soc.* 1993;41:811-817.

Clark F, Azen SP, Zemke R, et al. Occupational therapy for independent-living older adults: a randomized controlled trial. *JAMA.* 1997;278:1321-1326.

Downey L, Livingston R, Stopeck A. Diagnosing and treating breast cancer in elderly women: a call for improved understanding. *J Am Geriatr Soc.* 2007;55:1636-1644.

Fiatarone MA, O'Neil EF, Ryan ND, et al. Exercise training and nutritional supplementation for physical frailty in very elderly people. *N Engl J Med.* 1994;330:1769-1775.

Horrocks S, Anderson E, Salisbury C. Systematic review of whether nurse practitioners working in primary care can provide equivalent care to doctors. *BMJ.* 2002;324:819-823.

Kane RL. The chronic care paradox. *J Aging Soc Policy.* 2000;11(2/3):107-114.

Lerner MJ, Simmons CH. Observer's reaction to the 'innocent victim': compassion or rejection. *J Pers Soc Psychol.* 1966;4:203-210.

Morrison RS, Meier DC. Clinical practice. Palliative care. *N Engl J Med.* 2004;350(25): 2582-2590.

Mundinger M, Kane R, Lenz E, et al. Primary care outcomes in patients treated by nurse practitioners or physicians: a randomized trial. *JAMA.* 2000;283(1):59-68.

Pacala JT, Boult C, Boult L. Predictive validity of a questionnaire that identifies older persons at risk for hospital admission. *J Am Geriatr Soc* 1995;43:374-377.

Saliba D, Elliott M, Rubenstein LZ, et al. The vulnerable elders survey: a tool for identifying vulnerable older people in the community. *J Am Geriatr Soc.* 2001;49:1691-1699.

Stuck AE, Egger M, Hammer A, et al. Home visits to prevent nursing home admission and functional decline in elderly people: systematic review and meta-regression analysis. *JAMA.* 2002;287(8):1022-1028.

Stuck AE, Siu AL, Wieland GD, et al. Comprehensive geriatric assessment: a meta-analysis of controlled trials. *Lancet.* 1993;342:1032-1036.

Walter LC, Brand RJ, Counsell SR, et al. Development and validation of a prognostic index for 1-year mortality in older adults after hospitalization. *JAMA.* 2001;285:2987-2994.

Wenger NS, Shekelle PG. Measuring medical care provided to vulnerable elders: the assessing care of vulnerable elders-3 (ACOVE-3) quality indicators. *J Amer Geriat Assoc.* 2007;55(suppl):S247-S487.

PART II

DIFFERENTIAL DIAGNOSIS AND MANAGEMENT

CHAPTER 5

PREVENTION

GENERAL PRINCIPLES

The new and emerging generations of older people are increasingly interested in promoting healthy aging. The terms "health promotion" and "prevention" are used almost interchangeably. As noted in Chap. 4, prevention may take many forms in the context of chronic disease management. In essence, proactive primary care can be seen as a form of prevention (tertiary prevent as defined below). Some authors caution against the enthusiasm for single-disease approach to prevention among older persons, arguing that competitive risks will simply raise the rates for other diseases (Mangin, Sweeney, and Heath, 2007).

Ageism may lead people to discount the value of prevention in caring for older persons, but the evidence suggests that many preventive strategies are effective in this age group. To some extent, one's enthusiasm for preventive care for older persons may reflect concern about their future and the value of that future. Enthusiasm for prevention is based on beliefs about the following:

1. The efficacy of the intervention in preventing disease or dysfunction in the future. This includes an estimate of the likelihood of the patient's following the preventive regimen.
2. The value of the health gained. In the case of older patients, this includes concerns about the likelihood of other problems reducing the benefit.
3. The cost of the preventive activity. This includes both the direct cost and the indirect costs, such as anxiety, restricted lifestyle, and false-positive results.

Perhaps the most preventable problem connected with caring for older persons is iatrogenic disease. Here some of the major issues and strategies surrounding more conventional preventive activities are discussed. The major thesis here, as with much covered elsewhere in this volume, is that age alone should not be a predominant factor in choosing an approach to a patient. A number of preventive strategies deserve serious consideration in light of their immediate and future benefits for many elderly patients.

Preventive activities can be divided into three types. Primary prevention refers to some specific action taken to render the patient more resistant or the environment less harmful. The term "secondary prevention" has come to be used in two ways. One implies screening or early detection for asymptomatic disease or early disease. The idea here is that finding a problem early allows more effective treatment. The second meaning of secondary prevention involves using the techniques of primary prevention on people who already have the disease in an effort to delay progression. For example, getting people who have had a heart attack to stop smoking. That behavior will not prevent heart disease but it should reduce the risks of subsequent problems. Tertiary prevention is actually efforts to improve care to avoid later complications. All three areas are relevant to geriatric care. Table 5-1 offers examples of activities in each category. Not all the items indicated in this table are supported by clear research findings. Some cases—such as seat belts, exercise, and social support—are based on prudent judgment.

The federal government has set health goals for various population groups, including older people. Table 5-2 shows the indicators they have identified, which can be derived from available national data sources. Particularly distressing is the finding that the rate of preventive services decreases among physicians who derive a larger portion of their practice income from Medicare (Pham et al., 2005).

TABLE 5-1 PREVENTIVE STRATEGIES FOR OLDER PERSONS

PRIMARY	SECONDARY	TERTIARY
Immunization	Papanicolaou (Pap) smear	Comprehensive geriatric assessment
Influenza	Breast examination	Foot care
Pneumococcus	Breast self-examination	Dental care
Tetanus	Mammography	Toileting efforts
Blood pressure	Fecal blood, colonoscopy	
Smoking	Hypothyroidism	
Exercise	Depression	
Obesity	Vision	
Cholesterol	Hearing	
Sodium restriction	Oral cavity	
Social support	Tuberculosis	
Environment	PSA	
Seat belts		
Medication review		

PSA, prostate specific antigen.

TABLE 5-2 HEALTHY PEOPLE REPORT CARD ITEMS FOR SENIORS

Health status (minimize the following)
    Physically unhealthy days
    Frequent mental distress
    Complete tooth loss
    Disability (limitation in any way in physical, mental, or emotional
    problems; need for special equipment)

Health behaviors
    Leisure time physical activity
    Eating 5+ fruits and vegetables daily
    Obesity
    Smoking

Preventive care and screening
    Flu vaccine in past year
    Pneumonia vaccine ever
    Mammogram within past 2 years
    Sigmoidoscopy or colonoscopy ever
    Cholesterol checked within past 5 years

Injuries
    Hip fracture hospitalizations

Centers for Disease Control and Prevention and The Merck Company Foundation. The State of Aging and Health in America 2007. Whitehouse Station, NJ: The Merck Company Foundation; 2007.

In addressing prevention for older persons, it is important to bear in mind the goals pursued. The World Health Organization has provided a useful continuum, which progresses from disease to impairment to disability to handicap (although the latter term is no longer considered politically correct). Preventive efforts for older people can be productively targeted at several points along this spectrum. Efforts can seek to prevent disease, but they can also be designed to minimize its consequences, by reducing the progression to disability. Slowing that transition is, in essence, the heart of geriatrics.

Preventive efforts on behalf of elderly patients have special characteristics, beyond the emphasis on function. The narrowing of the therapeutic window, discussed in Chap. 4, means that older persons may be susceptible to the side effects of prevention as well as of treatment. Some risk factors that strongly predict the onset of disease in younger persons may not be appropriate for modification in older persons. Perhaps the condition has already become well established and is resistant to change, or the factor may have already exerted its influence at an earlier stage of life. Conversely, older people represent survivors. People exposed to a risk factor for many years and still living into old age may be affected differently than those who succumb younger. Thus, questions are repeatedly raised about how enthusiastic one should be to stop smoking or reduce cholesterol levels in the oldest of the old.

Clearly, primary prevention is the most desirable. But the nature of the changes required to achieve this end vary substantially. Some require a single brief contact (eg, immunization), but others imply sustained change in behaviors, such as changing eating habits or exercising. If a brief encounter can confer some form of long-lasting protection at minimal risk, such a strategy will be actively pursued.

Many risk reduction strategies, however, require major changes in behavior, many of which are pursued because they are pleasurable. Enthusiasm for attempting to change major health behaviors, especially those that are associated with either pleasure or addiction, is limited. At what point is the benefit worth the cost? How much quality of life should be sacrificed in the name of health? Conversely, how big a role does ageism play in deciding that it is not worth investing in prevention for older people? Just as with therapeutic decisions, thoughtful geriatricians struggle with the overall benefit of enforcing a major lifestyle change on someone who has both survived and has a finite life expectancy, with limited opportunities for pleasure. The task is made even harder when strong economic interests advertise the very products physicians seek to discourage.

One approach to risk reduction that fits with the predominant medical model is to transform the risk into a disease and treat it as such. For example, high blood pressure becomes hypertension; high cholesterol becomes hypercholesterolemia; thin bones become osteoporosis. When effective medications become available, as is the case in each of these scenarios, the drug companies now become active allies preaching to both the medical profession and the consumers. From a societal perspective, the question becomes one of cost-effectiveness. If the medications are expensive (especially over a lifetime), how much should be spent on this prevention? Many of the calculations suggest that those strategies that involve costly medications are not cost-effective, or that the strategy must be carefully targeted to those at highest risk. In some cases, older people are better (more cost-effective) targets than younger ones (Schousboe, 2005).

Because the number of activities that are both safe and effective is small, we must rely on the other two preventive strategies, each of which comes at a cost. Screening for one or another condition is useful where the disease process can be detected in advance of the condition's clinical appearance and there is evidence that earlier treatment produces real benefits (earlier diagnosis can create the appearance of longer survival simply by identifying the problem earlier); but such screening may be excessively costly if the number of treatable cases detected is low and the follow-up testing is expensive. Screening is usually judged on the criteria of sensitivity and specificity. The former refers to the proportion of actual cases correctly identified and the latter to the accuracy of labeling of noncases (normal individuals). Alas, the two factors are usually linked, so that an improvement in one comes at the cost of a decrement in the other. The decision about where to set them relative to each other depends on the expected prevalence of the problem and the consequences of a false-positive and a false-negative finding with respect to a given clinical condition.

Tertiary prevention is a central part of good geriatric care, which strives to minimize the progression of disease to disability. It requires a comprehensive effort to address both the physiologic and environmental factors that can create dependency.

While older persons have been traditionally excluded from preventive trials, that situation is changing. As it does, findings suggest that primary prevention is often appropriate for older persons as well, but the problems associated with translating the results of clinical trials into practice are at least as great as with younger persons. Active treatment of hypertension (both systolic and diastolic) is associated with reduced cardiovascular complications. Control of systolic blood pressure is associated with preventing heart failure.

Even more broadly, the value of geriatric assessment suggests that important problems in primary care of older persons are being ignored or undertreated. Reports that a yearly visit by a nurse practitioner to unselected persons aged 75 years and older can lead to substantial functional improvement and reduced nursing home admissions raise serious questions about how well the current primary care system is working (Stuck et al., 2002). Likewise a randomized trial showed that a home visit by an occupational therapist was shown to yield benefits for a cross-section of independent-living older adults (Clark et al., 1997). For older patients with already diagnosed complex problems, the concept of geriatric assessment has given way to a model of geriatric evaluation and management (GEM), which allows for the geriatric team to assume responsibility for the patient's care for a period sufficient to permit stabilization of the patient's condition and, in some instance, therapeutic trials. The problem still remains that when the patient is returned to the care of their primary care physician, the benefits of this rehabilitation may be lost unless provision is made to sustain the therapeutic changes. In the absence of this continuity, the investment represented by geriatric assessment may be threatened.

Clinicians' enthusiasm for prevention will be tempered by their ability to be paid for this work. Medicare's coverage of preventive services is modest. Table 5-3 shows the extent of this coverage.

EFFECTIVENESS OF PREVENTION IN OLDER PEOPLE

In evaluating the efficacy of preventive activities for older persons, we must confront a dilemma. Because older people were systematically excluded from many trials of prevention strategies, there are few hard data on which to base judgments. At the same time, there are strong feelings from both sides about the value of prevention. Active advocates for wellness among elderly people urge

TABLE 5-3 PREVENTIVE SERVICES COVERED BY THE MEDICARE PROGRAM AS OF JANUARY 2008

SERVICE	GROUPS COVERED	FREQUENCY OF SERVICE	COST-SHARING REQUIREMENTS[a]
IMMUNIZATIONS			
Pneumococcal	All beneficiaries	As needed (probably once per lifetime) (booster every 5 years recommended)	None
Hepatitis B	Beneficiaries at intermediate or high risk of contracting hepatitis B	As needed (probably once per lifetime)	Copayment after deductible
Influenza	All beneficiaries	Every year	None
SCREENING SERVICES			
Abdominal aortic aneurysm ultrasound screening	Beneficiaries at risk (referred by physician at Welcome to Medicare physical)	Once	Copayment after deductible
Cervical cancer—Papanicolaou (Pap) smear[h]	All female beneficiaries	Every 2 years if low risk, every year if high risk	Copayment with no deductible[b]
Breast cancer—mammography[h]	Female beneficiaries aged 40 and older	Every year	Copayment with no deductible[b]
Vaginal cancer—pelvic examination[h]	All female beneficiaries	Every 2 years[b]	Copayment with no deductible[b]

Service	Who is covered	Frequency	Cost
Colorectal cancer—fecal occult blood test[h]	Beneficiaries aged 50 and older	Every year	No copayment or deductible
Colorectal cancer—sigmoidoscopy[c]	Beneficiaries aged 50 and older	Every 4 years	Copayment after deductible[d]
Colorectal cancer—colonoscopy[c]	All beneficiaries	Every 10 years[e]	Copayment after deductible[d]
Osteoporosis—bone mass measurement[h]	Estrogen-deficient female beneficiaries at clinical risk for osteoporosis as well as other qualified individuals[f]	Every 2 years[g]	Copayment after deductible
Prostate cancer—prostate-specific antigen test and/or digital rectal examination	Men aged 50 and older	Every year	Copayment after deductible for examination; no cost for PSA test
Diabetes screening	Beneficiaries with risk factors	Twice a year	Copayment after deductible
Diabetic retinopathy examination	Diabetic beneficiaries	Yearly	Copayment after deductible
Glaucoma	Beneficiaries medically determined to be at high risk for glaucoma	Every year	Copayment after deductible
Hearing examination	If ordered by physician		Copayment after deductible

TABLE 5-3   PREVENTIVE SERVICES COVERED BY THE MEDICARE PROGRAM AS OF JANUARY 2008 (*Continued*)

SERVICE	GROUPS COVERED	FREQUENCY OF SERVICE	COST-SHARING REQUIREMENTS[a]
Physical examination (Welcome to Medicare)	Within first 6 months of getting Part B	Once	Copayment after deductible
OTHER			
Smoking cessation counseling	If ordered by physician (for smoking-related illness or taking medications that can be affected by tobacco)	Two attempts within a 12-month period	Copayment after deductible

a. Applicable Medicare cost-sharing requirements generally include a 20% copayment after a $135 per year deductible in 2008. Thereafter, beneficiaries are responsible for a copayment that is usually 20% of the Medicare-approved amount. For certain tests, the copayment may be higher.
b. The costs of the laboratory test portion of these services are not subject to copayment or deductible. The beneficiary is subject to a deductible and/or copayment for physician services only.
c. The doctor can decide to use a barium enema instead of a sigmoidoscopy or colonoscopy for beneficiaries aged 50 and older. The frequency of service is the same as the sigmoidoscopy or colonoscopy it substitutes for.
d. The copayment is increased from 20% to 25% for services rendered in an ambulatory surgical center.
e. Beneficiaries medically determined to be at high risk may receive a colonoscopy every 2 years.
f. The statute defines "other qualified individuals" as those who have vertebral abnormalities or primary hyperparathyroidism, or who are receiving long-term glucocorticoid steroid or osteoporosis drug therapy.
g. CMS permits coverage of a bone mass measurement at any time—sooner than 2 years—if the service is medically necessary.
h. Recommended by USPSTF
Centers for Medicare and Medicaid 2008. https://www.noridianmedicare.com/shared/parta/bulletins/2008/2066_jan/Preventive_Services_and_Screenings_for_Which_Medicare_Provides_Coverage.htm. Accessed July 9, 2008.

strenuous efforts to promote major life changes. They are allied with those who view many of the accoutrements of aging as acquired and hence capable of modification. They cite data showing that muscle strength and endurance can be regained with active training even at advanced ages.

Another group argues that older people have already reached a stage in life where they have demonstrated a capacity to cope. They would accept many of the consequences of aging and note that the demonstrated gains are less strongly associated with major improvements in morbidity and function than with values derived from testing.

The US Preventive Services Task Force attempted to assess available scientific information on the efficacy of preventive efforts for persons at all ages (US Preventive Services Task Force, 1996. *Guide to Clinical Preventive Services, 3rd Edition.* 2000). Updated online (www.ncbi.nlm.nih.gov/books/bv.fcgi?rid=hstat, accessed on November 03, 2007). Table 5-4 summarizes the major recommendations from the task force relevant to those aged 65 years and older. There is a considerable discrepancy in both directions between the services judged suitable and those covered by Medicare.

Appropriate treatment can do a great deal to keep such patients ambulatory and stable. The US Task Force avoided the debate about false-positive results with regard to screening for glaucoma by recommending that the decision be made by an ophthalmologist, but the importance of vision in the overall functioning of the elderly patient argues strongly for attention to this area. In a similar vein, the potential for improving function by replacing cataracts with implanted lenses mandates greater attention to visual problems as well as concern about the excess use of surgery. However, the functional benefit is not realized by cognitively impaired persons. More recent practice has shifted diabetes care attention from the usual concerns about eyes and feet to a greater appreciation about the importance of cardiovascular disease. Because of the vascular effects of diabetes, close attention should be paid to the lipid profiles of diabetics.

Some preventive interventions seem intuitively worthwhile, but occasionally data raise irksome questions. For example, vaccination against influenza is strongly recommended for older persons. Some studies show that immunization is associated with decreased use of hospitals (Nichol et al., 2007). Indeed, over the last several years the rate of such immunization has increased dramatically. However, ironically the rate of hospitalizations among older persons for influenza and pneumonia has also gone up during the same period, raising perplexing questions about the value of this widely lauded preventive measure (Simonsen et al., 2007).

Pneumococcal vaccines are now in widespread use, and many consider them to be useful in the care of elderly persons at risk, especially those in institutions, but there remains an active controversy about their cost-effectiveness. Tuberculosis remains a problem among older people, especially those living in institutions. Special care must be taken in interpreting a lack of reaction to tuberculin skin tests in elderly persons because of the risk of anergy.

TABLE 5-4   US PREVENTIVE SERVICES TASKFORCE RECOMMENDATIONS

USPSTF Recommendation	Level of Recommendation	Paid for by Medicare
Screening mammography, with or without clinical breast examination, every 1-2 years for women aged 40 and older.	B	√
Screen men and women 50 years of age or older for colorectal cancer.	A	√
Good evidence that periodic FOBT reduces mortality from colorectal cancer and fair evidence that sigmoidoscopy alone or in combination with FOBT reduces mortality.		
No direct evidence that screening colonoscopy is effective in reducing colorectal cancer mortality		
Women aged 65 and older be screened routinely for osteoporosis; routine screening begins at age 60 for women at increased risk for osteoporotic fractures.	B	√
Routinely screen men aged 35 years and older and women aged 45 years and older for lipid disorders and treat abnormal lipids in people who are at increased risk of coronary heart disease.	A	
Screening for lipid disorders include measurement of TC and HDL-C.	B	
Evidence is insufficient to recommend for or against triglyceride measurement as a part of routine screening for lipid disorders.	I	

Screening adults for depression in clinical practices that have systems in place to assure accurate diagnosis, effective treatment, and followup. — B

Evidence is insufficient to recommend for or against routine screening for dementia in older adults. — I

Evidence is insufficient to recommend for or against routinely screening asymptomatic adults for type 2 diabetes, impaired glucose tolerance, or impaired fasting glucose. — I

Screen adults aged 18 and older for high blood pressure. — A

Evidence is insufficient to recommend for or against routine screening for prostate cancer using PSA testing or DRE. Men 75+ should not be offered a PSA test routinely.* — I

Evidence is insufficient to recommend for or against routine behavioral counseling to promote a healthy diet in unselected patients in primary care settings. — I

Recommends intensive behavioral dietary counseling for adult patients with hyperlipidemia and other known risk factors for cardiovascular and diet-related chronic disease. Intensive counseling can be delivered by primary care clinicians or by referral to other specialists, such as nutritionists or dietitians. — B

Screen all adult patients for obesity and offer intensive counseling and behavioral interventions to promote sustained weight loss for obese adults. — B

Evidence is insufficient to recommend for or against the use of moderate- or low-intensity counseling together with behavioral interventions to promote sustained weight loss in obese adults. — I

TABLE 5-4 US PREVENTIVE SERVICES TASKFORCE RECOMMENDATIONS (*Continued*)

USPSTF RECOMMENDATION	LEVEL OF RECOMMENDATION	PAID FOR BY MEDICARE
Evidence is insufficient to recommend for or against the use of supplements of vitamins A, C, or E; multivitamins with folic acid; or antioxidant combinations for the prevention of cancer or cardiovascular disease.	I	
Recommends against the use of beta-carotene supplements, either alone or in combination, for the prevention of cancer or cardiovascular disease.	D	
Clinicians should discuss aspirin chemoprevention with adults who are at increased risk for CHD. Discussions with patients should address both the potential benefits and harms of aspirin therapy.	A	
Recommends against the routine use of estrogen and progestin for the prevention of chronic conditions in postmenopausal women.	D	
Evidence is insufficient to recommend for or against the use of unopposed estrogen for the prevention of chronic conditions in postmenopausal women who have had a hysterectomy.	I	
Strongly recommends screening for cervical cancer in women who have been sexually active and have a cervix.	A	√
Recommends against routinely screening women older than age 65 for cervical cancer if they have had adequate recent screening with normal Pap smears and are not otherwise at high risk for cervical cancer.	D	

Evidence is insufficient to recommend for or against the routine use of new
technologies to screen for cervical cancer.   I

Evidence is insufficient to recommend for or against routine screening by primary   I
care clinicians to detect suicide risk in the general population.

A. The USPSTF strongly recommends that clinicians routinely provide (the service) to eligible patients. The USPSTF found good evidence that (the
service) improves important health outcomes and concludes that benefits substantially outweigh harms.
B. The USPSTF recommends that clinicians routinely provide (the service) to eligible patients. The USPSTF found at least fair evidence that (the
service) improves important health outcomes and concludes that benefits outweigh harms.
C. The USPSTF makes no recommendation for or against routine provision of (the service). The USPSTF found at least fair evidence that (the service)
can improve health outcomes but concludes that the balance of benefits and harms is too close to justify a general recommendation.
D. The USPSTF recommends against routinely providing (the service) to asymptomatic patients. The USPSTF found at least fair evidence that (the
service) is ineffective or that harms outweigh benefits.
I. The USPSTF concludes that the evidence is insufficient to recommend for or against routinely providing (the service). Evidence that the (service)
is effective is lacking, of poor quality, or conflicting and the balance of benefits and harms cannot be determined.
* The USPHSTF has determined that the risks of PSA testing are greater than the benefits in men 75+ (http://www.ahrq.gov/clinic/uspstf/uspsrca.htm
Accessed August 5, 2008).
CHD, coronary heart disease; DRE, digital rectal examination; FOBT, fecal occult blood testing; HDL-C, high-density lipoprotein cholesterol; PSA,
prostate specific antigen; TC, total cholesterol.
Health Services Technology/Assessment Texts (HSTAT). Guide to Clinical Preventive Services, 3rd Edition. 2000. Updated online
(www.ncbi.nlm.nih.gov/books/bv.fcgi?rid=hstat), accessed on November 03, 2007.

Particularly in our current system, where Medicare Part B does not pay for many preventive services, it is important to appreciate that much can be done in prevention without special visits for that purpose. Most, if not all, of the procedures can be performed by an appropriately trained nonphysician.

The value of screening depends on the availability of an effective intervention and the likelihood that the intervention will change the clinical course. There is reason to believe that some cancers may perform differently in older persons. Although the incidence (and certainly the prevalence) increases with age, the rate of growth may be slower. Thus there is great controversy around the efficacy of active screening for prostate and breast cancer in older persons. The recent reanalysis of data from clinical trials of mammography illustrates just how confusing this literature can be. One analysis suggests that screening with mammography after age 69 leads to a small gain in life expectancy and is modestly cost-effective (Kerlikowske et al., 1999).

Some geriatricians question whether older women can tolerate treatment for cancer; others believe that cancer in the elderly progresses more slowly than younger patients. Cancer takes a toll on older people. The mean age of detection for the most common forms of cancer is about 68, and the mean age of death among those persons is about 72. Cancer foreshortens their lives. In the case of breast cancer, the median age of diagnosis is about 61 and the median age of death is around 69. Most recommendations call for stopping Pap smears at age 70 for women with no abnormalities. However, cervical cancer remains a serious risk for older women and studies show that the risk of cancer increases with longer intervals between tests (Sawaya et al., 2003). The issue of risk versus benefit becomes even more active when procedures like colonoscopy are considered (Lin et al., 2006).

At the same time, some areas are well served by increased clinical attention. Greater physician sensitivity to identifying depression in older persons can detect an often remediable condition. Detection of mental problems is greatly enhanced by structured screening data. Awareness of the likelihood of alcoholism can lead to recognizing a problem that can be corrected.

There is more controversy about the desirability of increasing the recognition of cognitive deficiency. Although standardized testing can detect cases that might otherwise be masked in older persons who have skillfully compensated for their loss, it is not immediately clear that there is great benefit in such early uncovering. Given the relatively small proportion of dementia cases that have reversible etiologies, screening for dementia would not seem to pass the first test of screening. However, some geriatricians suggest that the modest benefits of anticholinesterase therapy can gain at least months of function and postpone institutionalization, thus justifying an aggressive approach to screening. Others suggest that increasing the period of time when a person knows they have dementia may be a mixed blessing at best.

There is growing interest in various types of cognitive training. Basically extending the enthusiasm for physical activity, researchers have shown modest benefits from cognitive activity in maintaining cognitive prowess (Ball et al., 2002; Wolinsky et al., 2006). But it is too early to claim major victories.

By contrast, the benefits of aggressively identifying and bringing under treatment older persons with symptoms of depression have been demonstrated (Katon et al., 1995).

Routine screening for geriatric populations tends to uncover problems that are already known. Among a group of elderly persons coming for a health screening, 95% had at least one positive finding. Approximately 55% were referred to a physician for further evaluation and 15% were treated for the finding (Rubenstein et al., 1986). Routine annual laboratory testing of nursing home residents has received mixed reviews. A modest panel—including a complete blood count, electrolytes, renal and thyroid function tests, and a urinalysis—may be useful. (Levinstein et al., 1987)

Behavior change represents at once the most promising and the most frustrating component of prevention. While some may argue that you can't teach an old dog new tricks or that engrained habit patterns are hard to break, there is no evidence to support such pessimism. Quite to the contrary, anecdotal data about elderly people taking up exercise programs and changing their dietary habits provide reason for more optimism. The critical issue here is the degree to which such changes will sufficiently modify risk factors and change clinical courses to justify the disturbance.

In general, moderation seems safest. For example, data from the Alameda County study suggest that not smoking, modest physical activity, moderate weight, and regular meals are associated with lower mortality risks among older populations. As shown in Fig. 5-1, older persons' health habits are generally as good as or better than those of younger people. Although our data are scant, the

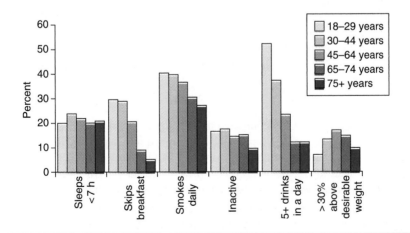

— FIGURE 5-1 — Personal health habits of people at different ages. From US Senate Committee on Aging. Aging America: trends and projections. DHHS Pub No. (FCoA)91-28001. 1991, Washington DC: US Department of Health and Human Services.

degree of enthusiasm for active modification will likely vary with the topic addressed.

The best preventive strategies for older persons are those associated with the least risk. The findings from the Treatment on Nonpharmacological Interventions in the Elderly (TONE) study, suggesting that weight loss and sodium restriction could effectively lower blood pressure in older persons, is a good example of such an approach. Reducing dietary salt intake was shown to lower blood pressure in another study as well. Along the same lines, antioxidant vitamins have been suggested by epidemiological evidence as a means of reducing cardiovascular disease. Several studies have shown protective benefits from using vitamin E to prevent Alzheimer disease, although the definitive data for either have not yet been seen. Taking broad-spectrum vitamin supplements is probably a good idea for most older people (Fletcher and Fairfield, 2002).

Low-dose aspirin seems like a good idea, although its use has been targeted to younger persons. It has been shown to reduce the incidence of myocardial infarction, but not stroke, in men, but to have the opposite result with women (Ridker et al., 2005).

Perhaps the greatest controversy around the value of epidemiological studies as the basis for preventive care recommendations has come in the area of hormone replacement therapy (HRT) in women. Based on observational studies, HRT was widely hailed as having multiple benefits including delaying osteoporosis, lowered cholesterol, and prevention of Alzheimer disease. However, subsequent findings from randomized clinical trials showed that many of these benefits were exaggerated, and that HRT (at least a combination of estrogen and progesterone; the treatment recommended to avoid risks of uterine cancer) may actually increase risks of heart disease and stroke, as well as of cancer. Now labeled a health hazard, instead of a preventive tool, its role in treating postmenopausal symptoms is still under evaluation, and will likely become a decision based on risk aversion.

OSTEOPOROSIS

A good example of the conflicted nature of prevention in older persons is the case of osteoporosis. (This topic is also addressed in Chap. 10.) Effective treatments are now available to delay the onset or halt the progression of this disease, which can lead to fractures and disabilities. Understanding the management of osteoporosis requires thinking systematically about the clinical goals. In this regard, the intellectual exercise is similar to that around hypertension. The real consideration is not necessarily attacking the primary disease but its ultimate effects. In the case of osteoporosis, the adverse outcomes are fractures of various types. However, once attention shifts to the actual outcomes of importance new strategies emerge. For example, if the goal is to prevent hip fractures, wearing hip protectors may be as effective, perhaps more so, than improving bone density, because hip fracture is the combined effect of falling and osteoporosis (Sawka et al., 2007). The studies on the actual effectiveness of such devices suggest that they do not work as well as one might hope (van Schoor, 2007). Part of the failure may be attributed to older peoples' reluctance to wear them. It is not easy to convince older patients, especially those with cognitive impairment, to wear such devices.

Drugs can be used to treat osteoporosis effectively, and with modest side effects, but these drugs can be expensive, especially over a lifetime. (A common bisphosphonate, alendronate, should be released in generic form in 2008.) The first line of defense against this disease is a regimen of calcium, vitamin D, and weight-bearing exercises; but this inexpensive and safe approach may be insufficient or hard to sustain. In these instances, drugs may be indicated (although the use of the big three should be continued).

The prime target for osteoporosis screening is postmenopausal women, but the disease can also affect men. Screening is done by bone mineral density testing. The World Health Organization standard for osteoporosis is a value of 2.5 standard deviations (SD) (often referred to as a T score) or more below the young adult mean value, but the National Osteoporosis Foundation recommends treating when T scores are ≤ 2 SD below the young adult mean value.

HRT is effective in delaying the course of osteoporosis, but the effects last only as long as the treatment. Given the new evidence of multiple disease risks associated with HRT, this option has effectively been removed from the osteoporosis treatment repertoire.

The class of bisphosphonates shows great promise in increasing bone density and reducing fracture rates. The major side effects are gastrointestinal disturbances and therefore these drugs must be taken on an empty stomach in an upright position. New monthly dosing regimens promise to reduce the side effects and the cost. The ultimate duration of this therapy is still not established. There is some evidence of a sustained effect for 5 years or more. A number of bisphosphonate products are emerging each year into this lucrative market, each with claims of improved benefits. In addition, other approaches are being actively explored. Nasally administered calcitonin is also approved by the Food and Drug Administration (FDA) for treatment of osteoporosis, but has weak fracture prevention efficacy. An intriguing finding has been that the statins, used to treat high cholesterol, have appeared to show a positive effect on bone mass density. This therapeutic effect has not yet been tested in randomized trials. Moreover, no clear fracture reduction benefit from statins has been demonstrated. Table 5-5 compares the effectiveness of the available bisphosphonates and other potential treatments. The fracture reduction benefit is disproportionately greater than the improvement in bone mineral density, and may be because of reduction of bone turnover from these drugs. Although parathyroid hormone is the most potent approach, it is not widely used because of the cost and administration problems, as well as concern regarding its long-term safety. Although PTH side effects are few, concern remains about the risk of osteosarcoma from its use.

TABLE 5-5   RELATIVE EFFECTIVENESS OF VARIOUS OSTEOPOROSIS TREATMENTS

	Mean% Change in Bone Mass Density at 12-18 Months‡		Rate of Fractures		
	Lumbar Spine	Femoral Neck	Vertebra	Nonspine	Hip
Alendronate (70 mg)*	+5	+3	↓	↓	↓
Risedronate (35 mg)*	+3	+2	↓	↓	↓
Ibandronate (150 mg)	+6	+3	↓	—	—
Ibandronate IV (3 mg)	+5	+3	↓	—	—
Zoledronate IV (5 mg)	+5	+3	↓	↓	↓
Raloxifene (60 mg)*	+3	+2	↓	—	—
Calcitonin (200 IU)*	+1	—	↓	—	—
Parathyroid hormone (20 mg)	+9	+4	↓	↓	—
Hormone replacement therapy†	+4	+1	↓	↓	↓

*FDA-approved agent for treating postmenopausal osteoporosis.
†No longer considered a realistic option.
‡Difference between drug and placebo.
⌐Direct evidence from randomized trials.
⌐Indirect evidence from observational studies.
Information provided by John Schousboe, MD.

GENERIC APPROACHES

It is generally not a good strategy to assume that one can simply impose a comprehensive approach to health promotion in a group on older people. Older persons often have their own agendas about what is important to them and what they believe will benefit them.

After smoking, the behavior with potentially the greatest benefit is exercise; but its record can create confusion in the minds of both older persons and their clinicians. Overall, there is widespread belief that exercise will benefit an older individual. However, exercise is not a unidimensional activity. There are various types, and each is directed at a specific target. Table 5-6 summarizes the major types of exercise and the intended benefits of each type. Different approaches to exercise should be pursued to achieve specific goals. Although its role in osteoporosis prevention remains controversial, exercise is generally recommended as a safe approach, with more possible benefits than risks. Less than a third of older persons report regular exercise, to say nothing of vigorous activity. Although evidence suggests that active aerobic exercise is necessary to reduce risk of cardiovascular accidents, even modest amounts of exercise will improve strength, keep joints more limber, promote a sense of well-being, and improve sleep. Even severely compromised nursing home residents can benefit from carefully supervised and graded strength-training exercise. Both the direct benefits (eg, improved muscle strength and activity tolerance) and indirect effects (eg, being treated with more esteem) allowed residents to function more autonomously (Fiatarone et al., 1994).

Exercise appears to improve both overall well-being and older persons' sense of self-worth, but it can be hard to recruit people to undertake it and to sustain such regimens (Pahor et al., 2006; Kerse et al., 2005). Likewise, occupational therapy has been shown to produce beneficial results for a group of independently

TABLE 5-6   TYPES OF EXERCISE

TYPE	PURPOSE/EXPECTED BENEFIT
Aerobic/Anaerobic	Cardiovascular conditioning
Resistance/Weights	Strength, tone, muscle mass
Antigravity	Prevent osteoporosis
Balance	Prevent falls
Stretching	Flexibility

living older adults (Clark et al. 1997). Modest efforts at exercise can yield substantial rewards in terms of improved function and reduced use of long-term care.

Epidemiological data suggest that even among persons in their seventies, cessation of smoking will reduce mortality to levels of nonsmokers in a sufficiently short time to justify actively encouraging quitting. Smoking cessation has rapid benefits for risks of both vascular and lung disease.

There is growing enthusiasm for controlling even modest levels of both diastolic and systolic hypertension among the elderly. The European Working Party on High Blood Pressure in the Elderly showed that treatment was associated with a significant reduction in cardiac mortality, a nonsignificant reduction in cerebrovascular mortality, but no reduction in overall mortality. The results from the Systolic Hypertension in the Elderly Program (SHEP) suggest that lowering isolated systolic hypertension can lead to reduced rates of fatal and nonfatal endpoints for stroke, coronary heart disease, and cardiovascular disease. However, the situation with those aged 80 and older becomes more complicated. Active treatment of hypertension may be associated with higher mortality (Goodwin, 2003).

It is important to distinguish carefully between the value of uncovering elevated blood pressure and the need to control it over a sustained period. Most older persons with hypertension are aware of it; the challenge is to maintain them in a safe range without producing significant side effects. Hypertension is very common among the elderly. Black females have the highest rates, and among white males the rate approaches 40%.

The effects of dietary changes are less certain. Weight loss for obese persons makes sense in terms of reducing cardiovascular load and in the management of adult-onset diabetes and hypertension, but hard data suggest that the benefit may be oversold, certainly for the former. The efficacy of changing diet, especially to reduce the amount of fat consumed, has not yet been clearly established.

Cholesterol and low-density lipoproteins (LDLs) are risk factors for heart disease for general populations, but have not been specifically tested in the elderly. However, elevated high-density lipoproteins have been shown to provide a protective factor for strokes in older people. More than 30% of white females have high-risk cholesterol levels (> 268 mg/dL). Cholesterol-lowering therapy works in older persons as well as in the middle-aged who were generally included in such trials. Recommendations for using lipid-lowering drugs in older patients with a history of cardiac or vascular disease are countered by other claims that cholesterol is not a significant risk factor in older persons. At the same time, only approximately 50% of older persons put on lipid-lowering medications remain on the regimen after 5 years. The preponderance of support now seems to favor more aggressive treatment of elevated LDL cholesterol, even in quite elderly persons (Aronow, 2002). However, many older patients do not remain on the statin therapy regimens long enough to benefit from them (Benner et al., 2002).

In areas such as weight, cholesterol, and blood pressure, the clinician must weigh the benefits of intervention against the costs (risks). There is a compelling argument that overzealous activity in the name of prevention may cost more in quality of life than it gains in quality years. Some have suggested that the survivor effect should be taken more seriously. Persons who survive to old age may have demonstrated a biological ability that deserves more respect. At the very least, any determination to change lifestyle at this stage of life should be made by the patient after suitable counseling. Nonetheless, older persons should not be denied the opportunity to actively consider the benefits of primary prevention. The growing body of evidence about at least the art of the possible imposes on clinicians a responsibility to provide them with such information.

One area of behavior with great theoretical promise but little immediate practical application is social support. There is some evidence to suggest that those older persons with strong social support systems, or at least perceived support, are at less risk for adverse events, but it is not yet clear how to build such a support system for those without one naturally. Social support likely plays at least two distinct roles: (1) Having (or perhaps just believing one has) a strong support system may reduce the risk of adverse events (through a yet-to-be-elucidated mechanism that likely involves stress). (2) For persons who are disabled and require assistance, having a real support system may prove the difference between staying in the community and needing to enter an institution. It is difficult to assess the availability of that support system in advance.

The perception, even the promise, of such support does not guarantee that the necessary support will be consistently and conveniently available when it is needed. Even well-intentioned family members may find the task too daunting to be able to maintain it.

PREVENTING DISABILITY

Although discussions of prevention tend to focus on the prevention of disease, the context of geriatrics—with its emphasis on functioning—urges a broader approach. When caring for older patients, equal attention must be paid to seeking means to keep them as active as possible. While there may be little that can be done to prevent the occurrence of a disease in an elderly person, much can be done to minimize the impact of that disease. Impairments cannot be allowed to become disabilities. Recent work in studying disability has raised new questions about the possible differences between transient and persistent disabled states. Studies that followed older people closely showed that many of them move in and out of transient states of disability. Hence, measures of disability over long periods may contain elements of both permanent and transient disability. This distinction is important because efforts to prevent disability may be falsely positive if they reflect transient conditions that would have improved on their own.

A major component of the efforts to avoid this transition is contained in geriatric assessment programs. The general approaches of such programs are reviewed in Chap. 3. It is important to note that these programs have been very varied in their composition. Table 3-1 in Chap. 3 summarizes the major randomized controlled trials using different approaches to assessment.

Work on demonstrated performance, especially when combined with timed measures, is promising. This additional component provides a way to achieve more variability and may lead to better prediction. It offers a means to detect more subtle change.

The overarching goal of geriatric practice is the improvement, or at least the preservation, of patients' function. In general, function can be thought of as being determined by three principal forces: (1) the patient's overall physical health, (2) the environment, and (3) the patient's motivation. Much of the discussion in this book deals with ways to maximize the patient's health status by proper diagnosis and treatment. Such steps are necessary but not sufficient for good geriatric care. It is essential to appreciate that a person's environment can play a critical role in affecting their functioning. Just imagine for a minute what it would be like to be in a country where you did not speak the language or even understand its symbols. Although your capabilities are intact, you cannot function effectively. By a similar token, even after therapy has achieved its maximal effect, a patient's environment can be crucial.

Environment in this case refers to both the physical and psychological setting. It is fairly easy to imagine the physical barriers to functioning. Narrow doorways, poor lighting, and stairs can all serve as barriers. The homes of older persons are often cluttered with obstacles and loose rugs, wires, and so on, which may increase the risk of tripping.

Occupational therapists can be especially helpful in assessing the patient's environment to suggest modifications and adaptive equipment. Environment refers to the ways patients are treated and, especially, the extent to which they are encouraged to do as much for themselves as they can.

The psychological barriers are more subtle, but perhaps more important. We noted earlier that a risk-averse environment can engender excessive dependency; so too can the pressure to be productive. As long as time is at a premium, care providers will be motivated to do things for patients, rather than encouraging them to perform those tasks themselves, especially if the latter course takes considerably longer. In the name of efficiency, we may be creating dependency. The efforts to encourage self-sufficiency are precisely what is usually called rehabilitation, even when it occurs in a plain wrapper.

The third element of functional effects is the patient's motivation. Today's older patients place especially high trust in their physicians, whom they view as figures of authority. Thus, one of the most subtle but nonetheless important aspect of this approach to prevention—the prevention of inactivity and despair—is the physician's attitude. For the patient, a gain in function or an ability to deal with a chronic problem is essential. It is surely no mean feat. Such behavior should be encouraged and rewarded. Indifference may be enough to discourage the patient from trying.

Other programs can be mobilized in the patient's behalf. Self-help groups are available in many communities to offer support with chronic illness, including stress management and drugless pain-control techniques. Social activity can play an essential role in maintaining function. Pets have proved to be very effective in improving morale and maintaining function.

Special efforts may be necessary to deal with members of the patient's family. Their concern over potentially dangerous accidents may lead them to become overprotective and thus exaggerate the condition of dependency.

IATROGENESIS

Probably the most important preventable problems faced by older persons today are those associated with treatment. Many iatrogenic problems result from the care that has been provided. In some cases, these problems can be traced to oversights and omissions. In other cases, overzealous care can be blamed. Some of the problems are attributable to lack of expertise in managing older persons, but a substantial portion is caused by the inevitable problems of trying to titrate therapy in an environment that is considerably less resilient to error. The more aggressive the treatment, the greater the chance that it will produce adverse effects. Figure 5-2 portrays in a conceptual manner this narrowing of the thera-peutic window (ie, the space between a therapeutic dose and a toxic dose) with age. As the response to therapy decreases, the susceptibility to toxic side effects

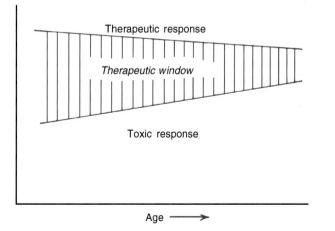

— FIGURE 5-2 — Narrowing of the therapeutic window. This diagram portrays in a conceptual manner how the space between a therapeutic dose and a toxic dose narrows with age.

increases. These changes are attributable to many factors, including the ability to metabolize drugs, changes in receptor behavior, and an altered chemical environment produced by other simultaneous drugs.

This narrowing of the therapeutic window is perhaps most easily recognized in the pharmacological treatment of older patients. In the face of reduced capacity for metabolizing and excreting many drugs, the older patient can develop high blood levels on "normal" dosages. Changes in receptors may alter sensitivity to chemicals in either direction.

Many older people are at risk of drug problems. A study of community-dwelling elders found that 20% of older people taking medications had inappropriate elements, such as potential drug–disease interactions and excessive duration of use. Another study found that more than 20% of older persons were taking drugs that an expert panel had identified as inappropriate for this age group. For example, several studies have shown that thrombolytics may have serious adverse consequences when used in elderly patients with acute myocardial infarctions. Although they are actively recommended for younger victims, their use in older persons must be monitored very closely.

Use of numerous drugs transforms the elderly patient into a living chemistry set. Because of their prevalence and importance, drugs are discussed separately in Chap. 14. There is good reason to believe older people are overmedicated (Hajjar et al., 2005). In this chapter, we focus attention on some of the more subtle ways in which other types of treatment can adversely affect older people. In general, many drugs can be discontinued safely. One caveat, however: In the fear of overmedicating older patients, doctors may be tempted to discontinue drugs that were begun at an earlier time. While such a reevaluation is prudent, the decision to discontinue should be made carefully. One study showed that stopping long-term diuretic medications in elderly patients resulted in an exacerbation of heart failure symptoms and a rise in their blood pressure (Walma et al., 1997).

On a more philosophical plane, one can think about aging as a continuously changing relationship between an organism and its environment. As noted in Chap. 1, aging is typified by a decreased capacity to respond to stress. A person's environment can do much to reduce or create stress. One of the signs of maturation is the person's ability to function independently of that environment and ultimately to influence that environment. Indeed, one of the attributes that distinguishes humans from other animals is precisely this capacity to shape the environment. In infancy, a person is readily influenced by their environment. Whereas a mature adult is likely to adapt to or alter the environment, the aged individual is greatly affected by changes of setting. With increased age, the delicate balance shifts again to the point where advanced age often means that the individual is heavily affected by the environment. It is hardly surprising, then, that the elderly patient is vulnerable to the variety of stresses imposed by modern medical care. Table 5-7 lists some of the iatrogenic problems elderly patients may suffer.

TABLE 5-7   COMMON IATROGENIC PROBLEMS OF OLDER PERSONS

Overzealous labeling
Dementia
Incontinence
Underdiagnosis
Bed rest
Polypharmacy
Enforced dependency
Environmental hazards
Transfer trauma

A few of these elements deserve special discussion. Hospital environments and other settings like nursing homes usually find it more efficient to do things for older people, who may be slow to perform these tasks, than to encourage them to do things for themselves. As a result, they encourage these older patients to become dependent. Older people, especially those who are already confused and disoriented, do not take well to change. They may become agitated and even develop exacerbations of their baseline states. This transfer trauma can be mitigated by taking extra pains to explain what is happening and easing the transition with extra support and attention.

SPECIAL RISKS OF HOSPITALS

Hospitals are dangerous places for any patient, as reflected in a report from the Institute of Medicine documenting the prevalence of medical errors (Kohn et al., 2000). Reports from the Institute of Medicine have called for more stringent efforts to make hospitals safer places and eliminate the many deaths associated with imperfect care. Older patients are at special risk. Most of us are resilient enough to enter an acute care hospital and suffer the vicissitudes of care with the expectation that we will emerge better (certainly in the long run). The calculation of benefits received for risks undertaken needs to be more carefully thought through with older patients.

Just a little thought reveals the litany of familiar hazards of hospitalization— from the risk of nosocomial infection to getting the wrong drug to the stress of major surgery or the danger of certain diagnostic procedures. One meta-analysis estimated the high rate of adverse drug reactions in hospitalized patients in general at almost 7% (Lazarou, Pomeranz, and Corey, 1998). All these are imposed on the general hazards of bed rest discussed in Chap. 10, Table 10-2. Table 5-8 offers some examples of potential hazards in the hospital. They include problems of both overtreatment and undertreatment.

TABLE 5-8   THE HAZARDS OF HOSPITALIZATION

Diagnostic procedures

Cardiac catheterization

Arteriography

Therapeutic procedures

Intravenous therapy

Urinary catheters

Nasogastric tube

Dialysis

Transfusion

Drugs

Medication error

Drug–drug interaction

Drug reaction

Drug side effect

Surgery

Anesthesia

Infection

Metabolic imbalance

Malnutrition

Hypovolemia

Bed rest

Hypovolemia and hypertension

Calcium metabolism

Fecal impaction

Urine incontinence

Thromboembolism

Nosocomial infection

Falls

TABLE 5-9   RISK FACTORS FOR IATROGENIC HOSPITALIZATION

Admission from nursing home or other hospital

Physician's assessment of overall condition on admission

Age

Number of drugs

Length of stay

Elderly patients are more likely to experience an untoward event during a hospital stay. In part, this is because they present with more physical problems; however, they are also more vulnerable. Table 5-9 lists patient characteristics associated with increased risk of hospital iatrogenic complications. Source of admission and condition on admission are especially salient. Because elderly patients are more likely to come from nursing homes and to be in poor condition on admission, they should be considered at high risk for iatrogenic complications.

In a study of patients hospitalized on a general medical service, the incidence of functional symptoms unrelated to diagnosis was over four times higher among patients aged 70 years and older than among younger patients. Younger patients were more likely to be treated for symptoms of confusion, but older patients were more likely to be treated for problems of not eating and incontinence (Gillick, Serrell, and Gillick, 1982). Table 5-10 provides a simple rapid screening test for identifying older patients at risk of functional decline in the hospital. Delirium can be a serious problem in elderly hospitalized patients (see Chap. 6 for a discussion of this condition).

TABLE 5-10   RISK FACTORS FOR FUNCTIONAL DECLINE IN ELDERLY
HOSPITALIZED PATIENTS

Age 75+

Missing >15 of the first 21 MMSE items

Dependence in 2+ IADL prior to admission

Pressure sore

Baseline functional dependency

History of low social activity

IADL, instrumental activities of daily living; MMSE, Mini-Mental State Examination.
Adapted from Inouye and Charpentier, 1996; Sager et al., 1996.

The elderly patient's vulnerability extends to a more subtle level. Admission to a hospital means entering an unfamiliar world. Moreover, the patient enters the hospital at a time of great stress. The anxiety of unknown consequences exists in addition to the physical stress of the illness.

The hospital presents physical and organizational barriers to which the patient must adapt. Not only the geography but the routines are different. The things we rely on to preserve our sense of identity—our clothing, our personal effects—are among the first things taken away. It is hardly surprising, then, that many elderly persons who are able to function in their familiar surroundings become disoriented and often agitated in the hospital. Just as a blind person can move flawlessly in familiar surroundings, an older person may have developed a host of adaptive mechanisms to function in their home situation, overcoming problems of memory loss and impaired vision.

Transferred into the sterile, rigid hospital room, such an individual may decompensate. The syndrome of "sundowning," whereby older patients in the hospital become agitated and disoriented as dusk falls, is likely a function of visual or hearing impairments, diminished sensory stimuli, and resultant disorientation.

The older person accustomed to coping with nocturia may wander at night in the dark to where the bathroom at home ought to be and wet the floor. In the crisis of urinary urgency, the patient may be unable to scale the side rails and make it to the bathroom in time. To label an individual who suffers such environmentally exacerbated accidents as incontinent is to inflict double jeopardy.

We fail to appreciate the dangers of bed rest for the elderly people. The bed is actually a very dangerous place for an older person! Besides the risk of falling out of bed, enforced immobility can produce much harm. Complications of bed rest are summarized in Table 5-11 and detailed in Chap. 10.

The hospital breeds dependency. Even with younger patients, hospital personnel are accustomed to performing basic functions for the patient. Use of the bathroom is by prescription only. Bathing is often a supervised event. Patients are transported from one location to another. Although most of us as patients may have enjoyed being indulged for a while, we soon begin to rail against the imposed dependency. In older patients who need to be urged, encouraged, and cajoled into doing as much for themselves as possible, such an atmosphere can be especially debilitating.

Encouraging patients to act independently necessitates patience and time; unfortunately, both are scarce in the acute care hospital. It is much faster and easier to do a task for a person who performs slowly and uncertainly than to take the time to encourage that person to do that task independently. Moreover, the result of a professionally performed task is usually neater and more in keeping with hospital standards. Thus, well-meaning staff bowing to the pressures for efficiency may be inclined to do things for elderly patients rather than urging the patients to do as much as possible for themselves. This well-intentioned behavior fosters dependency at a time when independent function is crucial.

TABLE 5-11 POTENTIAL COMPLICATIONS OF BED REST IN OLDER PERSONS

Pressure sores

Bone resorption

Hypercalcemia

Postural hypotension

Atelectasis and pneumonia

Thrombophlebitis and thromboembolism

Urinary incontinence

Constipation and fecal impaction

Decreased muscle strength

Decreased physical work capacity

Contractures

Depression and anxiety

Hospitals are notoriously averse to risk taking. Hospital policies are designed to err on the side of caution. Such behavior can further compromise the independent functioning of older patients. Patients who are not allowed to bathe themselves or who are wheeled rather than walked are likely to become less motivated to use their full capacities. Any fears about their ability are likely to increase.

In light of the multiple adverse consequences that may be associated with hospitalizing older people, we might pause to ask why we have not done more to make hospitals more hospitable for them.

Ironically, we have invested great care in minimizing the trauma of hospitalization for children. Creativity in architecture and programs has gone into making pediatric wards as nonthreatening and homelike as possible. Although children are rarely hospitalized and geriatric patients are frequently hospitalized, no similar investment of creativity has been devoted to making the hospital less stressful for frail elderly patients. We know enough about perceptual and functional problems of aging to recognize that even simple architectural modifications can make a hospital stay easier. Use of primary colors, windows at lower heights, better-designed furniture, use of textures and patterns, and better design of rooms can all help the older patient retain maximum functioning capacity.

Special units for managing geriatric patients are beginning to emerge. Staffed by an interdisciplinary team, which may include a social worker, physician, and physical or occupational therapist, and nurses, these units apply techniques of multidimensional functional evaluation to assess the diagnoses, needs, and capacity of the geriatric patient and develop treatment plans to address them.

Likewise, the reports of geriatric assessment units that took patients who had completed a course of acute care hospitalization and were otherwise destined for a nursing home and dramatically altered both their clinical state and their long-term care course, even reducing mortality rates, suggest that much more can be done for older persons while they are in a hospital. Such geriatric units can uncover treatable conditions, provide rehabilitation to improve functional capacity, and develop a plan of care that will allow elderly patients to remain in the community.

An iatrogenic danger to the elderly patient thus lies in underdiagnosis, especially of mundane but critical conditions involving hearing, vision, and dentition. In addition, even more clinically important problems such as thyroid disease or aortic aneurysms may be overlooked unless a careful examination is performed.

LABELING

Perhaps even more dangerous than the cases of underdiagnosis are those of overdiagnosis. The physician who too readily labels a disoriented patient as senile or demented, or who classifies a urinary accident as incontinence, may be sealing the fate of that patient unnecessarily. These two diagnoses are strongly associated with an increased likelihood of nursing home admission and thus should not be made lightly.

Physicians admitting patients to nursing homes are responsible for assuring both themselves and their patients on several scores:

1. The patient truly needs care in such a setting and cannot reasonably get such care elsewhere.
2. The institution is capable of providing the needed care.
3. The patient is prepared for a transfer to the nursing home.

Hospital discharge planners are often put under great stress to move patients out quickly, leaving little time for careful considerations, options, or even what goals the family and patient want to maximize. Too often the first train leaving the station is the best one to be on. Availability of placements trumps careful consideration of options. Because nursing home discharges are easier to arrange, they are frequently used. Earlier discharges from hospitals promote the concept of recuperation in a nursing home.

Too frequently, hospital discharge to the nursing home compounds the trauma. Discharge planning is often begun too late. There is insufficient time to find the best facility for the patient's needs or to allow the patient and the patient's family a sufficient role in making the decision for nursing home placement.

Good discharge planning includes at least six critical steps:

1. Adequate identification of those at risk of needing special arrangements on discharge
2. Assessment to identify problems and strengths
3. Clarification of what goals should be maximized
4. Determination of the risks and benefits associated with alternative modalities of care
5. Determination of the most suitable vendor among the modality of care selected
6. Transmission of adequate information to assure a successful transition

Patients and their families should play an active role in steps 3, 4, and 5. Ideally, they should make the choice after the information has been provided by professionals. In practice, this is rarely the case. Often, getting family members to agree on what are the most important goals for posthospital care (ie, Do concerns about recovery trump those of autonomy? Where does safety factor?) can be very time consuming and requires great skill. Older patients and their families may not agree. Old family histories may intrude.

Adequate information about the risks and benefits of alternative modalities is not presented (it may not be known). No encouragement or assistance is provided to help patients and families determine precisely what outcomes they seek to maximize. Little time is allowed to weigh the complexities of the choice. When it comes to choosing among vendors of a given service, real choices may not exist because of the constraints of payment arrangements, including managed care.

As discussed in Chap. 16, the nature of nursing home care is changing. The pressure for earlier discharges from hospitals has created a new demand for what has been termed subacute care—in essence, care that was formerly provided in hospitals.

SUMMARY

Many useful steps can be taken to improve and protect the health of elderly patients. The elderly patient represents a different risk-benefit ratio than the younger patient. Actions well tolerated in others may produce serious consequences in the old. A bed is a dangerous place for the older patient; confinement to bed rest should be avoided whenever possible.

The physician must guard against several potential iatrogenic problems with elderly patients. Diagnostic labels implying incurable problems (such as dementia and incontinence) should not be used until a careful search for correctable causes has been undertaken. Special attention should be given to the tendency to create dependency through well-intentioned care. By keeping in mind the need to maintain the patient's functioning, the physician can remain sensitive to the effects of the environment to enhance or impede such activity.

References

Aronow WS. Should hypercholesterolemia in older persons be treated to reduce cardio-vascular events? *J Gerntol A Biol Sci Med Sci.* 2002;57A:M411-M413.

Ball K, Berch DB, Helmers KF, et al. Effects of cognitive training interventions with older adults: a randomized controlled trial. *JAMA.* 2002;288(18):2271-2281.

Benner JS, Glynn RJ, Mogun H, et al. Long-term persistence in use of statin therapy in elderly patients. *JAMA.* 2002;288:455-461.

Clark F, Azen SP, Zemke R, et al. Occupational therapy for independent-living older adults: a randomized controlled trial. *JAMA.* 1997;278(16):1321-1326.

Fiatarone MA, O'Neill EF, Ryan ND, et al. Exercise training and nutritional supplementa-tion for physical frailty in very elderly people. *N Engl J Med.* 1994;330(25):1769-1775.

Fletcher RH, Fairfield KM. Vitamins for chronic disease prevention in adults. *JAMA.* 2002;287:3127-3129.

Gillick MR, Serrell NA, Gillick LS. Adverse consequences of hospitalization in the elderly. *Soc Sci Med.* 1982;16:1033-1038.

Goldberg TH, Chavin SI. Preventive medicine and screening in older adults. *J Am Geriatr Soc.* 1997;43:344-354.

Goodwin JS. Embracing complexity: a consideration of hypertension in the very old. *J Gerontol A Biol Sci Med Sci.* 2003;58(7):653-658.

Gorbien M, Bishop J, Beers M, et al. Iatrogenic illness in hospitalized elderly people. *J Am Geriatr Soc.* 1992;40:1031-1042.

Hajjar ER, Hanlon JT, Sloane RJ, et al. Unnecessary drug use in frail older people at hos-pital discharge. *J Am Geriatr Soc.* 2005;53(9):1518-1523.

Inouye SK, Charpentier PA. Precipitating factors for delirium in hospitalized elderly persons. *JAMA.* 1996;275:852-857.

Katon W, Von Korff M, Lin E, et al. Collaborative management to achieve treatment guide-lines. Impact on depression in primary care. *JAMA.* 1995;273(13):1026-1031.

Kerlikowske K, Salzmann P, Phillips KA, et al. Continuing screening mammography in women aged 70 to 79 years. *JAMA.* 1999;282:2156-2163.

Kerse N, et al. Is physical activity counseling effective for older people? A cluster randomized, controlled trial in primary care. *J Am Geriatr Soc.* 2005;53(11):1951-1956.

Kohn LT, Corrigan JM, Donaldson MS, eds. *To Err Is Human: Building a Safer Health System.* Washington, DC: National Academy Press; 2000.

Lazarou J, Pomeranz BH, Corey PN. Incidence of adverse drug reactions in hospitalized patients: a meta-analysis of prospective studies. *JAMA.* 1998;279:1200-1205.

Levinstein MR, Ouslander JG, Rubenstein, LZ, et al. Yield of routine annual laboratory tests in a skilled nursing home population. *JAMA.* 1987;258(14):1919-1915.

Lin OS, Kozarek RA, Schembre DB, et al. Screening colonoscopy in very elderly patients: prevalence of neoplasia and estimated impact on life expectancy. *JAMA.* 2006; 295(20):2357-2365.

Mangin D, Sweeney K, Heath I. Preventive health care in elderly people needs rethinking. *BMJ.* 2007;335(7614):285-287.

Nichol KL, Nordin JD, Nelson DB, et al. Effectiveness of influenza vaccine in the community-dwelling elderly. *N Engl J Med.* 2007;357(14):1373-81.

Pahor M, Blair SN, Espeland M, et al. Effects of a physical activity intervention on measures of physical performance: results of the lifestyle interventions and independence for Elders Pilot (LIFE-P) study. *J Gerontol A Biol Sci Med Sci.* 2006; 61(11): 1157-1165.

Pham HH, Schrag D, Hargraves JL, et al. Delivery of preventive services to older adults by primary care physicians. *JAMA.* 2005;294(4):473-481.

Ridker PM, Cook NR, Lee IM, et al. A randomized trial of low-dose aspirin in the primary prevention of cardiovascular disease in women. *N Engl J Med.* 2005;352(13):1293-1304.

Rubenstein LZ, Josephson KR, Nichol-Seamans M, et al. Comprehensive health screening of well elderly adults: an analysis of a community program. *Journal of Gerontology.* 1986;41(3):342-352.

Sager MA, Rudberg MA, Jalaloddin M, et al. Hospital admission risk profile (HARP): identifying older patients at risk for functional decline following acute medical illness and hospitalization. *J Am Geriatr Soc.* 1996;44:251-257.

Sawaya GF, McConnell KJ, Kulasingam SL, et al. Risk of cervical cancer associated with extending the interval between cervical-cancer screenings. *N Engl J Med.* 2003; 349(16):1501-1509.

Sawka AM, Boulos P, Beattie K, et al. Hip protectors decrease hip fracture risk in elderly nursing home residents: a Bayesian meta-analysis. *J Clin Epidemiol.* 2007;60(4): 336-344.

Scheitel SM, Fleming KC, Chutka DS, et al. Geriatric health maintenance. *Mayo Clin Proc.* 1996;71:289-302.

Schousboe JT, Ensrud KE, Nyman JA, et al. Universal bone densitometry screening combined with alendronate therapy for those diagnosed with osteoporosis is highly cost-effective for elderly women. *J Am Geriatr Soc.* 2005; 53(10):1697-1704.

Simonsen L, Taylor RJ, Viboud C, et al. Mortality benefits of influenza vaccination in elderly people: an ongoing controversy. *Lancet Infect Dis.* 2007;7(10):658-666.

Stuck AE, Egger M, Hammer A, et al. Home visits to prevent nursing home admission and functional decline in elderly people: systematic review and meta-regression analysis. *JAMA.* 2002;287(8):1022-1028.

Srivastava M, Deal C. Medical management and prevention of fragility fractures. *Adv Osteoporotic Fracture Manage.* 2001;1(2):34-40.

US Preventive Services Task Force. *Guide to Clinical Preventive Services: Report of the US Preventive Services Task Force, 2nd ed.* Baltimore, MD: Williams & Wilkins; 1996.

van Schoor NM, Smit JH, Bouta LM, et al. Maximum potential preventive effect of hip protectors. *J Am Geriatr Soc.* 2007;55(4):507-10.

Walma EP, Hoes AW, van Dooren C, et al. Withdrawal of long-term diuretic medication in elderly patients: a double-blind randomised trial. *BMJ.* 1997;315:464-468.

Wolinsky FD, Unverzagt FW, Smith DM, et al. The ACTIVE cognitive training trial and health-related quality of life: protection that lasts for 5 years. *J Gerontol A Biol Sci Med Sci.* 2006;61(12):1324-1329.

Suggested Readings

Gill TM, Williams CS, Mendes de Leon CF, et al. The role of change in physical performance in determining risk for dependence in activities of daily living among nondisabled community-living elderly persons. *J Clin Epidemiol.* 1997;50:765-777.

Hanlon JT, Schmader KE, Boult C, et al. Use of inappropriate prescription drugs by older people. *J Am Geriatr Soc.* 2002;50:26-34.

Institute of Medicine. *Disability in America: Toward a National Agenda for Prevention.* Washington, DC: National Academy Press; 1991.

Ross KS, Carter HB, Pearson JD, et al. Comparative efficiency of prostate-specific antigen screening strategies for prostate cancer detection. *JAMA.* 2000;284:1399-1405.

Singh MAF. Exercise comes of age: rationale and recommendations for a geriatric exercise prescription. *J Gerontol A Biol Sci Med Sci.* 2002;57A:M262-M282.

Walter LC, Covinsky KE. Cancer screening in elderly patients: a framework for decision making. *JAMA.* 2001;285:2750-2756.

Winawer SJ, Fletcher RH, Miller L. Colorectal screening clinical guidelines and rationale. *Gastroenterol.* 1997;112:59-62.

CHAPTER 6

CONFUSION: DELIRIUM AND DEMENTIA

Diagnosis and management of geriatric patients exhibiting symptoms and signs of confusion can make a critical difference to their overall health and the ability to function independently. Confusion can be acute in onset, or it can be manifest by slowly progressive cognitive impairment. The major causes of confusion in the geriatric population are delirium and dementia. As more people live into the tenth decade of life, the chance that they will develop some form of dementia increases substantially. Community-based studies report a prevalence of dementia as high as 47% among those 85 years of age and older. Prevalence rates are, however, highly dependent on the criteria used to define dementia. Between 25% and 50% of older patients admitted to acute care medical and surgical services are delirious on admission or develop delirium during their hospital stay. In nursing homes, 50% to 80% of those older than age 65 years have some degree of cognitive impairment. Delirium is often superimposed on dementia in both hospital and community settings, and is a risk factor for functional decline and mortality.

Misdiagnosis and inappropriate management of syndromes leading to confusion in geriatric patients can cause substantial morbidity among the patients, hardship to their families, and excess health-care expenditures. This chapter provides a practical framework for diagnosing and managing geriatric patients who demonstrate confusion. We focus on the most common causes of confusion in the geriatric population—delirium and dementia—although a variety of other disorders can cause confusion.

CONFUSION

Imprecise definition of the abnormalities of cognitive function in older patients labeled as "confused" has led to problems in the diagnosis and management of these patients. Confusion has been defined as a mental state in which reactions to environmental stimuli are inappropriate because the person is bewildered, perplexed, or unable to orientate himself (Stedman's Medical Dictionary, 2000). This type of definition, although descriptive, is too broad and imprecise to be clinically useful. Descriptions such as impairment of cognitive function or cognitive impairment coupled with careful documentation of the timing and nature of specific abnormalities provide more precise and clinically useful information. Such documentation is best accomplished by screening and a thorough mental status examination, if indicated.

Screening for delirium can be accomplished with the confusion assessment method (CAM). The Mini-Cog is useful in screening for cognitive impairment and dementia. Both of these screening tests are discussed later in the chapter.

A thorough mental status examination has several basic components that are essential in diagnosing dementia, delirium, or other syndromes (Table 6-1). Attention should focus on each of these components in a systematic manner. Recording observations in each area is helpful in recognizing and evaluating changes over time. Standardized and validated measures of cognitive function (see appendix) can be helpful in diagnosis and subsequent monitoring. Several factors may, however, influence performance and interpretation of standard mental status tests, such as prior educational level, primary language other than English, severely impaired hearing, or poor baseline intellectual function. Thus, scores on these tests should not be used to replace a more comprehensive examination such as that in Table 6-1.

Important information can be gleaned unobtrusively from simply observing and interacting with the patient during the history. Is the patient alert and attentive? Does the patient respond appropriately to questions? How is the patient dressed and groomed? Does the patient repeat oneself or give an imprecise social

TABLE 6-1 KEY ASPECTS OF MENTAL STATUS EXAMINATION

State of consciousness

General appearance and behavior

Orientation

Memory (short- and long-term)

Language

Visuospatial functions

Executive control functions (eg, planning and sequencing of tasks)

Other cognitive functions (eg, calculations, proverb interpretation)

Insight and judgment

Thought content

Mood and affect

or medical history, suggesting memory impairment? Orientation, insight, and judgment can sometimes be assessed during the history as well.

Questions relating to specific areas of cognitive functioning should be introduced in a nonthreatening manner, because many patients with early deficits respond defensively. Each of the three basic components of memory should be tested: immediate recall (eg, repeating digits), recent memory (eg, recalling three objects after a few minutes), and remote memory (eg, ability to give details of early life). Language and other cognitive functions should be carefully evaluated. Is the patient's speech clear? Can the patient read (and understand) and write? Does there seem to be a good general fund of knowledge (eg, current events)? Other cognitive functions that can be tested easily include the ability to perform simple calculations (eg, one that relates to making change while shopping) and to copy diagrams. The ability to interpret proverbs abstractly and to list the names of animals (12 names in 1 min is normal) are sensitive indicators of cognitive function and are easy to test.

Judgment and insight can usually be assessed during the examination without asking specific questions, though input from family members or other caregivers can be helpful and sometimes necessary. Any abnormal thought content should also be noted during the examination; bizarre ideas, mood-incongruent thoughts, and delusions (especially paranoid delusions) may be prominent in older patients with cognitive impairment and are important both diagnostically and therapeutically. Observations during the examination may also detect abnormalities of executive control. Executive function involves the planning, sequencing, and executive of goal-directed activities. These functions are critical to the ability to perform instrumental activities of daily living (IADL). Screening tests for executive dysfunction include a clock-drawing test, which is a component of the Mini-Cog (see later paragraphs).

Throughout the examination, the patient's mood and affect should be assessed. Depression, apathy, emotional liability, agitation, and aggression are common in older patients with cognitive impairment (Lyketsos et al., 2002) and failure to recognize these abnormalities can lead to improper diagnosis and management. In some patients—such as those who are very intelligent or poorly educated, or have low intelligence, as well as those in whom depression is suspected—more detailed neuropsychological testing by an experienced psychologist is helpful in more precisely defining abnormalities in cognitive function and in differentiating between the many and often interacting underlying causes.

Differential Diagnosis of Confusion

The causes of confusion in the geriatric population are myriad. The differential diagnosis in an older patient who presents with confusion includes disorders of the brain (eg, stroke, dementia), a systemic illness presenting atypically (eg, infection, metabolic disturbance, myocardial infarction, congestive heart failure), sensory impairment (eg, hearing loss), and adverse effects of a variety of drugs or alcohol.

Similar to many other disorders in geriatric patients, confusion often results from multiple interacting processes rather than a single causative factor. Accurate diagnosis depends on specifically defining abnormalities in mental status and cognitive function and on consistent definitions for clinical syndromes. Disorders causing confusion in the geriatric population can be broadly categorized into three groups:

1. Acute disorders usually associated with acute illness, drugs, and environmental factors (ie, delirium)
2. More slowly progressive impairment of cognitive function as seen in most dementia syndromes
3. Impaired cognitive function associated with affective disorders and psychoses

Older patients are often labeled "senile" because they are unable to answer a question or because they are not given adequate time to respond. Other age-associated disorders such as impaired hearing and Parkinson disease can also lead to mislabeling an older patient as confused or senile. Old age alone does not cause impairment of cognitive function of sufficient severity to render an individual dysfunctional. Slowed thinking and reaction time, mild recent memory loss, and impaired executive function can occur with increasing age and may or may not progress to dementia. Mild cognitive impairment (MCI) and cognitive impairment, not dementia (CIND) have been used to describe these deficits. The definitions, prognosis, and treatment of MCI are currently being studied (Petersen et al., 2001; Ravaglia et al., 2008 and therapeutic implications of MCI are subjects of intensive research.

Three questions are helpful in making an accurate diagnosis of the underlying cause(s) of confusion:

1. Has the onset of abnormalities been acute (ie, over a few hours or a few days)?
2. Are there physical factors (ie, medical illness, sensory deprivation, drugs) that may contribute to the abnormalities?
3. Are psychological factors (ie, depression and/or psychosis) contributing to or complicating the impairments in cognitive function?

These questions focus on identifying treatable conditions, which, when diagnosed and treated, might result in substantially improved cognitive function.

DELIRIUM

Delirium is an acute or subacute alteration in mental status especially common in the geriatric population. The prevalence of delirium in hospitalized geriatric patients is approximately 15% on admission, and the incidence in this

TABLE 6-2   DIAGNOSTIC CRITERIA FOR DELIRIUM

1. Disturbance of consciousness (ie, reduced clarity of awareness of the environment) in conjunction with reduced ability to focus, sustain, or shift attention

2. A change in cognition (such as memory deficit, disorientation, or language disturbance) or the development of a perceptual disturbance that is not better accounted for by a preexisting, established, or evolving dementia

3. Development of the disturbance during a brief period (usually hours to days) and a tendency for fluctuation during the course of the day

4. Evidence from the history, physical examination, or laboratory findings that the disturbance is caused by
   a. A general medical condition
   b. A substance intoxication, side effect, or withdrawal

Reproduced with permission from the American Psychiatric Association, 2000.

---

setting may be up to one-third. Delirium may persist for days or weeks, and is therefore common in postacute care settings. Many factors predispose geriatric patients to the development of delirium, including impaired sensory functioning and sensory deprivation, sleep deprivation, immobilization, and transfer to an unfamiliar environment.

The *Diagnostic and Statistical Manual of Mental Disorders* (DSM-IV-TR) (American Psychiatric Association, 2000) defines diagnostic criteria for delirium (Table 6-2). The key features of this disorder include the following:

- Disturbance of consciousness
- Change in cognition not better accounted for by dementia
- Symptoms and signs developing over a short period of time (hours to days)
- Fluctuation of the symptoms and signs
- Evidence that the disturbances are caused by the physiological consequences of a medical condition

The disturbances of consciousness and attention, with the suddenness of onset and the fluctuating cognitive status, are the major features that distinguish delirium from other causes of impaired cognitive function. Delirium is characterized by difficulty in sustaining attention to external and internal stimuli, sensory misperceptions (eg, illusions), and a fragmented or disordered stream of thought. Disturbances of psychomotor activity (such as restlessness, picking at bedclothes, attempting to get out of bed, sluggishness, drowsiness, and generally decreased psychomotor activity) and emotional disturbances (anxiety, fear, irritability, anger, apathy) are common in delirious patients. Neurological signs (except asterixis) are uncommon in delirium.

Among hospitalized geriatric patients, several factors are associated with the development of delirium (Inouye and Charpentier, 1996), including

- Age greater than 80 years
- Male sex
- Preexisting dementia
- Fracture
- Symptomatic infection
- Malnutrition
- Addition of three or more medications
- Use of neuroleptics and narcotics
- Use of restraints
- Bladder catheters

Rapid recognition of delirium is critical because it is often related to other reversible conditions and its development may be a poor prognostic sign for adverse outcomes including nursing home placement and death. CAM is a validated tool to identify delirium (Inouye et al., 1990). The diagnosis of delirium by the CAM requires the presence of

- Acute onset and fluctuating course *and*
- Inattention *and*
- Disorganized thinking *or*
- Altered level of consciousness

Differentiating delirium from dementia is important, because the latter is not immediately life threatening, and inappropriately labeling a delirious patient as demented may delay the diagnosis of serious and treatable underlying medical conditions. It is not possible to make the diagnosis of dementia when delirium is present in a patient with previously normal or unknown cognitive function. The diagnosis of dementia must await the treatment of all of the potentially reversible causes of delirium, as discussed later. Table 6-3 shows some of the key clinical features that are helpful in differentiating delirium from dementia. *Sundowning* is a term that describes an increase in confusion which commonly occurs in geriatric patients, especially those with preexisting dementia, at night. This condition is probably related to sensory deprivation in unfamiliar surroundings (such as the acute care hospital) and patients who sundown may actually meet the criteria for delirium.

A complete list of conditions that can cause delirium in the geriatric population would be too long to be useful in a clinical setting. Table 6-4 lists some of the common causes of this disorder. Several of them deserve further attention. Each geriatric patient who becomes acutely confused should be evaluated to rule out treatable conditions such as metabolic disorders, infections, and causes for

TABLE 6-3   KEY FEATURES DIFFERENTIATION DELIRIUM FROM DEMENTIA

FEATURE	DELIRIUM	DEMENTIA
Onset	Acute, often at night	Insidious
Course	Fluctuating, with lucid intervals, during day; worse at night	Generally stable over course of day
Duration	Hours to weeks	Months to years
Awareness	Reduced	Clear
Alertness	Abnormally low or high	Usually normal
Attention	Hypoalert or hyper-alert, distractible; fluctuates over course of day	Usually normal
Orientation	Usually impaired for time, tendency to mistake unfamiliar for familiar place and persons	Often impaired
Memory	Immediate and recent impaired	Recent and remote impaired
Thinking	Disorganized	Impoverished
Perception	Illusions and halluci-nations (usually visual) relatively common	Usually normal
Speech	Incoherent, hesitant, slow or rapid	Difficulty in finding words
Sleep–wake cycle	Always disrupted	Often fragmented sleep
Physical illness or drug toxicity	Either or both present	Often absent, especially in Alzheimer disease

Reproduced with permission from Lipkowski, 1987.

TABLE 6-4   COMMON CAUSES OF DELIRIUM IN GERIATRIC PATIENTS

Metabolic disorders
  Hypoxia
  Hypercarbia
  Hypo- or hyperglycemia
  Hyponatremia
  Azotemia

Infections

Decreased cardiac output
  Dehydration
  Acute blood loss
  Acute myocardial infarction
  Congestive heart failure

Stroke (small cortical)

Drugs (see Table 6-5)

Intoxication (alcohol, other)

Hypo- or hyperthermia

Acute psychoses

Transfer to unfamiliar surroundings (especially when sensory input is
  diminished)

Other
  Fecal impaction
  Urinary retention

decreased cardiac output (ie, dehydration, acute blood loss, heart failure). The evaluation should include vital signs (including pulse oximetry and a finger-stick glucose determination in diabetics), a careful physical examination, a complete blood count and basic metabolic panel, and other diagnostic tests as indicated by the findings and the patient's comorbidities.

Sometimes this workup is unrevealing. Small cortical strokes, which do not produce focal symptoms or signs, can cause delirium. These events may be difficult or impossible to diagnose with certainty, but there should be a high index of suspicion for this diagnosis in certain subgroups of patients—especially those with a history of hypertension, previous strokes, transient ischemic attacks, or cardiac arrhythmias. If delirium recurs, a source of emboli should be sought and associated conditions (such as hypertension) should be treated optimally. Fecal impaction and urinary retention, common in geriatric patients in acute care hospitals, can have dramatic effects on cognitive function and may be causes of acute confusion. The response to relief from these conditions can be just as impressive.

Drugs are a major cause of acute as well as chronic impairment of cognitive function in older patients (Medical Letter, 2002). Table 6-5 lists commonly prescribed drugs that can cause or contribute to delirium. Every attempt should be made to avoid or discontinue any medication that may be worsening cognitive function in a delirious geriatric patient. Environmental factors, especially rapid changes in location (such as being hospitalized, going on vacation, or entering a nursing home) and sensory deprivation, can precipitate delirium. This is especially true of those with early forms of dementia (see below). Measures such as preparing older patients for changes in location; placing familiar objects in the surroundings; and maximizing sensory input with lighting, clocks, and calendars may help prevent or manage delirium in some patients. A Hospital Elder Life Program has been described that may help prevent delirium, and cognitive and functional decline among high-risk older patients in acute hospitals (Inouye et al., 1999; Inouye et al., 2000). This program incorporates several strategies for identifying potentially reversible causes of delirium and medical behavioral and environmental interventions for patients who develop delirium.

TABLE 6-5   DRUGS THAT CAN CAUSE OR CONTRIBUTE TO DELIRIUM AND DEMENTIA*

Analgesics	Cardiovascular
Narcotic	Antiarrhythmics
Non-narcotic	Digoxin
Nonsteroidal anti-inflammatory agents	
Anticholinergics/Antihistamines	H_2 receptor antagonists
Anticonvulsants	Psychotropic drugs
Antihypertensives	Antianxiety drugs
Antipsychotics	Antidepressant drugs
Antimicrobials	Sedatives/Hypnotics
Antiparkinsonism drugs	Skeletal muscle relaxants
Alcohol	Steroids

*See Medical Letter, 2002 for a more complete list.

DEMENTIA

Dementia is a clinical syndrome involving a sustained loss of intellectual functions and memory of sufficient severity to cause dysfunction in daily living. Loss of functional ability is the key feature that distinguishes dementia from MCI. Its key features include

- A gradually progressing course (usually over months to years)
- No disturbance of consciousness

Dementia in the geriatric population can be grouped into two broad categories:

1. Reversible or partially reversible dementias
2. Nonreversible dementias

Reversible Dementias

While it is especially important to rule out treatable and potentially reversible causes of dementia in individual patients, these dementias account for a very small proportion of dementias (Clarfield, 2003). Moreover, finding a reversible cause does not guarantee that the dementia will improve after the putative cause has been treated.

Table 6-6 lists causes of reversible dementia. These disorders can be detected by careful history, physical examination, and selected laboratory studies. Drugs known to cause abnormalities in cognitive function (see Table 6-5) should be discontinued whenever feasible. There should be a high index of suspicion regarding excessive alcohol intake in older patients. The incidence of alcohol consumption varies considerably in different populations but is easily missed and can cause dementia as well as delirium, depression, falls, and other medical complications.

One particular disorder, depressive pseudodementia, deserves special emphasis. This term has been used to refer to patients who have reversible or partially reversible impairments of cognitive function caused by depression. Depression may coexist with dementia in more than one-third of outpatients with dementia, and in an even greater proportion in nursing homes. The interrelationship between depression and dementia is complex. Many patients with early forms of dementia become depressed. Sorting out how much of the cognitive impairment is caused by depression and how much by an organic factor(s) can be difficult. Some clinical characteristics can be helpful in diagnosis including prominent complaints of memory loss, patchy and inconsistent cognitive deficits on examination, and frequent "don't know" answers. Detailed neuropsychological testing, performed by a psychologist or other health-care professional skilled in the use

TABLE 6-6 CAUSES OF POTENTIALLY REVERSIBLE DEMENTIAS

Neoplasms	Autoimmune disorders
Metabolic disorders	Central nervous system vasculitis, temporal arteritis
Trauma	Disseminated lupus erythematosus
Toxins	Multiple sclerosis
Alcoholism	Drugs (see Table 6-5)
Heavy metals	Nutritional disorders
Organic poisons	Psychiatric disorders
Infections	Depression
Viral, including HIV	Other disorders (eg, normal-pressure hydrocephalus)

Reproduced with permission from Costa et al., 1996; Katzman, Lasker, and Bernstein, 1988. HIV, human immunodeficiency virus.

of these tools, can be helpful in many patients. At times, even after a complete assessment, uncertainty still exists regarding the role of depression in producing intellectual deficits. Under these circumstances, a careful trial of an antidepressant is justified to facilitate the diagnosis and may help improve overall functioning and quality of life. Older patients who develop reversible cognitive impairment while depressed appear at relatively high risk for developing dementia over the following few years, and their cognitive function should be followed closely over time.

Nonreversible Dementias

Several different classifications have been recommended for the nonreversible dementias. The Agency for Health Care Policy and Research (AHCPR) guideline on Alzheimer and related dementias (Costa et al., 1996) lists four basic categories, based on the work of Katzman, Lasker, and Bernstein (1988) can be defined as given in Table 6-7.

1. Degenerative diseases of the central nervous system
2. Vascular disorders
3. Trauma
4. Infections

TABLE 6-7   CAUSES OF NONREVERSIBLE DEMENTIAS

Degenerative diseases
  Alzheimer disease
  Dementia associated with Lewy bodies
  Parkinson disease
  Pick disease
  Huntington disease
  Progressive supranuclear palsy
  Others
Vascular dementias
  Occlusive cerebrovascular disease (multi-infarct dementia)
  Binswanger disease
  Cerebral embolism(s)
  Arteritis
  Anoxia secondary to cardiac arrest, cardiac failure of carbon monoxide
    intoxication
Traumatic dementia
  Craniocerebral injury
  Dementia pugilistica
Infections
  Acquired immunodeficiency syndrome
  Opportunistic infections
  Creutzfeldt-Jakob disease
  Progressive multifocal leukoencephalopathy
  Postencephalitic dementia

Adapted from Katzman, Lasker, and Bernstein, 1988.

Alzheimer disease (AD), other degenerative disorders, and vascular dementias account for a vast majority of dementias in the geriatric population, and are the focus of discussion in this chapter.

Alzheimer and Other Degenerative Diseases   AD and multi-infarct dementia account for the vast majority of dementias in the geriatric population. They frequently coexist in the same patient (Snowden et al., 1997; Langa, Foster, and Larson, 2004). Dementia with Lewy bodies (DLB) accounts for up to 25% of dementias in some series, and may overlap with Alzheimer and Parkinson dementias (McKeith et al., 1996; Small et al., 1997). In addition to the characteristic pathological findings, DLB is characterized by

- Detailed visual hallucinations
- Parkinsonian signs
- Alterations of alertness and attention

Table 6-8 lists the diagnostic criteria for AD. Family history and increasing age are its primary risk factors. Approximately 6% to 8% of persons older than age 65 have AD. The prevalence doubles every 5 years, so that nearly 30% of the population older than age 85 has AD. By the age of 90, almost 50% of persons with a

TABLE 6-8   DIAGNOSTIC CRITERIA FOR ALZHEIMER DEMENTIA

A. The development of multiple cognitive deficits manifested by both
   1. Memory impairment (impaired ability to learn new information or to recall previously learned information)
   2. One (or more) of the following cognitive disturbances:
      a. Aphasia (language disturbance)
      b. Apraxia (impaired ability to perform motor activities despite intact motor function)
      c. Agnosia (failure to recognize or identify objects despite intact sensory function)
      d. Disturbance in executive functioning (ie, planning, organizing, sequencing, abstracting)

B. The cognitive deficits cause severe impairment in social or occupational functioning and represent a major decline from a previous level of functioning

C. The course is characterized by gradual onset and continuing cognitive decline

D. The cognitive deficits are not because of any of the following:
   1. Other central nervous system conditions that cause progressive deficits in memory and cognition (eg, cerebrovascular disease, Parkinson disease, Huntington disease, subdural hematoma, normal-pressure hydrocephalus, brain tumor)
   2. Systemic conditions known to cause dementia (eg, hypothyroidism, vitamin deficiencies, hypercalcemia, neurosyphilis, HIV infection)

E. The deficits do not occur exclusively during the course of a delirium

F. The disturbance is not better accounted for by another axis I disorder (eg, major depressive disorder, schizophrenia)

Reproduced with permission from the American Psychiatric Association, 2000.

first-degree relative suffering from AD might develop the disease themselves. Rare genetic mutations on chromosomes 1, 14, and 21 cause early-onset familial forms of AD, and some forms of late-onset AD are linked to chromosome 12 (Small et al., 1997). The strongest genetic linkage with late-onset AD identified thus far is the apolipoprotein E epsilon4 (apo E-E4) allele on chromosome 19. The relative risk of AD associated with one or more copies of this allele in whites is approximately 2.5. However, apo E-E4 does not appear to confer increased risk for AD among African Americans or Hispanics. One study suggests, however, that the cumulative risks of AD to age 90 in the general population, adjusted for education and sex, are four times higher for African Americans and two times higher for Hispanics than for whites (Tang et al., 1998). Because the presence of one or more apo E-E4 alleles is neither sensitive nor specific, there is disagreement on recommending it as a screening test for AD (Small et al., 1997; Mayeux et al., 1998). Thus, routine screening, even among high-risk populations, is generally not recommended.

Other possible risk factors for AD include previous head injury, female sex, lower education level, and other yet-to-be-identified susceptibility genes. Possible protective factors include the use of estrogen, antioxidants, and non-steroidal anti-inflammatory drugs. The clinical significance of these possible protective effects, however, remains to be proven.

Vascular Dementias   Vascular dementias predominately caused by multiple infarcts (multi-infarct dementia) are common in the geriatric population. Multi-infarct dementia can occur alone or in combination with other disorders that cause dementia (Zekry et al., 2002). Autopsy studies suggest that cerebrovascular disease may play an important role in the presence and severity of symptoms of AD (Snowdon et al., 1997). Multi-infarct dementia results when a patient has sustained recurrent cortical or subcortical strokes. Many of these strokes are too small to cause permanent or residual focal neurological deficits or evidence of strokes on computed tomography (CT). Magnetic resonance imaging (MRI) may be more sensitive in detecting small infarcts, but there has been a tendency to overinterpret some of these findings as more MRI scans are being done. Table 6-9 identifies characteristics of patients likely to have multi-infarct dementia and compares the clinical characteristics of primary degenerative and multi-infarct dementias. A key feature of multi-infarct dementia is the stepwise deterioration in cognitive functioning, as illustrated in Fig. 6-1. Another form of vascular form of dementia has been described, termed senile dementia of the Binswanger type, which may be impossible to differentiate clinically from multi-infarct dementia. It has become increasingly important to differentiate vascular from other dementias because patients with the former may benefit from more aggressive treatment of hypertension and other cardiovascular risk factors (Forette et al., 2002; Murray et al., 2002), whereas some of the newer pharmacological treatments for AD may not help patients with vascular forms of dementias.

TABLE 6-9   ALZHEIMER DISEASE VERSUS MULTI-INFARCT DEMENTIA: COMPARISON OF CLINICAL
CHARACTERISTICS

CHARACTERISTICS	ALZHEIMER DISEASE	MULTI-INFARCT DEMENTIA
Demographic		
Sex	Women more commonly affected	Men more commonly affected
Age	Generally over age 75 years	Generally over age 60 years
History		
Time course of deficits	Gradually progressive	Stuttering or episodic, with stepwise deterioration
History of hypertension	Less common	Common
History of stroke(s), transient ischemic attack(s), or other focal neurological symptoms	Less common	Common
Examination		
Hypertension	Less common	Common
Focal neurological signs	Uncommon	Common
Signs of atherosclerotic cardiovascular disease	Less common	Common
Emotional liability	Less common	More common

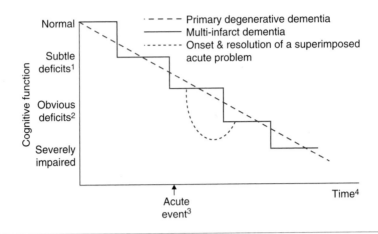

— FIGURE 6-1 — Primary degenerative dementia versus multi-infarct dementia: comparison of time courses. (1) Recognized by patient, but only detectable on detailed testing. (2) Deficits recognized by family and friends. (3) See text for explanation. (4) Exact time courses are variable; see text.

EVALUATION

A consensus statement of the American Association of Geriatric Psychiatry, the Alzheimer's Association, and the American Geriatrics Society (Small et al., 1997) and other recommendations (Costa et al., 1996; Feil, MacLean, and Sultzer, 2007; Lyketsos et al., 2006) have updated recommendations for the evaluation of patients suspected of having a dementia syndrome. The first step is to recognize clues that dementia may be present. The Mini-Cog assessment is a useful screening tool in identifying patients who should undergo further assessment. It screens both memory (3-item recall) and executive function (clock drawing) (Borson et al., 2003).

Table 6-10 lists symptoms that should suggest further evaluation. Patients suspected of having dementia should undergo the following:

- Focused history and physical examination, including assessment for delirium and depression and identification of comorbid conditions (eg, sensory impairment)
- A functional status assessment (see Chap. 3)
- A mental status examination (see Table 6-1)
- Selected laboratory studies to rule out reversible dementia and delirium

TABLE 6-10 SYMPTOMS THAT MAY INDICATE DEMENTIA

* Learning and retaining new information
  Is repetitious; has trouble remembering recent conversations, events, appointments; frequently misplaces objects
* Handling complex tasks
  Has trouble following a complex train of thought or performing tasks that require many steps, such as balancing a checkbook or cooking a meal
* Reasoning ability
  Is unable to respond with a reasonable plan to problems at work or home, such as knowing what to do if the bathroom is flooded; shows uncharacteristic disregard for rules of social conduct
* Spatial ability and orientation
  Has trouble driving, organizing objects around the house, finding their way around familiar places
* Language
  Has increasing difficulty with finding the words to express what they want to say and with following conversations
* Behavior
  Appears more passive and less responsive, is more irritable than usual, is more suspicious than usual, misinterprets visual or auditory stimuli

Reproduced with permission from Costa et al., 1996.

Table 6-11 outlines key aspects of the history. Because many physical illnesses and drugs can cause cognitive dysfunction, active medical problems and use of prescription and nonprescription drugs (including alcohol) should be reviewed. The nature and severity of the symptoms should be characterized. What are the deficits? Does the patient admit to them or is the family member describing them? How is the patient reacting to the problems? The responses to these questions can be helpful in differentiating between dementia, depressive, or mixed condition. The onset of symptoms and the rate of progression are particularly important. The sudden onset of cognitive impairment (over a few days) should prompt a search for one of the underlying causes of delirium listed in Table 6-4. Irregular, stepwise decrements in cognitive function (as opposed to a more even and gradual loss) favor a diagnosis of multi-infarct dementia (see Table 6-9 and Fig. 6-1). Patients with dementia are often brought for evaluation

TABLE 6-11   EVALUATING DEMENTIA: THE HISTORY

Summarize active medical problems and current physical complaints

List drugs (including over-the-counter preparations and alcohol)

Cardiovascular and neurological history

Characterize the symptoms
    Nature of deficits (memory vs. other cognitive functions)
    Onset and rate of progression
    Impaired function (eg, managing money or medications)
    Associated psychological symptoms
        Depression
        Anxiety or agitation
        Paranoid ideation
        Psychotic thought processes (delusions and/or hallucinations)

Ask about special problems
    Wandering (and getting lost)
    Dangerous driving and car crashes
    Disruptive or self-endangering behaviors
    Verbal agitation
    Physical aggression
    Insomnia
    Poor hygiene
    Malnutrition
    Incontinence

Assess the social situation
    Living arrangements
    Social supports
    Availability of relatives and other caregivers
    Employment and health of caregivers

at a time of sudden worsening of cognitive function (as illustrated by the broken line in Fig. 6-1) and may even meet the criteria for delirium. These sudden changes may be triggered by a number of acute events (a small stroke without focal signs, acute physical illness, drugs, changes in environment, or personal loss such as the death or departure of a relative). Only a careful history (or familiarity with the patient) will help to determine when an acute event has been superimposed on a preexisting dementia. Appropriate management of the acute event will, in many instances, result in improvement in cognitive function (see Fig. 6-1, broken line).

The history should also include specific questions about common problems requiring special attention in patients with dementia. These problems may include wandering, dangerous driving and car crashes, disruptive behavior (eg, verbal agitation, physical aggression, and nighttime agitation), delusions or hallucinations, insomnia, poor hygiene, malnutrition, and incontinence. They require careful management and most often substantial involvement of family or other caregivers.

A social history is especially important in patients with dementia. Living arrangements and social supports should be assessed. Along with functional status, these factors play a major role in the management of patients with dementia and are of critical importance in determining the possible necessity for institutionalization. A patient with dementia and weak social supports may require institutionalization at a higher level of function than a patient with strong social supports. In addition to the lack of availability of a spouse, child, or other relative who can serve as a caregiver, the caregiver's employment and/or poor health can play an important role in determining the need for institutional care.

A general physical examination should focus particularly on cardiovascular and neurological assessment. Hypertension and other cardiovascular findings and focal neurological signs (such as unilateral weakness or sensory deficit, hemianopsia, Babinski reflex) favor a diagnosis of multi-infarct dementia. Pathological reflexes (such as the glabellar and palmomental reflexes) are nonspecific and occur in many forms of dementia as well as in a small proportion of normal-aged persons. These frontal lobe release signs—as well as impaired stereognosis or graphesthesia, gait disorder, and abnormalities on cerebellar testing—are significantly more common in patients with AD than in age-matched controls. Parkinsonian signs (tremor, bradykinesia, muscle rigidity) should be sought because they may indicate either dementia associated with Lewy bodies or frank Parkinson disease.

A careful mental status examination (see Table 6-1) and a standardized mental status test should be performed. Although practice guidelines indicate that no single test is clearly superior, the Mini-Cog is useful for screening, and the Mini-Mental State Examination and the Time and Change Test are rapid tests that can be used in clinical practice to get an objective score related to cognitive function (see appendix). Neuropsychological testing can be helpful when there is a normal mental status score but also functional and/or behavioral changes (this can occur in patients with high baseline intelligence) or when there is a low score without functional deficits (this can occur in patients with lower educational levels). Neuropsychological testing can also be helpful in differentiating depression and dementia and in pinpointing specific cognitive strengths and weaknesses for patients, families, and health providers.

Selected diagnostic studies are useful in ruling out reversible forms of dementia (Table 6-12). Although CT and MRI scans of the head are expensive, many clinicians and experts order one of these tests for patients with dementia of recent onset in whom no other clinical findings explain the dementia and in those with focal neurological signs or symptoms. Cerebral atrophy on one of these scans does not establish the diagnosis of AD; it can occur with normal aging as well as with several specific disease processes. The scan is thus recommended to rule out treatable causes (eg, subdural hematoma, tumors, normal-pressure hydrocephalus). CT and MRI each have advantages and disadvantages. They are roughly equivalent in the detection of most remediable structural lesions. MRI will demonstrate more lesions than CT in patients with multi-infarct dementia, but will also demonstrate white matter changes of uncertain clinical significance (Small et al., 1997). Position emission tomography (PET) scan abnormalities can precede the development of clinical deficits by several years in patients at risk for AD. However, PET scanning remains largely a research rather than a clinical practice tool. The blood tests recommended are directed at finding common comorbidities as opposed to identifying the cause of the underlying dementia. For example, thyroid hormone and/or vitamin B_{12} replacement may be important for a patient's health, but have not been shown to reverse cognitive deficits (Clarfield, 2003; Balk et al., 2007).

TABLE 6-12   EVALUATING DEMENTIA: RECOMMENDED DIAGNOSTIC STUDIES

Blood studies
    Complete blood count
    Glucose
    Urea nitrogen
    Electrolytes
    Calcium and phosphorous
    Liver function tests
    Thyroid stimulating hormone
    Vitamin B_{12} and folate
    Serologic test for syphilis
    Human immunodeficiency virus antibodies (if suspected)

Radiographic studies
    Computed tomography (or magnetic resonance imaging) of the head

Other studies
    Neuropsychological testing (selected patients; see text)

MANAGEMENT OF DEMENTIA

General Principles

Table 6-13 outlines key principles for the management of dementia. Although complete cure is not available for the vast majority of dementias, optimal management can provide improvements in the ability of these patients to function, as well as in their overall well-being and that of their families and other caregivers.

If causes of reversible or partially reversible forms of dementia are identified (see Table 6-6), they should be specifically treated. Small strokes (lacunar infarcts), which can cause further deterioration of cognitive function in patients with AD, as well as those with vascular dementia may be prevented by controlling hypertension; thus hypertension should be aggressively treated in patients with dementia as long as side effects can be avoided (Forette et al., 2002). Other specific diseases such as Parkinson disease should be optimally managed. The treatment of these and other medical conditions is especially challenging because treatment (usually drugs) may have adverse effects on cognitive function.

Pharmacological Treatment of Dementia

There are three basic approaches to the pharmacological treatment of dementia:

1. Agents that enhance cognition and function
2. Drug treatment of coexisting depression
3. Pharmacological treatment of complications such as paranoia, delusions, psychosis, and agitation (verbal and physical)

Drug treatment of depression may provide substantial benefits in patients with dementia (Lyketsos et al., 2003) and is discussed in detail in Chap. 7. The use of antipsychotics to treat the neuropsychiatric symptoms of dementia is highly controversial (Sink, Holden, and Yaffe, 2005; Wang et al., 2005; Schneider et al., 2005; Schneider et al., 2006; Ayalon et al., 2006). Pharmacological treatments including antipsychotics and sedatives are discussed in Chap. 14.

The primary pharmacological approach to the treatment of AD has been the use of cholinesterase inhibitors. Their effectiveness in improving function and quality of life remain controversial, and the potential benefits of these drugs versus their risks and costs must be weighed carefully in individual patients. Some evidence suggests that these drugs may also have some efficacy for multi-infarct dementia and DLB. There are four approved drugs of this class on the market:

TABLE 6-13 KEY PRINCIPLES IN THE MANAGEMENT OF DEMENTIA

Optimize the patient's physical and mental function through physical activity and mind plasticity principals and activities
   Treatment underlying medical and other conditions (eg, hypertension, Parkinson disease, depression [Chap. 7])
   Avoid use of drugs with central nervous system side effects (unless required for management of psychological or behavioral disturbances—see Chap. 14)
   Assess the environment and suggest alterations, if necessary
   Encourage physical and mental activity
   Avoid situations stressing intellectual capabilities; use memory aids whenever possible
   Prepare the patient for changes in location
   Emphasize good nutrition
Identify and manage behavioral symptoms and complications
   Wandering
   Dangerous driving
   Behavioral disorders
   Depression (see Chap. 7)
   Agitation or aggressiveness
   Psychosis (delusions, hallucinations)
   Malnutrition
   Incontinence (see Chap. 8)
Provide ongoing care
   Reassessment of cognitive and physical function
   Treatment of medical conditions
Provide medical information to patient and family
   Nature of the disease
   Extent of impairment
   Prognosis
Provide social service information to patient and family
   Local Alzheimer's Association
   Community health-care resources (day centers, homemakers, home health aides)
   Legal and financial counseling
   Use of advance directives
   Provide family counseling for
   Identification and resolution of family conflicts
   Handling anger and guilt
   Decisions on respite or institutional care
   Legal concerns
   Ethical concerns (see Chap. 17)

tacrine, donepezil, rivastigmine, and galantamine. Randomized placebo-controlled clinical trials suggest that these drugs can have positive effects on cognitive function, and may improve or prevent decline in overall function and potentially delay nursing home admission (Ritchie et al., 2004; Santaguida et al., 2004; Winblad et al., 2006). The clinical importance of these improvements may be marginal in many patients (Raina et al., 2008). Tacrine is potentially hepatotoxic and is generally not prescribed for this reason. Gastrointestinal side effects can be problematic and include nausea, vomiting, and diarrhea and nightmares can be bothersome as well. On the other hand, the benefits of these drugs include slight improvements in cognitive function, and up to a several-month delay in the progression of cognitive impairment and the development of related behavioral symptoms. One large trial has shown that adding vitamin E to donepezil does not improve outcomes for patients with MCI (Peterson et al., 2005). While these drugs have been used to help manage behavioral symptoms associated with dementia, at least one controlled study of one of them (donepezil) failed to demonstrate efficacy for this purpose (Howard et al., 2007).

Other drugs, including estrogen (in women), vitamin E, ginkgo biloba, and nonsteroidal anti-inflammatory agents have been used to prevent dementia. There is, however, no evidence that these drugs are effective in preventing or treating dementia (most evidence suggests they are not). There is also no evidence that vitamin B_{12}, B_6, or folic acid supplementation improves cognitive function (Balk et al., 2007).

▓ Nonpharmacological Management

A variety of supportive measures and other nonpharmacological management techniques are useful in improving the overall function and well-being of patients with dementia and their families (see Table 6-13). These interventions range from specific recommendations for caregivers, such as alterations in the physical environment, the use of memory aids, the avoidance of stressful tasks, and preparation for the patient's move to another living setting with a higher level of care, to more general techniques, such as providing information and counseling services (AGS/AAGP Position Statement, 2003; Ayalon et al., 2006). Many nursing homes have developed special care units for dementia patients. With few exceptions, however (Rovner et al., 1996), there is little evidence that such units improve outcomes (Phillips et al., 1997). Nonpharmacologic treatment of agitation can, however, be effective in this setting (Cohen-Mansfield et al., 2007). Assisted-living facilities have also developed specialized dementia units, with specially designed environments, trained staff, and intensive activities programming, and without the more hospital-like environment typical of many nursing homes. The effectiveness of such units and whether people with advanced dementia can optimally be cared for in them has not been well studied.

Symptoms commonly associated with moderate to severe cognitive impairment (CI), such as memory loss, aphasia, motor apraxia, visual agnosia, and apathy make it challenging for caregivers to interact, motivate, and implement restorative care interventions (Rabins, Lyketsos, and Steele, 2006). In addition to functional and motivational challenges, problematic behavioral symptoms, such as verbal and physical aggression, sleep disturbance, depression, delusions, hallucinations, and resistance to care occur in at least 50% to 80% of individuals diagnosed with dementia at some time during the course of their illness. Nursing assistants, who provide the majority of hands-on care in long-term care settings, are frequently challenged by the agitated and uncooperative behaviors of cognitively impaired residents. There are, however, a variety of techniques that have been shown to be effective in engaging these individuals in functional activities while managing behavioral problems. These include such things as getting to know individual and drawing on their past experiences and patterns (eg, giving a housewife household activities to do), using humor, providing simply repetitive activities, encouraging mimicking by demonstrating the behavior/activity that you want the individual to perform, communicating face on and using multiple sources of input (eg, verbal and written).

The provision of ongoing care is especially important in the management of dementia patients. Reassessment of the patient's cognitive abilities can be helpful in identifying potentially reversible causes for deteriorating function and in making specific recommendations to family and other caregivers. The family is the primary target of strategies to help manage dementia patients in noninstitutional settings. Caring for relatives with dementia is physically, emotionally, and financially stressful. Information on the disease itself and the extent of impairment and on community resources helpful in managing these patients can be of critical importance to family and caregivers. The local chapter of the Alzheimer's Association and the Area Agency on Aging are examples of community resources that can provide education and linkages with appropriate services. Anticipating and teaching family members strategies to cope with common behavioral problems associated with dementia—such as wandering, incontinence, day–night reversal, and nighttime agitation—can be of critical importance. Hazardous driving that can result in car crashes is an especially troublesome problem. Several states require reporting patients with dementia who maintain drivers' licenses. There remain, however, no validated methods of assessing driving capabilities and safety among individuals with early dementia. Wandering may be especially hazardous for the dementia patient's safety and is associated with falls. Incontinence is common and often very difficult for families to manage (see Chap. 8). Books providing information and suggestions for family management techniques are very useful (see Suggested Readings). Support groups for families of patients with AD through the Alzheimer's Association are available in most large cities. Family counseling can be helpful in dealing with a variety of issues such as anger, guilt, decisions on institutionalization, handling the patient's assets, and terminal care. Dementia patients and their families should also be encouraged to discuss and document their wishes, using a durable power of attorney for health care or an equivalent mechanism early in the course of the illness (see Chap. 17). Family members should be encouraged to seek respite care periodically to provide time for themselves. Some communities have formal respite care programs available. In the absence of such programs, informal arrangements can often be made to relieve the primary family caregivers for short periods of time at regular intervals. Such relief will help the caregiver to cope with what is generally a very stressful situation. Often a multidisciplinary group of health professionals—made up of a physician, a nurse, a social worker, and, when needed, rehabilitation therapists, a lawyer, and a clergy member—must coordinate efforts to manage these patients and provide support to family and caregivers.

EVIDENCE SUMMARY

Do's

- Assess for correctable underlying causes of delirium and dementia.
- Carefully review medication regimens to determine if one or more medication can affect cognitive function and try to eliminate potential offenders.
- Screen for behaviors and symptoms that put demented patients at risk (eg, trying to cook unattended, driving, wandering at night).
- Screen older patients with dementia for depression, which can exacerbate cognitive impairment.
- Pay attention to the health and emotional status of caregivers.

Don'ts

- Automatically do brain imaging in every patient with cognitive impairment.
- Use psychoactive drugs or narcotics if they can be avoided in patients with cognitive impairment.
- Use physical restraints in hospitalized older patients with delirium or dementia unless essential for their safety and medical care.

Consider

- Formal neuropsychological testing if the diagnosis is uncertain, or if the patient or family wants to better understand cognitive capabilities
- A trial of a cholinesterase inhibitor for older patients with dementia
- Judicious use of antidepressants and antipsychotics for dementia patients with concomitant depression or psychosis respectively
- Referring family members for support groups, in-home help, and respite programs when appropriate

References

American Geriatrics Society, American Association for Geriatric Psychiatry. Consensus statement on improving the quality of mental health care in U.S. nursing homes: management of depression and behavioral symptoms associated with dementia. *JAGS.* 2003;51:1287-1298.

American Psychiatric Association. *Diagnostic and Statistical Manual of Mental Disorders,* Text Revision 4th ed. Washington, DC: APA; 2000.

Ayalon L, Gum AM, Feliciano L, et al. Effectiveness of nonpharmacological interventions for the management of neuropsychiatric symptoms in patients with dementia. *Arch Intern Med.* 2006;166:2182-2188.

Balk EM, Raman G, Tatsioni A, et al. Vitamin B_6, B_{12}, and folic acid supplementation and cognitive function. *Arch Intern Med.* 2007;167:21-30.

Borson S, Scanlan JM, Chen P, et al. The mini-cog as a screen for dementia: validation in a population-based sample. *JAGS.* 2003;51:1451-1454.

Carson S, McDonagh MS, Peterson K. A systematic review of the efficacy and safety of atypical antipsychotics in patients with psychological and behavioral symptoms of dementia. *JAGS.* 2006;54:354-361.

Clarfield AM. The reversible dementias: do they reverse? *Ann Intern Med.* 1988;109:476-486.

Clarfield AM. The decreasing prevalence of reversible dementias: an updated meta-analysis. *Arch Intern Med.* 2003;163:2219-2229.

Cohen-Mansfield J, Libin A, Marx MS. Nonpharmacological treatment of agitation: a controlled trial of systematic individualized intervention. *J Gerontol Med Sci.* 2007;62A:908-916.

Costa PT Jr, Williams TF, Somerfield M, et al. *Recognition and Initial Assessment of Alzheimer's Disease and Related Dementias.* Clinical Practice Guideline No. 19. Rockville, MD: US Department of Health and Human Services, Public Health Service, Agency for Health Care Policy and Research; November 1996; AHCPR Publication No. 97–0702.

Cummings JL. Alzheimer's disease. *N Engl J Med.* 2004;351:56-67.

Feil DG, MacLean C, Sultzer D. Quality indicators for the care of dementia in vulnerable elders. *JAGS.* 2007;55:S293-S301.

Forette F, Seux ML, Staessen JA, et al. The prevention of dementia with antihypertensive treatment. *Arch Intern Med.* 2002;162:2046-2052.

Howard RJ, Juszczak E, Ballard CG, et al. Donepezil for the treatment of agitation in Alzheimer's disease. *N Engl J Med.* 2007;357:1382-1392.

Inouye SK, van Dyck CH, Alessi CA, et al. Clarifying confusion: the confusion assessment method: a new method for detection of delirium. *Ann Intern Med.* 1990;113:941-948.

Inouye SK, Charpentier PA. Precipitating factors of delirium in hospitalized elderly persons: predictive model and interrelationship with baseline vulnerability. *JAMA.* 1996;275:852-857.

Inouye SK, Bogardus ST Jr, Charpentier PA, et al. A multicomponent intervention to prevent delirium in hospitalized older patients. *N Engl J Med.* 1999;340:669-676.

Inouye SK, Bogardus ST, Baker DI, et al. The hospital elder life program: a model of care to prevent cognitive and functional decline in older hospitalized patients. *J Am Geriatr Soc.* 2000;48:1697-1706.

Inouye SK. Delirium in older persons. *N Engl J Med.* 2006;354:1157-1165.

Katzman R, Lasker B, Bernstein N. Advances in the diagnosis of dementia: accuracy of diagnosis and consequences of misdiagnosis of disorders causing dementia. In: Terry RD, ed. *Aging and the Brain.* New York, NY: Raven Press; 1988:17-62.

Lipowski ZJ. Delirium (acute confusional states). *JAMA.* 1987;258:1789-1792.

Langa KM, Foster NL, Larson EB. Mixed dementia: emerging concepts and therapeutic implications. *JAMA.* 2004;292:2901-2908.

Lyketsos CG, Lopez O, Jones B, et al. Prevalence of neuropsychiatric symptoms in dementia and mild cognitive impairment. *JAMA.* 2002;288:1475-1483.

Lyketsos CG, DelCampo L, Steinberg M, et al. Treating depression in Alzheimer disease: efficacy and safety of sertraline therapy, and the benefits of depression reduction: the DIADS. *Arch Gen Psychiatry.* 2003;60:737-746.

Lyketsos G, Colenda CC, Beck C, et al. Position statement of the American Association for Geriatric Psychiatry regarding principles of care for patients with dementia resulting from Alzheimer disease. *Am J Geriatr Psychiatry.* 2006;14:561-573.

Mayeux R, Saunders AM, Shea S, et al. Utility of the apolipoprotein E genotype in the diagnosis of Alzheimer's disease. *N Engl J Med.* 1998;338:506-511.

Medical Letter. Drugs that may cause psychiatric symptoms. *Med Lett.* 2002;44(1134): 59-62.

McKeith LG, Galasko D, Kosaka K, et al. Consensus guidelines for the clinical and pathologic diagnosis of dementia with Lewy bodies (DLB): report on the consortium of DLB international workshop. *Neurology.* 1996;47:1113-1124.

Mitchell SL. A 93-year-old man with advanced dementia and eating problems. *JAMA.* 2007;298:2527-2536.

Murray MD, Lane KA, Gao S, et al. Preservation of cognitive function with antihypertensive medications. *Arch Intern Med.* 2002;162:2090-2096.

Petersen RC, Stevens JC, Ganguli M, et al. Practice parameter: mild cognitive impairment (an evidence-based review). Report of the Quality Standards Subcommittee of the American Academy of Neurology. *Neurology.* 2001;56:113-1142.

Peterson RC, Thomas RG, Grundman M, et al. Vitamin E and donepezil for the treatment of mild cognitive impairment. *N Engl J Med.* 2005;352:2379-2388.

Phillips C, Sloane P, Hawes C, et al. Effects of residence in Alzheimer disease special care units on functional outcomes. *JAMA.* 1997;278:1340-1344.

Rabins P, Lyketsos C, Steele C. *Practical Dementia Care.* New York, NY: Oxford University Press; 2006.

Raina P, Santaguida P, Ismaila A, et al. Effectiveness of cholinesterase inhibitors and memantine for treating dementia: evidence review for clinical practice guideline. *Ann Intern Med.* 2008;148:379-397.

Ravaglia G, Forti P, Montesi F, et al. Mild cognitive impairment: epidemiology and dementia risk in an elderly Italian population. *JAGS.* 2008;56:51-58.

Ritchie CW, Ames D, Clayton T, et al. Metaanalysis of randomized trials of the efficacy and safety of donepezil, galantamine, and rivastigmine for the treatment of Alzheimer disease. *Am J Geriat Psychiatry.* 2004;12:358-369.

Roman GC, Royall DR. Executive control function: a rational basis for the diagnosis of vascular dementia. *Alzheimer Dis Assoc Disord.* 1999;13:S69-S80.

Rovner BW, Steele CD, Shmuely Y, et al. A randomized trial of dementia care in nursing homes. *J Am Geriatric Soc.* 1996;44:7-13.

Santaguida PS, Raina P, Booker L, et al. *Pharmacological Treatment of Dementia. Summary, Evidence, Report/Technology Assessment No. 97.* Rockville, MD: Agency for Healthcare Research Quality (AHRQ); 2004.

Schneider LS, Dagerman KS, Insel P. Risk of death with atypical antipsychotics drug treatment for dementia: meta-analysis of randomized placebo-controlled trials. *JAMA.* 2005;294:1934-1943.

Schneider LS, Tariot PN, Dagerman KS, et al. Effectiveness of atypical antipsychotic drugs in patients with Alzheimer's disease. *N Engl J Med.* 2006;355:1525-1538.

Sink KM, Holden KF, Yaffe K. Pharmacological treatment of neuropsychiatric symptoms of dementia: a review of the evidence. *JAMA.* 2005;293:596-608.

Small GW, Rabins PV, Barry PP, et al. Diagnosis and treatment of Alzheimer disease and related disorders. *JAMA.* 1997;278:1363-1371.

Snowden DA, Greiner LH, Mortimer JA, et al. Brain infarction and the clinical expression of Alzheimer's disease: the nun study. *JAMA.* 1997;277:813-817.

Pugh MB, ed. *Stedman's Medical Dictionary.* New York, NY: Lippincott Williams & Wilkins; 2000.

Tang MX, Stern Y, Marder K, et al. The ApoE-E4 allele and the risk of Alzheimer disease among African Americans, whites, and Hispanics. *JAMA.* 1998;279:751-755.

Wang PS, Schneweiss S, Avorn J, et al. Risk of death in elderly users of conventional vs. atypical antipsychotic medications. *N Engl J Med.* 2005;353:2335-2341.

Wenger NS, Solomon DH, Roth CP, et al. Application of assessing care of vulnerable elders-3 quality indicators to patients with advanced dementia and poor prognosis. *JAGS.* 2007;55:S457-S463.

Winblad B, Kilander L, Erikson S, et al. Donepezil in patients with severe Alzheimer's disease: double-blind, parallel-group, placebo-controlled study. *Lancet.* 2006;367:1057-1165.

Zekry D, Hauw JJ, Gold G. Mixed dementia: epidemiology, diagnosis, and treatment. *JAGS.* 2002;50:1431-1438.

Suggested Readings

Gomez-Tortosa E, Ingraham AO, Irizarry MC, et al. Dementia with Lewy bodies. *J Am Geriatr Soc.* 1998;46:1449-1458.

Holsinger T, Deveau J, Boustani M, et al. Does this patient have dementia? *JAMA.* 2007;297:2391-2404.

Selected Web Sites (Accessed on March 16, 2008)

http://www.healthinaging.org/agingintheknow/chapters_ch_trial.asp?ch=57
http://www.healthinaging.org/agingintheknow/chapters_ch_trial.asp?ch=59
http://www.alz.org
http://www.nia.nih.gov/alzheimers

Tools

Mini-Cog
http://www.hospitalmedicine.org/geriresource/toolbox/mini_cog.htm (Accessed on April 12, 2008)
Confusion assessment method
http://www.ohsu.edu/sgimhartford/toolbox/Card2bCAM.pdf (Accessed on April 12, 2008)

CHAPTER 7

DIAGNOSIS AND MANAGEMENT OF DEPRESSION

Depression in older adults is a persistent or recurrent disorder resulting from psychosocial stress or the physiologic effects of disease. This psychological problem can lead to disability, cognitive impairment, exacerbation of medical problems, increased use of health-care services, and increased suicide (Ahmed, Lefante, and Alam, 2007; Blazer, Sachs-Ericsson, and Hybels, 2007; Kirchner et al., 2007; Roriz-Cruz et al., 2007). It complicates the treatment of other physiological problems. It is severely under-recognized and undertreated. Unfortunately, the signs and symptoms of depression are easily missed in older adults, or assumed to be because of normal age changes and responses to life events or medical problems. These individuals do not present with the typical symptoms of depression, such as depressed mood, or sadness. The signs and symptoms that are reported may be related to a physical illness and exacerbated or exaggerated by the depression. While it is sometimes a slow and difficult diagnostic process, it is critical to rule out medical problems (acute or chronic) prior to a definitive diagnosis of depression.

Sorting out the complex interrelationships between symptoms and signs of depression caused by physical illnesses and those caused primarily by an affective disorder or related psychiatric diagnosis is challenging for health-care providers. Recognition and appropriate management of depression are critical, however, to optimize the management of comorbidities, maintain function and quality of life, reduce the need for health-care resources, and prevent further morbidity and even mortality. This chapter addresses these issues from the perspective of the nonpsychiatrist, highlighting diagnostic techniques and initial management options. It should be recognized, however, that the management of some older adults will best be done by involving psychiatrists and psychologists, and possibly an integrated care model approach (Skultety and Zeiss, 2006).

AGING AND DEPRESSION

The prevalence of major depression among older adults actually decreases with age, with this rate being 6.5% to 9% among those living in the community (Lyness et al., 2002). While an additional 2% of older individuals experience dysthymia (a chronic depressive disorder characterized by functional impairment and at least 2 years of depressive symptoms), this also consistently has decreased with age (Ahmed, Lefante, and Alam, 2007). Major depression is found in 16% to 50% of older adults in nursing homes or acute care settings (Davison et al., 2007; McCusker et al., 2005). The generally lower rate of major depression among older individuals may be caused by selective mortality, institutionalization, missed diagnoses, and/or cohort effects (ie, that older individuals tend to deny mental health problems such as depression) (Koenig, 2007). The prevalence of subsyndromal depression (ie, symptoms of depression that do not meet standard criteria for major depression), however, steadily increases with age and ranges from 10% to 25% among community dwelling and increases to 50% among those in nursing homes or acute care settings (Speer and Schneider, 2003). Dysthymia, in contrast, is a chronic depressive disorder characterized by functional impairment and at least 2 years of depressive symptoms. The implications of depression are substantial and include increased mortality and morbidity including increased incidences of metabolic syndrome (Roriz-Cruz et al., 2007), weight changes (Forman-Hoffman et al., 2007), and declines in function and impaired cognition (Amore et al., 2007). When depression is associated with other medical problems (eg, hip fracture or osteoarthritis), there is often an exacerbation of associated pain, poor compliance and motivation, and impaired recovery and function. Persons aged 65 and over account for 25% of all suicides, and as many as 75% of older adults who commit suicide were suffering from depression (Ruckenbauer, Yazdani, and Ravaglia, 2007). Several factors are associated with suicide in the geriatric population (Table 7-1).

Bipolar affective disorder is not uncommon in the elderly (Aziz, Lorberg, and Tampi, 2006); these disorders account for 10% to 25% of all geriatric patients with mood disorders and 5% of patients admitted to geropsychiatric inpatient units. A diagnosis of bipolar disease is based on a distinct period of persistently elevated mood lasting for 1 or more weeks and three additional symptoms that may include inflated self-esteem or grandiosity, hypersexuality, increased activity, decreased need for sleep, pressured speech, racing thoughts or flight of ideas, and distractibility. Grandiose or paranoid delusions may be present. Although the criteria for diagnosing bipolar disorder in younger and older patients are identical, some differences in phenomenology have been noted. Elderly patients with bipolar disorder are more likely to have a mixture of depression and marked irritability. Pressured speech that tends to go off on tangents is common, although the

TABLE 7-1   FACTORS ASSOCIATED WITH SUICIDE IN THE GERIATRIC POPULATION

FACTOR	HIGH RISK	LOW RISK
Sex	Male	Female
Religion	Protestant	Catholic or Jewish
Race	White	Nonwhite
Marital status	Widowed or divorced Recent death of a spouse	Married
Occupational background	Blue-collar low-paying job	Professional or white-collar job
Current employment status	Retired or unemployed	Employed full- or part-time
Living environment	Urban Living alone Isolated Recent move	Rural Living with spouse or other relatives Living in close-knit neighborhood
Physical health	Poor health Terminal illness Pain and suffering Multiple comorbid conditions	Good health
Mental health	Depression (current or previous) Alcoholism Low self-esteem Loneliness Feeling rejected, unloved Poor quality of life	Happy and well adjusted Positive self-concept and outlook Sense of personal control over life
Personal background	Broken home Dependent personality History of poor interpersonal relationships	Intact family of origin Independent, assertive, flexible personality History of close friendships

TABLE 7-1   FACTORS ASSOCIATED WITH SUICIDE IN THE GERIATRIC POPULATION (*Continued*)

FACTOR	HIGH RISK	LOW RISK
	Family history of mental illness	No family history of mental illness
	Poor marital history	No previous suicide attempts
	Poor work record	No history of suicide in family
		Good marital history
		Good work record

Adapted with permission from Osgood NJ: *Suicide in the Elderly.* Rockville, MD, Aspen, 1985.

severity of thinking disturbance is less pronounced than in young adults and flight of ideas is less common. Hypersexuality and grandiosity may be present but also tend to be less prominent in older adults. Manic-like syndromes in late life are distinguished by a greater likelihood of confusion, often a reflection of an underlying cognitive disturbance, such as an incipient dementia.

Several biological, physical, psychological, and sociological factors predispose older persons to depression (Table 7-2). Aging changes in the central nervous system, such as changes in neurotransmitter concentrations (especially catecholaminergic neurotransmitters), may play a role in the development of geriatric depression. Vascular depression, commonly seen in about 30% of stroke survivors (Blazer and Hybels, 2006), is linked to white-matter hyperintensities, which are bright regions seen in the brain parenchyma on T2-weighted magnetic resonance imaging (MRi). Inflammatory markers such as interleukin 6 (IL-6) have likewise been associated with depression (Kiecolt-Glaser et al., 2007), as has vitamin D deficiency (Wilkins et al., 2006). Other physical problems such as impaired vision (Evans, Fletcher, and Wormald, 2007) and chronic pain (Sawyer et al., 2007) and mild cognitive impairment (Han et al., 2006; Solfrizzi et al., 2007) are similarly associated with depression.

Losses, whether real or perceived, are common in the geriatric population and can be a contributory factor to depression (Windsor et al., 2007). Loss of job, income, and social supports (especially the death of family members and friends) increase with age and can result in social isolation and subsequent ongoing bereavement and frank depression. Loss of independence which occurs with the loss of a driving license or acute declines in function can further cause

TABLE 7-2   FACTORS PREDISPOSING OLDER PEOPLE TO DEPRESSION

Biological
    Family history (genetic predisposition)
    Prior episode(s) of depression
    Aging changes in neurotransmission
Physical
    Specific diseases (see Table 7-5)
    Chronic medical conditions (especially with pain or loss of function)
    Exposure to drugs (see Table 7-6)
    Sensory deprivation (loss of vision or hearing)
    Loss of physical function
Psychological
    Unresolved conflicts (eg, anger, guilt)
    Memory loss and dementia
    Personality disorders
Social
    Losses of family and friends (bereavement)
    Isolation
    Loss of job
    Loss of income

depression. Other psychosocial factors such as impaired spiritual well-being (Bekelman et al., 2007) and a perceived sense of unmet needs (Blazer, Sachs-Ericsson, and Hybels, 2007) have similarly been noted to contribute to depression.

SYMPTOMS AND SIGNS OF DEPRESSION

Major depression typically is diagnosed by evidence of depressed mood and/or loss of interest or pleasure. There may also be an associated appetite change, insomnia or hypersomnia, psychomotor agitation or retardation, loss of energy and fatigue, feelings of worthlessness, difficulties with concentration, and/or recurrent thoughts of death or suicide. In older depressed patients, it is more likely that they will present with a preoccupation with somatic and cognitive symptoms and less frequently report depressed mood and guilty preoccupations.

They may commonly report poor self-perception of health and complain repeatedly about constipation or urinary frequency. These individuals may not acknowledge sustained feelings of sadness. They will, however, report a persistent loss of pleasure and interest in previously enjoyable activities (anhedonia). Generally, older individuals do not exhibit the signs and symptoms of depressed mood that meet the criteria for a major depressive disorder.

Minor, or subsyndromal, depression is more common than major depression. It is defined as one or more periods of depressive symptoms that are identical to major depressive episodes in duration (2 weeks or longer) but that involves fewer symptoms and less impairment. An episode of subsyndromal depression involves either a sad/depressed mood or loss of interest/pleasure in nearly all activities.

The diagnosis of depression, whether major or minor, in older persons is complicated by the overlap of physical illness. Patients with serious medical illness may be preoccupied, for example, with thoughts about death or worthlessness because of concomitant disability. Older adults with depression also tend to have a higher rate of anxiety, nervousness, and irritability than their younger counterparts. They may engage in somatization and put themselves as at risk for iatrogenic disease that occur owing to unnecessary tests and treatments. As noted earlier, rigorous steps must be taken to exclude any possible cause of their symptoms prior to concluding that depression is the primary diagnosis. This workup must consider, however, the risks and benefits of any procedure or test for each individual.

Recognizing the signs and symptoms of depression and identifying depression disorders in older adults is complicated by many factors including

- The presence of common medical conditions (eg, Parkinson disease, congestive heart failure) which can result in the individual appearing depressed, even when depression is not present.
- Nonspecific physical symptoms (such as fatigue, weakness, anorexia, diffuse pain) which are commonly associated with comorbid conditions.
- Specific physical symptoms, relating to every major organ system, can represent depression as well as physical illness in geriatric patients.
- Depression can exacerbate symptoms of coexisting physical illnesses such as exacerbation of memory changes or pain associated with arthritis.

The physical appearance of older patients suspected of being depressed should be interpreted cautiously. Normal age changes such as pale, thin, wrinkled skin; loss of teeth; kyphosis; and a wide-based slow gait, alone or in addition to the presence of diseases such as anemia or Parkinson disease may make the older individual look depressed. Parkinson disease which manifests itself by masked facies, bradykinesia, and stooped posture can be misinterpreted as depression. Patients with sensory changes resulting in impaired vision and hearing may appear withdrawn and disinterested simply because they cannot see or hear you or others and therefore withdraw from social interactions. The psychomotor retardation of hypothyroidism may offer the physical appearance of depression. Systemic illnesses such as malignancy, dehydration, malnutrition, or chronic obstructive pulmonary disease can produce a depressed appearance with a flat affect or decreased energy. It is possible that the older individual will present with both medical problems and associated depression. In this scenario, it is critical that the medical management be optimized for each of the underlying problems, and the depression treated so that the quality of life and symptom management of the medical problems are optimized. Table 7-3 provides an overview of some common examples of somatic symptoms that may actually represent, or be exacerbated by, depression in older patients.

Insomnia

Older adults with mental health problems such as undiagnosed depression or anxiety may initially present with complaints of sleep disorders. Those with underlying shortness of breath, paroxysmal nocturnal dyspnea, anxiety and restlessness, and gastroesophageal reflux disease are likely to suffer from insomnia as these medical problems are exacerbated with a recumbent posture and may interfere with falling or staying asleep. Although it is one of the key symptoms in diagnosing different forms of depression, a variety of factors may underlie insomnia (Table 7-4). Insomnia can also be caused by the effects of (or withdrawal from) several medications or use of alcohol or late-night caffeine.

Older adults may complain of sleep problems caused by underlying physiological or psychological problems such as pain, anxiety, depression, shortness of breath, gastritis, or unrealistic sleep expectations (ie, belief in the need to sleep for a straight 8 h). In addition, there are a number of specific sleep disorders which are known to present more frequently in older individuals. Obstructive sleep apnea (OSA), which results in abnormal breathing, is the most common sleep-related problem. The development of OSA seems to be age dependent and male dominant. The incidence is also higher in those individuals who are obese and have enlarged neck circumferences. The risks associated with untreated OSA include nighttime hypoxia with associated risks for cardiac arrhythmias and myocardial and cerebral infarction. Specific signs such as loud snoring, which are often elicited from the bed partner, should prompt the provider to refer the older individual to a sleep center for further workup. Once diagnosed, the treatment for OSA includes continuous positive airway pressure, dental appliances, and uvulopalatopharyngoplasty. Another common sleep disorder that can cause insomnia is restless leg syndrome (RLS). The incidence of RLS increases to 20% of those 80 years of age or older (Barthlen, 2002). Patients with RLS have uncomfortable sensations in the lower extremities which they attempt to relieve by moving their legs during sleep, or rising and walking around. Managing restless legs is challenging but can be achieved with medications. Even without disease, aging is

TABLE 7-3   EXAMPLES OF PHYSICAL SYMPTOMS THAT CAN
             REPRESENT DEPRESSION

SYSTEM	SYMPTOM
General	Fatigue
	Weakness
	Anorexia
	Weight loss
	Anxiety
	Insomnia (see Table 7-4)
	"Pain all over"
	Apathy
Cardiopulmonary	Chest pain
	Shortness of breath
	Palpitations
	Dizziness
Gastrointestinal	Abdominal pain
	Constipation
	Diarrhea
Genitourinary	Frequency
	Urgency
	Incontinence
Musculoskeletal	Diffuse pain
	Back pain
Neurological	Headache
	Memory disturbance
	Dizziness
	Paresthesias

associated with changes in sleep patterns, such as daytime naps, early bedtime, increased time until onset of sleep, decreases in the absolute and relative amounts of the deeper stages of sleep, and increased periods of wakefulness, all of which contribute to the complaint of insomnia. Insomnia is a good example of how a primary symptom of depression must be evaluated to first determine that there is not an important and treatable underlying cause. It is important to avoid

TABLE 7-4   KEY FACTORS IN EVALUATING THE COMPLAINT OF
INSOMNIA

Sleep disturbance should be carefully characterized
   Delayed sleep onset
   Frequent awakenings
   Early morning awakenings

Physical symptoms can underlie insomnia (from patient and bed partner)
   Symptoms of physical illnesses
      Pain from musculoskeletal disorders
      Orthopnea, paroxysmal nocturnal dyspnea, or cough
      Nocturia
      Gastroesophageal reflux
   Symptoms suggestive of periodic leg movements
   Uncomfortable sensations in legs with a desire to move the legs
   Symptoms suggestive of sleep apnea
      Loud or irregular snoring
      Awakening sweating, anxious, tachycardiac
      Excessive movement
      Morning drowsiness

Aging changes occurring in sleep patterns
   Increased sleep latency
   Decreased time in deeper stages of sleep
   Increased awakenings

Behavioral factors can affect sleep patterns
   Daytime naps > 30 min
   Earlier bedtime
   Increased time spent in bed not sleeping

Medications can affect sleep
   Hypnotic withdrawal
   Caffeine
   Alcohol (causes sleep fragmentation)
   Certain antidepressants
   Diuretics
   Steroids

assuming or blaming the symptom on age or depression before a comprehensive medical workup has been completed.

DEPRESSION ASSOCIATED WITH MEDICAL CONDITIONS

Medical disorders that may imitate depression are particularly important to consider in elderly patients because of the increased vulnerability of this population to physical illnesses. Hyperthyroidism, for example, may present with apathy and diminished energy that mimics depression.

Symptoms and signs of depression are associated with medical conditions in the geriatric population as evidenced by the following:

- Some diseases can result in the physical appearance of depression, even when depression is not present (eg, Parkinson disease).
- Many diseases can either directly cause depression or elicit a reaction of depression. The latter is especially true of conditions that cause or produce fear of chronic pain, disability, and dependence.
- Drugs used to treat medical conditions can cause symptoms and signs of depression.
- The environment, such as entering a nursing home, can predispose to depression.

A wide variety of physical illnesses can present with or be accompanied by symptoms and signs of depression (Table 7-5). Any medical condition associated with systemic involvement and metabolic disturbances can have profound effects on mental function and affect. The most common among these are fever, dehydration, decreased cardiac output, electrolyte disturbances, and hypoxia. Hyponatremia (whether from disease process or drugs) and hypercalcemia (associated with malignancy) may also cause older patients to appear depressed. Systemic diseases, especially malignancies and endocrine disorders such as diabetes, are often associated with symptoms of depression. Depression— accompanied by anorexia, weight loss, and back pain—is commonly present in patients with cancer of the pancreas. Among the endocrine disorders, thyroid and parathyroid conditions are most commonly accompanied by symptoms of depression. Most hypothyroid patients manifest psychomotor retardation, irritability, or depression. Hyperthyroidism may also present as withdrawal and depression in older patients—so-called apathetic thyrotoxicosis. Hyperparathyroidism with attendant hypercalcemia can simulate depression and is often manifest by apathy, fatigue, bone pain, and constipation. Other systemic physical conditions, such as infectious diseases, anemia, and nutritional deficiencies, can also have prominent manifestations of depression in the geriatric population.

TABLE 7-5   MEDICAL ILLNESSES ASSOCIATED WITH DEPRESSION

Metabolic disturbances
  Dehydration
  Azotemia, uremia
  Acid–base disturbances
  Hypoxia
  Hypo- and hypernatremia
  Hypo- and hyperglycemia
  Hypo- and hypercalcemia
Endocrine
  Hypo- and hyperthyroidism
  Hyperparathyroidism
  Diabetes mellitus
  Cushing disease
  Addison disease
Infections
Cardiovascular
  Congestive heart failure
  Myocardial infarction
Pulmonary
  Chronic obstructive lung disease
  Malignancy
Gastrointestinal
  Malignancy (especially pancreatic)
  Irritable bowel
Genitourinary
  Urinary incontinence
Musculoskeletal
  Degenerative arthritis
  Osteoporosis with vertebral compression or hip fracture
  Polymyalgia rheumatica
  Paget disease
Neurologic
  Dementia (all types)
  Parkinson disease
  Stroke
  Tumors
Other
  Anemia (of any cause)
  Vitamin deficiencies
  Hematologic or other systemic malignancy

Adapted with permission from Levenson AJ, Hall RCW (eds): *Neuropsychiatric Manifestations of Physical Disease in the Elderly.* New York, Raven Press, 1981.

Because cardiovascular and nervous system diseases are among the most threatening and potentially disabling, they can precipitate symptoms of depression. Myocardial infarction, with attendant fear of shortened life span and restricted lifestyle, commonly precipitates depression. Stroke is often accompanied by depression, although the depression may not always correlate with the extent of physical disability. Patients in whom stroke has produced substantial disability (eg, hemiparesis, aphasia) can become depressed in response to their loss of function; others post stroke may become depressed because of vascular depression (Blazer and Hybels, 2006). Other causes of brain damage, especially in the frontal lobes, such as tumors and subdural hematomas, can likewise be associated with depression. Older individuals with dementia, both Alzheimer and multi-infarct dementia, may have prominent symptoms of depression (see Chap. 6). Patients with Parkinson disease also have a high incidence of clinically diagnosed depression.

Symptoms of depression associated with medical problems may simply be a response to the disease. For example, hospitalizations associated with medical illnesses can result in feelings of isolation, sensory deprivation, and immobilization and contribute or cause depressive symptoms. Likewise, iatrogenic complications such as constipation and fecal impaction, a urinary tract infection or urinary retention that causes new-onset incontinence can also cause depression. Drugs are the most common cause of treatment-induced depression. Although a wide variety of pharmacologic agents can produce symptoms of depression (Table 7-6), antihypertensive agents, antilipids, antiepilepsy medications, selective estrogen receptor modulators, H_2-receptor antagonists, corticosteroids, and in some cases, nonsteroidal anti-inflammatory agents, and sedative-hypnotics are the most common groups of drugs that cause depression among older adults (Kotlyar, Dysken, and Adson, 2005). The true impact of medications on the development depression is inconsistent, however, and it has been projected that there may be genetic differences among individuals that impact the side effects of these medications (Kotlyar, Dysken, and Adson, 2005). Given the individual impact of medication, whenever possible, drugs that can potentially exacerbate depression should be discontinued.

DIAGNOSING DEPRESSION

The interrelationship between depression and its signs and symptoms, medical illnesses, and treatment effects make diagnosing depression particularly challenging. The following are some general guidelines to help with the differential diagnosis between depression and other causes of the associated signs and symptoms reported by older adults:

- Screening tools (eg, Geriatric Depression Scale) that screen for depressive symptoms may be helpful in identifying depressed geriatric patients. However, somatic components of many depression scales are less useful in

TABLE 7-6   DRUGS THAT CAN CAUSE SYMPTOMS OF DEPRESSION

Antihypertensives	Meprobamate
Angiotensin-converting enzyme	Antipsychotics
inhibitors	Chlorpromazine
Calcium channel blockers (verapamil)	Haloperidol
Clonidine	Thiothixene
Hydralazine	Hypnotics
β-Blockers (eg, propranolol)	Chloral hydrate
Reserpine	Benzodiazepines
Analgesics	Steroids
Narcotics	Corticosteroids
Antiparkinsonism drugs	Estrogens
Levodopa	Anticonvulsants
Bromocriptine	Celontin
Antimicrobials	Zarontin
Sulfonamides	Antiviral
Isoniazid	Zovirax
Cardiovascular preparations	Antibiotics
Digitalis	Ciprofloxacin
Diuretics	Statins
Lidocaine	Pravachol
Hypoglycemic agents	Others
Psychotropic agents	Alcohol
Sedatives	Cancer chemotherapeutic
Barbiturates	agents
Benzodiazepines	Cimetidine

Adapted with permission from Levenson AJ, Hall RCW (eds): *Neuropsychiatric Manifestations of Physical Disease in the Elderly.* New York, Raven Press, 1981; Medical Letter: Drugs that may cause phychiatric symptoms. *Med Lett.* 44(1134):59-62,2002.

older patients because of the high prevalence of physical symptoms and medical illnesses.

- Nonspecific or multiple somatic symptoms that are suggestive of depression should not be diagnosed as such until physical illnesses have been excluded.
- Somatic symptoms unexplained by physical findings or diagnostic studies, especially those of relatively sudden onset in an older person who is not usually hypochondriacal, should raise the suspicion of depression.

- Drugs used to treat medical illnesses (see Table 7-6), sedative-hypnotics, and alcohol abuse should be considered as potential causes for symptoms and signs of depression.
- Standard diagnostic criteria should be the basis for diagnosing various forms of depression in the geriatric population, but several differences may distinguish depression in older, as opposed to younger, patients.
- Major depressive episodes should be differentiated from other diagnoses such as uncomplicated bereavement, bipolar disorder, dysthymic disorder, minor depression, and adjustment disorders with a depressed mood.
- Consultation with experienced geriatric psychiatrists, psychologists, or psychiatric nurse practitioners should be obtained whenever possible to help diagnose and manage depressive disorders.
- Whenever there is uncertainty about the diagnosis, or while medical workup is being initiated, the depression and associated symptoms should be treated with a judicious (but adequate) therapeutic trial of an antidepressant.

Several differences in the presentation of depression can make the diagnosis much more challenging and difficult in older people, as compared to younger people (Table 7-7). The most common clinical problem is differentiating major depressive episodes from other forms of depression. Table 7-8 outlines the criteria for major depression based on the *Diagnostic and Statistical Manual of Mental Disorders* (DSM-IV) (American Psychiatric Association, 1994). The DSM-IV criteria require that the depressive symptoms are not a direct effect of a general medical condition or medication and that patients have at least one core symptom (depressed mood or loss of interest or

TABLE 7-7 SOME DIFFERENCES IN THE PRESENTATION OF DEPRESSION IN THE OLDER POPULATION, AS COMPARED WITH THE YOUNGER POPULATION

1. Somatic complaints, rather than psychological symptoms, often predominate in the clinical picture
2. Older patients often deny having a dysphoric mood
3. Apathy and withdrawal are common
4. Feelings of guilt are less common
5. Loss of self-esteem is prominent
6. Inability to concentrate with resultant impairment of memory and other cognitive functions is common (see Chap. 6)

TABLE 7-8   SUMMARY CRITERIA FOR MAJOR DEPRESSIVE EPISODE*

A. Five (or more) of the following symptoms have been present nearly every day during the same 2-week period and represent a change from previous functioning; at least one is either (1) depressed mood or (2) loss of interest or pleasure. Symptoms that are clearly caused by a general medical condition should not be counted

   (1) Depressed mood most of the day*
   (2) Markedly diminished interest or pleasure in all, or almost all, activities most of the day†
   (3) Significant weight loss when not dieting or weight gain, or decrease or increase in appetite
   (4) Insomnia or hypersomnia
   (5) Psychomotor agitation or retardation
   (6) Fatigue or loss of energy
   (7) Feelings of worthlessness or excessive or inappropriate guilt (which may be delusional)
   (8) Diminished ability to think or concentrate, or indecisiveness
   (9) Recurrent thoughts of death (not just fear of dying), recurrent suicidal ideation without a specific plan, or a suicide attempt or a specific plan for committing suicide

The symptoms

B. Do not meet criteria for a mixed episode.

C. Cause clinically significant stress or impairment in social, occupational, or other important areas of functioning

D. Are not due to the direct physiological effects of a substance or a general medical condition

E. Are not better accounted for by bereavement; the symptoms persist for longer than 2 months or are characterized by marked functional impairment, morbid preoccupation with worthlessness, suicidal ideation, psychotic symptoms, or psychomotor retardation

*Core symptom: For a diagnosis of major depression, the individual must have at least one core symptom and that five or more symptoms have occurred nearly every day for most of the day for at least 2 weeks. The symptoms must be causing significant distress or impaired functioning and must not be due to a direct physiologic cause.
Data from the American Psychiatric Association. Diagnostic and Statistical Manual of Mental Disorders. 4th ed. Washington, DC: American Psychiatric Association; 1994.

pleasure) and that five or more symptoms have occurred nearly every day for most of the day for at least 2 weeks. The symptoms must be causing significant distress or impaired functioning. DSM-V is currently under development and consideration for the addition of laboratory values is in process. Table 7-9 lists some of the key features that can aid in distinguishing major depression from other conditions.

There are several valid and reliable measures to screen older adults for depression. Table 7-10 provides a listing of these measures. Most commonly used is the Geriatric Depression Scale which is available in a longer 30-item measure, a 15-item and a 5-item measure, and has even been tested as a single item tool. It is particularly important to differentiate between depression and dementia in many patients and screening tools can help guide that process. Several resources, such as the Mental Health Toolkit (National Conference of Gerontological Nurse Practitioners, 2007) provide a stepped approach to this process. In addition, screening tools for depression have been specifically developed for individuals with comorbid conditions. The Cornell Depression Scale (Alexopoulos et al., 1988) was developed to screen for depression in older adults with dementia. The Stroke Aphasic Depression Questionnaire, Signs of Depression Scale, and the Visual Analogue Mood Scale have all been used to assess for depression in older adults with stroke (Bennett et al., 2007). For the primary care setting, the Primary Care Evaluation of Mental Disorders (PRIME-MD) (Spitzer, Williams, and Kroenke, 1994) was developed. This measure consists of five questions that address the diagnostic categories of the DSM-IV. Given the high prevalence of depression, and the risk for missing a diagnosis, screening should be incorporated into all routine examinations.

Because of the overlap of symptoms and signs of depression and physical illness and the close association between many medical conditions and depression, older patients presenting with what appears to be a depression should have physical illnesses carefully excluded. This is important as well to develop trust with the patient and their family, and assure these individuals that a comprehensive evaluation of the symptoms has been done. This evaluation can usually be accomplished by a thorough history, physical examination, and basic laboratory studies (Table 7-11). Complains of fatigue, for example, could be explored by checking the thyroid-stimulating hormone (TSH) level. Sometimes the assurance that there are no acute medical problems will help the individual recognize that the symptoms may be caused by mood and the focused depression treatment can be initiated. Other diagnostic studies can provide helpful objective data, in particularly difficult to distinguish persistent somatic symptoms/complains such as shortness of breath or fatigue. For example, echocardiography (ECG) and radionuclide cardiac scans can help rule out organic heart disease as a basis for these symptoms.

TABLE 7-9   MAJOR DEPRESSION VERSUS OTHER FORMS OF
              DEPRESSION

DIAGNOSTIC CLASSIFICATION	KEY FEATURES DISTINGUISHING FROM MAJOR DEPRESSION
Bipolar disorder	The patient may meet, or have met in the past, criteria for major depression but is having or has had one or more manic episode; the latter are characterized by distinct periods of a relatively persistent elevated or irritable mood and other symptoms such as increased activity, restlessness, talkativeness, flight of ideas, inflated self-esteem, and distractibility
Cyclothymic disorder	There are numerous periods during which symptoms of depression and mania are present but not of sufficient severity or duration to meet the criteria for a major depressive or manic episode; in addition to a loss of interest and pleasure in most activities, the periods of depression are accompanied by other symptoms such as fatigue, insomnia or hypersomnia, social withdrawal, pessimism, and tearfulness
Dysthymic disorder	Patient usually exhibits a prominently depressed mood, marked loss of interest or pleasure in most activities, and other symptoms of depression; the symptoms are not of sufficient severity or duration to meet the criteria for a major depressive episode, and the periods of depression may be separated by up to a few months of normal mood
Adjustment disorder with depressed mood	The patient exhibits a depressed mood, tearfulness, hopelessness, or other symptoms in excess of a normal response to an identifiable psychosocial or physical stressor; the response is not an exacerbation of another psychiatric condition, occurs within 3 months of the

TABLE 7-9   MAJOR DEPRESSION VERSUS OTHER FORMS OF
DEPRESSION (*Continued*)

DIAGNOSTIC CLASSIFICATION	KEY FEATURES DISTINGUISHING FROM MAJOR DEPRESSION
	onset of the stressor, eventually remits after the stressor ceases (or the patient adapts to the stressor), and does not meet the criteria for other forms of depression or uncomplicated bereavement
Uncomplicated bereavement	This is a depressive syndrome that arises in response to the death of a loved one—its onset is not more than 2-3 months after the death, and the symptoms last for variable periods of time; the patient generally regards the depression as a normal response—guilt and thoughts of death refer directly to the loved one; morbid preoccupation with worthlessness, marked or prolonged functional impairment, and marked psychomotor retardation are uncommon and suggest the development of major depression

TABLE 7-10   EXAMPLES OF SCREENING TOOLS FOR DEPRESSION

1. Centers for Epidemiological Studies Depression Scale
   (http://patienteducation.stanford.edu/research/cesd.pdf)
2. Geriatric Depression Scale
   (http://www.stanford.edu/~yesavage/GDS.html)
3. Beck Depression Scale
   (http://www.fpnotebook.com/Psych/Exam/BckDprsnInvntry.htm)
4. Cornell Scale for Depression in Dementia (http://www.
   thedoctorwillseeyounow.com/articles/behavior/depressn_12/)

TABLE 7-11   DIAGNOSTIC STUDIES HELPFUL IN EVALUATING DEPRESSED GERIATRIC PATIENTS WITH SOMATIC SYMPTOMS

BASIC EVALUATION
History
Physical examination
Complete blood count
Erythrocyte sedimentation rate
Serum electrolytes, glucose, and calcium
Renal function tests
Liver function tests
Thyroid function tests
Calcium and vitamin D
Serum B_{12} or methylmalonic acid
Folate
Syphilis serology
Urinalysis

EXAMPLES OF OTHER POTENTIALLY HELPFUL STUDIES	
SYMPTOM OR SIGN	DIAGNOSTIC STUDY
Pain	Evaluation for underlying cause (eg, appropriate radiologic procedure such as bone film, bone scan, GI series)
Chest pain	ECG, noninvasive cardiovascular studies (eg, exercise stress test, echocardiography, radionuclide scans)
Shortness of breath	Chest films, pulmonary function tests, pulse oximetry arterial blood gases
Constipation	Test for occult blood in stool, colonoscopy, abdominal x-ray, thyroid function tests
Focal neurological signs or symptoms	CT or MRI scan, EEG

CT, computed tomography; ECG, electrocardiography; EEG, electroencephalography; GI, gastrointestinal; MRI, magnetic resonance imaging.

MANAGEMENT

General Considerations

Several treatment modalities are available to manage depression in older persons (Table 7-12). Pharmacological and behavioral interventions and psychotherapy have some effectiveness in mild to moderate depression in the outpatient geriatric population (Brenes GA et al., 2007; Skultety and Zeiss, 2006). A recent Cochrane review on pharmacological management of depression concluded that selective serotonin reuptake inhibitors (SSRIs) and tricyclic antidepressants (TCAs) are equally effective (Mottram, Wilson, and Strobl, 2006). There are, however, more side effects and risks associated with use of TCAs when compared to SSRIs. Behavioral interventions such as the use of exercise and cognitive behavioral therapy have been noted to be effective. Most recently, the successful treatment of depression has focused on the use of interdisciplinary treatment models. Programs such as (Burns et al., 2000; Unutzer et al. 2002) Improving Mood Promoting Access to Collaborative Treatment (IMPACT) which used a stepped care model in the primary care setting have been noted to successfully manage depression in older adults. A depression clinical specialist guided the patient through the steps of treatment which combined behavioral interventions with drug management. The choice of treatment(s) for an individual patient depends on many factors, including the primary disorder causing the depression, the severity of symptoms, the availability and practicality of the various treatment modalities, and underlying conditions that might contraindicate a specific form of treatment (eg, cognitive issues that may make psychotherapy more difficult, underlying medical problems that increase the risk of medication management).

The first step in any treatment approach is to remove the underlying cause of depression, whether this is medical or situational. For example, if a specific pharmacological treatment is being given that may cause depression, attempts should be made to remove this agent. While difficult to achieve, strategies to alleviate multiple losses (such as death of loved ones and pets or change in living locations) can be considered. Likewise attempts to resolve acute illness, or exacerbations of chronic illness, are needed to assure that the individual is at his or her optimal state of health. These interventions should be implemented before other therapies are initiated unless the depression is severe enough to warrant immediate treatment (eg, the patient is delusional or suicidal).

The course of treatment for depression, particularly major depression, should proceed as follows: acute treatment to reverse the current episode, continuation of treatment to prevent relapse, and maintenance treatment to prevent recurrence.

TABLE 7-12   EVIDENCE-BASED TREATMENT MODALITIES FOR DEPRESSION

Treatment	Evidence Level	Description of the Intervention	Reference (Selected Examples)
Cognitive behavior therapy	A	Active time limited therapy that aims to change the thinking and behavior of individuals that influences their depression. Effective when compared to no treatment	(Conradi et al., 2007) (Unutzer et al., 2002)
Medication	A	Tricyclic antidepressants Selective serotonin reuptake inhibitors Monoamine oxidase inhibitors can all effectively treat depression	(Wilson et al., 2001) (Mittmann et al., 1997)
Hormone therapy	C	Estrogen use in females given as a patch, cream, injection, implant or suppository Was effective only in women post hysterectomy	(Carranza-Lira et al., 2002)
		Use of testosterone in men orally, by injection, as skin patches or as a gel Single group study showed decrease in depression among a small group of older men	(Perry, Uates, and Williams, 2002)
Exercise	B	Two main types of exercise: aerobic activity such as running or brisk walking and resistance training focused on muscle strengthening activity	(Singh, Clements, and Singh, 2001) (Penninx et al., 2002) (McNeil, LeBlanc, and Joyner, 1991)

TABLE 7-12 EVIDENCE-BASED TREATMENT MODALITIES FOR DEPRESSION (*Continued*)

TREATMENT	EVIDENCE LEVEL	DESCRIPTION OF THE INTERVENTION	REFERENCE (SELECTED EXAMPLES)
		Aerobic activity was found to be more effective than education in lowering depression scores	
		Resistance exercise alone has been less effective	
ECT	A	Involves delivering a brief electric current to the brain to produce a cerebral seizure	(van der Wurff FB, 2003, 56; van der Wurff FB et al., 2003, 57)
		ECT was better than placebo (sham ECT)	
St John's wort	B	Herb available as a table, capsule, or liquid forms	(Anghelescu et al., 2006)
		Reduces symptoms equally when compared to antidepressants, although the effectiveness may only be short term	(Kasper et al., 2006)

A, supported by one or more high quality randomized trials; B, supported by one or more high-quality nonrandomized cohort studies or low-quality RCTs; C, supported by one or more case series and/or poor quality cohort and/or case-control studies; D, supported by expert opinion and/or extrapolation from studies in other populations or settings; X, evidence supports the treatment being ineffective or harmful.
There is insufficient evidence to support multiple herbal remedies (with the exception of St. John's wort), acupuncture, music therapy, or vitamins.
ECT, electroconvulsive therapy; RCT, randomized controlled trials.

Continuation treatment to stabilize the recovery involves ongoing antidepressant therapy for an additional 6 months. Maintenance treatment (≥ 3 years) is provided to patients with a history of recurrent depression. The duration of maintenance therapy should be based on the individual's prior history of recurrent episodes. Psychotherapy and other behavioral interventions, antidepressant medications, and electroconvulsive therapy (ECT) are all empirically proven treatments for depression in older persons (Table 7-12).

Nonpharmacological Management

Psychotherapy   Cognitive behavior therapy (CBT) is one of the most commonly used therapies for older adults with dementia. CBT proposed that the symptoms of anxiety and depression are caused by inaccurate thoughts and maladaptive behaviors. The goal of CBT is to help the individuals change these thoughts and behavior. CBT techniques can be implemented into the primary care visit by all health-care providers (Kraus, Kunik, and Stanley, 2007). As shown in Table 7-12, numerous other types of therapeutic interventions can be provided. Problem-solving therapy involves working with the patient to identify practical life difficulties that are causing distress and providing guidance to help the patient identify solutions. The treatment is delivered generally in six to eight meetings spaced 1 to 2 weeks apart. Cognitive and interpersonal psychotherapy are also time limited but less highly structured. Psychotherapy for minor depression has been promising, with efficacy demonstrated particularly in persons who have suffered a loss. Also, caregivers of older persons may develop minor or major depressive syndromes that benefit from psychotherapy. Psychotherapy may be combined with an antidepressant, and the combination has been associated with a longer period of remission following recovery from the acute episode. Psychotherapy combined with antidepressant medication is recommended for all patients with severe or suicidal depression.

Exercise   Multiple intervention studies have demonstrated that exercise interventions and ongoing physical activity can improve depression in older adults (Brenes et al., 2007; Sims et al., 2006). These studies have used aerobic activities to effectively decrease depression in individuals who did not respond to medication alone and when compared to medication alone. Currently the Treatment with Exercise Augmentation for Depression (TREAD) study, a National Institute of Mental Health (NIMH)-funded, randomized controlled trial (RCT) is being implemented to assess the relative efficacy of two doses of aerobic exercise to augment SSRI treatment of major depression. The advantage of exercise in the treatment of depression among older adults is that they will be likely to increase their physical and functional health which may also improve mood.

Pharmacological Treatment

When symptoms and signs of depression are of sufficient severity and duration to meet the criteria for major depression (see Table 7-8), if the depression is producing marked functional disability, interfering with recovery from other illnesses (eg, not participating in rehabilitation services), or when the patient is not responding to nonpharmacological interventions alone, drug treatment should be considered.

The choice of agent depends on the patient's comorbid medical conditions, the side effect profile of the antidepressant, and the individual patient's sensitivity to these effects. Potential interactions with other medications and prior use of antidepressant medications also should be considered. Current complaints of sleep disturbance, anxiety, poor appetite or weight changes, or psychomotor retardation help to further direct the practitioner's choice of a therapeutic agent. For individuals who do not sleep well, for example, a drug that is more sedating would be appropriate. Providers may find it helpful to use a staged approach to drug initiation and management (Steffens, McQuoid, and Krishnan, 2002).

SSRIs and TCAs are comparably effective for treating mild to moderate major depression, but SSRIs are often better tolerated. Citalopram, mirtazapine, bupropion, escitalopram, paroxetine, sertraline, venlafaxine, and duloxetine have been described as preferred agents for older adults based on efficacy and side effect profiles. Table 7-13 provides a detailed summary of dosing, formulations, precautions, and advantages of the individual SSRIs. Although the SSRIs are generally free of severe side effects, a small proportion of elderly patients develop hyponatremia because of the syndrome of inappropriate antidiuretic hormone secretion and some experience anxiety, sleep disturbance, or agitation. Sexual side effects and weight gain or loss occur commonly with all SSRIs and may be a reason for poor treatment adherence.

SSRIs inhibit the hepatic isoenzyme *CYP2D6*, which can interfere with the oxidative metabolism of many drugs. The most frequent interactions involving the *CYP2D6* system involve fluoxetine and fluvoxamine, whereas drug interactions are less common with citalopram. SSRIs may increase the anticoagulant effects of medications such as warfarin, potentially through cytochrome isoenzyme inhibition or the inhibition of platelet activity. Careful monitoring of blood clotting is indicated following the introduction of an SSRI to patients being treated with warfarin. Fluoxetine causes substantial inhibition of *CYP2C19* and consequently inhibits the metabolism of alprazolam, quinidine, calcium channel blockers, TCAs, and carbamazepine via the cytochrome P-450 (CYP) 3A4 subsystem.

Serotonin syndrome is a potentially life-threatening adverse reaction to use of SSRIs. Symptoms include mental status changes, agitation, myoclonus, hyperreflexia, tachycardia, sweating, shivering, tremor, diarrhea, lack of coordination, fever, and even death. The risk of serotonin syndrome is increased in individuals

TABLE 7-13   ANTIDEPRESSANTS FOR GERIATRIC PATIENTS

DRUG GROUP GENERIC NAME (BRAND NAME)	DRUG GROUP SIDE EFFECTS	SPECIAL CONCERNS WITH OLDER ADULTS
TRICYCLIC ANTIDEPRESSANTS		
Amitriptyline (Elavil)	Dry mouth	These drugs are best avoided because of the side effects
Amoxapine (Asendin)	Blurred vision	Amoxapine can cause extrapyramidal effects
Clomipramine (Anafranil)	Constipation	
Desipramine (Norpramin or Pertofrane)	Difficulty urinating	
Doxepin (Sinequan or Adapin)	Increased heart rate	
Imipramine (Tofranil)	Loss of sex drive and erectile failure	
Maprotiline (Ludiomil)	Increased sensitivity to the sun	
Nortriptyline (Pamelor or Aventyl)	Weight gain	
Protriptyline (Vivactil)	Drowsiness	
Trimipramine (Surmontil)	Dizziness and nausea	
MAOIs		
Phenelzine (Nardil)	Light-headedness upon standing	All foods and drinks containing tyramine must be avoided or the patient may experience a hypertensive crisis, stroke or, myocardial infarction
Tranylcypromine (Parnate)	Dizziness	
Isocarboxazid (Marplan)	Insomnia	
Selegiline (Emsam)	Weight gain	

TABLE 4-13 ANTIDEPRESSANTS FOR GERIATRIC PATIENTS (*Continued*)

DRUG GROUP GENERIC NAME (BRAND NAME)	DRUG GROUP SIDE EFFECTS	SPECIAL CONCERNS WITH OLDER ADULTS
	Headaches Insomnia Sexual problems such as impotence Sleepiness	
SSRIs Fluoxetine (Prozac) Fluvoxamine (Luvox) Sertraline (Zoloft) Paroxetine (Paxil) Escitalopram (Lexapro) Citalopram (Celexa) Duloxetine (Cymbalta) Mirtazapine (Remeron)	Nausea Insomnia Anxiety and restlessness Decreased sex drive Dizziness Weight gain or weight loss Tremors Sweating Drowsiness or fatigue Dry mouth Diarrhea or constipation Headaches Nausea Nervousness	SSRIs can cause an increase in suicidal thoughts and behaviors SSRIs also carry a risk for increased hostility, agitation, and anxiety SSRIs should not be taken at the same time as MAOIs Taking an SSRI within 2 weeks of an MAOI can cause a fatal reaction In adults 65 and older, SSRIs increase the risk for falls, fractures, and bone loss Mirtazapine cause significant sedation and weight gain so is effective for those with sleep disorders and weight loss

Atypical Antidepressants

Bupropion (Wellbutrin)	Sexual dysfunction	Venlafaxine should not be used in
Trazodone (Desyrel)	Dry mouth	those with hypertension
Venlafaxine (Effexor)	Fatigue	Duloxetine may be effective in those
Nefazodone (Serzone)	Sleepiness	suffering from both depression and
	Weight gain	pain
	Blurred vision	Nefazodone may cause hepatotoxicity

MAOIs, monoamine oxidase inhibitors; SSRIs, selective serotonin reuptake inhibitors.

with deficits in peripheral 5-HT metabolism from cardiovascular, liver, or pulmonary diseases; or tobacco use; or when SSRIs are used with nefazodone, venlafaxine, mirtazapine, and monamine oxide inhibitors, TCAs, SSRIs, meperidine, opioids, St. John's wort, or tramadol. Following the discontinuation of an SSRI there have been reports of a serotonergic withdrawal syndrome. This may last for 2 to 3 weeks and is characterized by light-headedness, insomnia, agitation, nausea, headache, and sensory disturbances. Mood disturbance may also occur. The shorter-acting SSRIs (sertraline, paroxetine) appear to induce this syndrome, but venlafaxine and other SSRIs have also been implicated. Therefore, these agents should be tapered rather than stopped abruptly.

Tricyclic Antidepressants   The TCAs nortriptyline and desipramine are the most appropriate for use in older persons. Table 7-13 provides a detailed summary of drug names, side effects, and special issues concerning usage in older adults. They are effective but are associated with anticholinergic side effects and have a quinidine-like effect that delays ventricular conduction. For nortriptyline, therapeutic response is associated with blood levels between 50 and 150 ng/mL and for desipramine, levels above 120 ng/mL. Over 60% of patients with non-psychotic major depression or with depression that is not associated with dementia respond within 6 weeks to levels in these ranges. Although 5% of the population requires lower dosing because of the absence of the enzyme required to metabolize secondary amine tricyclics, most patients achieve target concentrations at dosages of 50 to 75 mg/day of nortriptyline and 100 to 150 mg/day of desipramine.

Other Antidepressants   Table 7-14 provides a detailed summary of dosing, formulations, precautions, and advantages of other pharmacological agents used to treat depression. Bupropion is generally safe, free of sexual side effects, and well tolerated when used at recommended doses. Bupropion can be activating in some individuals and has been associated with a 0.4% risk of seizures, which is much higher when recommended doses are exceeded. Bupropion, therefore, is contraindicated in persons with a seizure disorder. Bupropion appears to act by increasing the activity of dopamine and norepinephrine and therefore has stimulant-like qualities. Venlafaxine acts as an SSRI at lower doses while also inhibiting the reuptake of norepinephrine at the high end of the therapeutic range of 75 to 225 mg/day. Venlafaxine is effective for both generalized anxiety and major depression. Blood pressure should be monitored in individuals receiving high dosages of this drug. Patients requiring doses at the high end of the therapeutic range should have blood-pressure monitoring. Venlafaxine should be discontinued by gradual tapering to avoid the risk of flu-like discontinuation symptoms.

TABLE 7-14   CHARACTERISTICS OF SELECTED ANTIDEPRESSANTS FOR GERIATRIC PATIENTS

DRUG*	RECOMMENDED STARTING DAILY DOSAGE	DAILY DOSAGE RANGE	LEVEL OF SEDATION	ELIMINATION HALF-LIFE[†]	COMMENTS
SELECTIVE SEROTONIN REUPTAKE INHIBITORS					
Citalopram (Celexa)	10-20 mg	20-30 mg	Very low	Very long	Less inhibition of hepatic cytochrome P-450 May cause somnolence, insomnia, anorexia
Escitalopram (Lexapro)	10 mg	10 mg	Very low	Very long	Side effects as for citalopram
Fluoxetine (Prozac)	5-10 mg	20-60 mg	Very low	Very long	Inhibits hepatic cytochrome P-450[‡] Must be discontinued 6 weeks before initiating monamine oxidase inhibitor
Paroxetine (Paxil)	10 mg	10-50 mg	Very low	Long	Inhibits hepatic cytochrome P-450[‡] Has anticholinergic side effects
Sertraline (Zoloft)	25 mg	50-200 mg	Very low	Very long	Less inhibition of cytochrome P-450
SEROTONIN–NOREPINEPHRINE REUPTAKE BLOCKERS					
Venlafaxine (Effexor)	25 mg	75-225 mg	Very low	Intermediate	Reduced clearance with renal or hepatic impairment

TABLE 7-14 CHARACTERISTICS OF SELECTED ANTIDEPRESSANTS FOR GERIATRIC PATIENTS (*Continued*)

DRUG*	RECOMMENDED STARTING DAILY DOSAGE	DAILY DOSAGE RANGE	LEVEL OF SEDATION	ELIMINATION HALF-LIFE [†]	COMMENTS
					Can cause dose-related hypertension Must be tapered over 1-2 weeks when discontinuing
TRICYCLIC ANTIDEPRESSANTS					
Nortriptyline (Pamelor, others)	10-30 mg	25-150 mg	Mild	Long	Lower but still substantial anti-cholinergic effects [§] Blood levels can be monitored
OTHER AGENTS [†]					
Bupropion (Wellbutrin)	50-100 mg	150-450 mg	Mild	Intermediate	Divided doses necessary
Mirtazapine (Remeron)	15 mg	15-45 mg	Mild	Long	Reduced clearance with renal impairment May cause or exacerbate hypertension

| Nefazodone (Serzone) | 100 mg | 200-400 mg | Mild | Short | Potent inhibitor of cytochrome P-450 ‡
Can increase concentrations of terfenadine, astemizole, and cisapride
Has antianxiety effects |
| Trazodone (Desyrel) | 25-50 mg | 75-400 mg | Moderate–high | Short | Can cause hypotension
May be useful in low doses as a hypnotic |

* Other less commonly used antidepressants are discussed in the text.
† Short = <8 h; intermediate = 8-20 h; long = 20-30 h; very long = >30 h. Half-lives may vary in older patients and some drugs have active metabolites.
‡ See text for drug interactions.
§ See text for anticholinergic side effects.

Duloxetine is a newer antidepressant medication that has been approved for the treatment of both depression and neuropathic pain secondary to diabetes mellitus. Duloxetine is a serotonin- and norepinephrine-reuptake inhibitor, and its pharmacodynamic characteristics are generally like those of venlafaxine, although it is structurally unique. Because of its effects of increasing neural sphincter activity and bladder capacity, it has also been approved for the treatment of urinary incontinence and has been shown to reduce stress incontinence in women. These features may make duloxetine advantageous for the older patient.

Mirtazapine is a norepinephrine, 5-HT$_2$, and 5-HT$_3$ antagonist, and consistently has the side effects of sedation and weight gain. Therefore, this drug is often used to treat depression while managing associated symptoms. The monoamine oxidase inhibitors (MAOIs) are an older group of antidepressants that have significant side effects such as orthostatic hypotension and require careful food restriction of those foods with tyramine (eg, cheese), and avoidance of pseudoephedrine or pressor amines as these can cause a life-threatening hypertensive crisis. The use of MAOIs with an SSRI or meperidine can cause a fatal serotonin syndrome associated with delirium and hyperthermia. Methylphenidate and other stimulants have been used to treat major depression in older adults. There is limited evidence to support the effectiveness of this treatment and generally use is on a case by case basis.

Electroconvulsive Shock Treatment   Although generally reserved for individuals with severe depression, electroconvulsive shock treatment (ECT) has been shown to be effective for decreasing symptoms of depression in older adults (Frazer, Christensen, and Griffiths, 2005). ECT involves delivering a brief electric current to the brain to produce a cerebral seizure. Potential side effects of ECT, however, are a major drawback. These include possible memory changes with associated confusion, cardiovascular problems, and increased risk of falls as well as the risks associated with general anesthesia.

Management of Bipolar Disorders   Most persons with bipolar disorders have a history of episodes in early adulthood and often receive chronic treatment with antimanic medication. Occasionally this regimen may need adjustment if a new episode of mania emerges. In a comprehensive review of interventions to treat bipolar disorders in the elderly, it was noted that treatment with lithium, divalproex sodium, carbamazepine, lamotrigine, atypical antipsychotics, and antidepressants has been found to be beneficial. Although there are no specific guidelines for the treatment of these patients, monotherapy followed by combination therapy of the various classes of drugs may help with the resolution of symptoms. ECT and psychotherapy may be useful in the treatment of refractory disease.

SUMMARY EVIDENCE-BASED RECOMMENDATIONS FOR DEPRESSION INTERVENTIONS

DO'S

- Individual cognitive behavioral therapy
- Depression care management with medications either in the home or clinic setting

DON'T DO

- Physical rehabilitation and occupational therapy
- Nutrition interventions
- Peer support

CONSIDER

- Individual therapy other than cognitive behavioral therapy
- Group psychotherapy there was not evidence to support the effectivness of group psychotherapy but we can take out..i know it is done
- Exercise interventions
- Combined exercise with medications when either is ineffective alone
- Suicide prevention
- Geriatric health evaluation and skills training
- Bereavement therapy

References

Ahmed A, Lefante CM, Alam N. Depression and nursing home admission among hospitalized older adults with coronary artery disease: a propensity score analysis. *Am J Geriatr Cardiol.* 2007;16(2):76-83.

Alexopoulos GA, Abrams RC, Young RC, et al. Cornell scale for depression in dementia. *Biol Psych.* 1988;23:271-284.

American Psychiatric Association. *Diagnostic and Statistical Manual of Mental Disorders.* 4th ed. Washington, DC: APA; 1994.

Amore M, Tagariello P, Laterza C, et al. Beyond nosography of depression in elderly. *Arch Gerontol Geriatr.* 2007;suppl 1:13-22.

Anghelescu IG, Kohnen R, Szegedi A, et al. Comparison of Hypericum extract WS 5570 and paroxetine in ongoing treatment after recovery from an episode of moderate to severe depression: results from a randomized multicenter study. *Pharmacopsychiatry.* 2006;39(6):213-219.

Aziz R, Lorberg B, Tampi RR. Treatments for late-life bipolar disorder. *Am J Geriatr Pharmacother.* 2006 Dec;4(4):347-364.

Barthlen GM. Sleep disorders. Obstructive sleep apnea syndrome, restless legs syndrome, and insomnia in geriatric patients.*Geriatrics.* 2002; 57(11):34-9.

Bekelman DB, Dy SM, Becker DM, et al. Spiritual well-being and depression in patients with heart failure. *J Gen Intern Med.* 2007;22(4):470-477.

Bennett HE, Thomas SA, Austen R, et al. Validation of screening measures for assessing mood in stroke patients. *Br J Clin Psychol.* 2007;46(3):367-376.

Blazer DG, Hybels C. Origin of depression in later life. *Psychol Med.* 2006;35:1241-1252.

Blazer DG, Sachs-Ericsson N, Hybels CF. Perception of unmet basic needs as a predictor of depressive symptoms among community-dwelling older adults. *J Gerontol A Biol Sci Med Sci.* 2007;62(2):191-195.

Brenes GA, Williamson JD, Messier SP, et al. Treatment of minor depression in older adults: a pilot study comparing sertraline and exercise. *Aging Ment Health.* 2007;11(1):61-68.

Burns R, Nichols LO, Martindale-Adams J, et al. Interdisciplinary geriatric primary care evaluation and management: two year outcomes. *J Am Geriatr Soc.* 2000;48:8-13.

Carranza-Lira S, Najera Mojica JL, Herrera J, et al. Changes in hormones, lipids and symptoms after the administration of a commercial preparation with dehydroepiandrosterone in postmenopausal women. *Proc West Pharmacol Soc.* 2002;45:181-183.

Conradi HJ, de Jonge P, Kluiter H, et al. Enhanced treatment for depression in primary care: long-term outcomes of a psycho-educational prevention program alone and enriched with psychiatric consultation or cognitive behavioral therapy. *Psychol Med.* 2007;37(6):849-862.

Davison TE, McCabe MP, Mellor D, et al. The prevalence and recognition of major depression among low-level aged care residents with and without cognitive impairment. *Aging Ment Health.* 2007;11(1):82-88.

Evans JR, Fletcher AE, Wormald RP. Depression and anxiety in visually impaired older people. *Ophthalmology.* 2007;114(2):283-288.

Forman-Hoffman VL, Yankey JW, Hillis SL, et al. Weight and depressive symptoms in older adults: direction of influence? *J Gerontol B Psychol Sci Soc Sci.* 2007 Jan;62(1): S43-S51.

Frazer CJ, Christensen H, Griffiths KM. Effectiveness of treatments for depression in older people. *Med J Aust.* 2005;182(12):627-632.

Han L, McCusker J, Abrahamowicz M, et al. The temporal relationship between depression symptoms and cognitive functioning in older medical patients: prospective or concurrent? *J Gerontol A Biol Sci Med Sci.* 2006;61(12):1319-1323.

Kasper S, Anghelescu IG, Szegedi A, et al. Superior efficacy of St John's wort extract WS 5570 compared to placebo in patients with major depression: a randomized, double-blind, placebo-controlled, multi-center trial. *BMC Med.* 2006;4:14-18.

Kiecolt-Glaser JK, Belury MA, Porter K, et al. Depressive symptoms, omega-6: omega-3 fatty acids, and inflammation in older adults. *Psychosom Med.* 2007;69(3):217-224.

Kirchner JE, Zubritsky C, Cody M, et al. Alcohol consumption among older adults in primary care. *J Gen Intern Med.* 2007;22(1):92-978.

Koenig HG. Physician attitudes toward treatment of depression in older medical inpatients. *Aging Ment Health.* 2007;11(2):197-204.

Kotlyar M, Dysken M, Adson DE. Update on drug-induced depression in the elderly. *Am J Geriatr Pharmacother.* 2005 Dec;3(4):288-300.

Kraus CA, Kunik ME, Stanley MA. Use of cognitive behavioral therapy in late life psychiatric disorders. *Geriatrics.* 2007;62(6):7-8.

Levenson AJ, Hall RCW, eds. *Neuropsychiatric Manifestations of Physical Disease in the Elderly.* New York, NY: Raven Press; 1981.

Lyness JM, Caine ED, King DA, et al. Depressive disorders and symptoms in older primary care patients: one year outcomes. *Am J Geriatr Psychiatry.* 2002;1:275-282.

McCusker J, Cole M, Dufouil C, et al. The prevalence and correlates of major and minor depression in older medical inpatients. *J Am Geriatr Soc.* 2005;53(8):1344-1355.

McNeil JK, LeBlanc EM, Joyner M. The effect of exercise on depressive symptoms in the moderately depressed elderly. *Psychol Aging.* 1991;6(3):487-488.

Medical Letter. Drugs that may cause psychiatric symptoms. *Med Lett.* 2002;44(1134): 59-62.

Mittmann N, Herrmann N, Einarson TR, et al. The efficacy, safety and tolerability of antidepressants in late life depression: a meta-analysis. *J Affect Disord.* 1997;46(3): 191-217.

Mottram P, Wilson K, Strobl J. Antidepressants for depressed elderly. *Cochrane Database Syst Rev.* 2006;25(1):CD003491.

National Conference of Gerontological Nurse Practitioners. Mental Health Toolkit (electronic version). www.ncgnp.org. Accessed on July 9, 2008.

Osgood NJ. *Suicide in the Elderly.* Rockville, MD: Aspen; 1985.

Penninx BW, Rejeski WJ, Pandya J, et al. Exercise and depressive symptoms: a comparison of aerobic and resistance exercise effects on emotional and physical function in older persons with high and low depressive symptomatology. *J Gerontol B Psychol Sci Soc Sci.* 2002;57(2):124-132.

Perry PJ, Uates WR, Williams R. Testosterone therapy in late life major depression in males. *J Clin Psychiatry.* 2002;63:1096-1101.

Roriz-Cruz M, Rosset I, Wada T, et al. Stroke-independent association between metabolic syndrome and functional dependence, depression, and low quality of life in elderly community-dwelling Brazilian people. *J Am Geriatr Soc.* 2007;55(3):374-382.

Ruckenbauer G, Yazdani F, Ravaglia G. Suicide in old age: illness or autonomous decision of the will? *Arch Gerontol Geriatr.* 2007;44(1):355-358.

Sawyer P, Lillis JP, Bodner EV, et al. Substantial daily pain among nursing home residents. *J Am Med Dir Assoc.* 2007;8(3):158-165.

Sims J, Hill K, Davidson S, et al. Exploring the feasibility of a community-based strength training program for older people with depressive symptoms and its impact on depressive symptoms. *BMC Geriatr.* 2006 Nov 30;6:6-18.

Singh N, Clements KM, Singh MA. The efficacy of exercise as a long-term antidepressant in elderly subjects: a randomized, controlled trial. *J Gerontol A Biol Sci Med Sci.* 2001;56(8):M497-M504.

Skultety KM, Zeiss A. The treatment of depression in older adults in the primary care setting: an evidence-based review. *Health Psychol.* 2006;25(6):665-674.

Solfrizzi V, D'Introno A, Colacicco AM, et al. Incident Occurrence of Depressive Symptoms among Patients with Mild Cognitive Impairment: the Italian Longitudinal Study on Aging. *Dement Geriatr Cogn Disord.* 2007;24(1):55-64.

Speer DC, Schneider MG. Mental health needs of older adults and primary care: opportunity for interdisciplinary geriatric team practice. *Clin Psychol: Sci Pract.* 2003;21:85-101.

Spitzer RL, Williams JB, Kroenke K. Utility of a New Procedure for Diagnosing Mental Disorders in Primary Care: the PRIME-MD 1000 study. *JAMA.* 1994;272(22):1749-1756.

Steffens DC, McQuoid DR, Krishnan KR. The Duke Somatic Treatment Algorithm for Geriatric Depression (STAGED) approach. *Psychopharmacol Bull.* 2002;36(2):58-68.

Stewart AL, Hays RD, Ware JE. The MOS short-form general health survey: reliability and validity in a patient population. *Med Care.* 1988;26:724-735.

Unutzer J, Katon W, Callahan CM, et al. Collaborative care management of late life depression in the primary care setting: a randomized controlled trial. *JAMA.* 2002;288(22):2836-2845.

Wilkins CH, Sheline YI, Roe CM, et al. Vitamin D deficiency is associated with low mood and worse cognitive performance in older adults. *Am J Geriatr Psychiatry.* 2006;14(1):1032-1040.

Wilson K, Mottram P, Sivanranthan A, et al. Antidepressant versus placebo for depressed elderly. *Cochrane Database Syst Rev.* 2001;2:CD000561.

Windsor TD, Anstey KJ, Butterworth P, et al. The role of perceived control in explaining depressive symptoms associated with driving cessation in a longitudinal study. *Gerontologist.* 2007;47(2):215-223.

Suggested Readings

Ayers CR, Sorrell JT, Thorp SR, et al. Evidence-based *psychological* treatments for late-life anxiety. *Psychol Aging.* 2007;22(1):8-17.

Gatz M. Commentary on evidence-based psychological treatments for older adults. *Psychol Aging.* 2007;22(1):52-55.

Frazer CJ, Christensen H, Griffiths KM. Effectiveness of treatments for depression in older people. *Med J Aust.* 2005;182(12):627-632.

Unutzer J. Late-life depression. *N Engl J Med.* 2007;357:2269-2276.

Van der Wurff FB, Stek ML, Hoogendijk WJ, Beekman AT. The efficacy and safety of ECT in depressed older adults: a literature review. *Int J Geriatr Psychiatry.* 2003 Oct;18(10):894-904

Van der Wurff FB, Stek ML, Hoogendijk WL, Beekman AT. Electroconvulsive therapy for the depressed elderly. *Cochrane Database Syst Rev.* 2003;(2):CD003593.

Web References

Review of the Geriatric Depression Scale
http://www.stanford.edu/~yesavage/GDS.html. Accessed on July 9, 2008.
Preventing Chronic Disease
Centers for Disease Control: Review of treatment interventions for depression
http://www.cdc.gov/Pcd/issues/2008/jan/pdf/07_0154.pdf. Accessed on July 9, 2008.
Depression and Older Adults: Patient and family educational materials familydoctor.
    org/online/famdocen/home/seniors/mental-health/588.html
Depression in Older Adults: Patient and family educational materials
http://nihseniorhealth.gov/depression/toc.html
Tools
Geriatric Depression Scale
http://www.stanford.edu/~yesavage/GDS.html
Center for Epidemiologic Studies Depression Scale (CES-D)
counsellingresource.com/quizzes/cesd/index.html
Beck Depression Scale
http://www.fpnotebook.com/Psych/Exam/BckDprsnInvntry.htm. Accessed on July 9. 2008
Cornell Scale for Depression in Dementia
Dementiahttp://www.michigan.gov/documents/mdch/bhs_CPG_Depression_Appendix_2
    _206523_7.pdf. Accessed on July 9, 2008.

CHAPTER 8

INCONTINENCE

Incontinence is a common, bothersome, and potentially disabling condition in the geriatric population. It is defined as the involuntary loss of urine or stool in sufficient amount or frequency to constitute a social and/or health problem. Figure 8-1 illustrates the prevalence of urinary incontinence across various settings. Incontinence ranges in severity from occasional episodes of dribbling small amounts of urine to continuous urinary incontinence with concomitant fecal incontinence.

Approximately 1 in 3 women and 15% to 20% of men older than 65 years have some degree of urinary incontinence. Between 5% and 10% of community-dwelling older adults have incontinence more often than weekly and/or use a pad for protection from urinary accidents. The prevalence is as high as 60% to 80% in many long-term care institutions, where patients often have both urinary and stool incontinence. In both community and institutional settings, incontinence is associated with both impaired mobility and poor cognition.

Physical health, psychological well-being, social status, and the costs of health care can all be adversely affected by incontinence (Table 8-1). Urinary incontinence is curable in many geriatric patients, especially those who have adequate mobility and mental functioning. Even when it is not curable, incontinence can always be managed in a manner that will keep patients comfortable, make life easier for caregivers, and minimize the costs of caring for the condition and its complications.

Despite some change in the social perception of incontinence because of television advertisements and public media and educational efforts, many older patients are embarrassed and frustrated by their incontinence and either deny it or do not discuss it with a health professional. It is therefore essential that specific questions about incontinence be included in periodic assessments and that incontinence be noted as a problem when it is detected in institutional settings. Examples of such questions include the following:

"Do you have trouble with your bladder?"
"Do you ever lose urine when you don't want to?"
"Do you ever wear padding to protect yourself in case you lose urine?"

This chapter briefly reviews the pathophysiology of geriatric incontinence and provides detailed information on the evaluation and management of this condition. Although most of the chapter focuses on urinary incontinence, much of the pathophysiology also applies to fecal incontinence, which is briefly addressed at the end of the chapter.

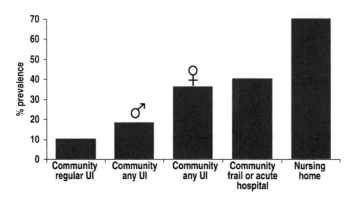

— FIGURE 8-1 —   Prevalence of urinary incontinence in the geriatric population. "Regular UI" is more often than weekly and/or the use of a pad. (Percentages range in various studies; those shown reflect approximate average's from multiple sources.)

TABLE 8-1   POTENTIAL ADVERSE EFFECTS OF URINARY INCONTINENCE

Physical heath
 Skin irritation and breakdown
 Recurrent urinary tract infections
 Falls (especially with nighttime incontinence)

Psychological health
 Isolation
 Depression
 Dependency

Social consequences
 Stress on family, friends, and caregivers
 Predisposition to institutionalization

Economic costs
 Supplies (padding, catheters, etc)
 Laundry
 Labor (nurses, housekeepers)
 Management of complications

NORMAL URINATION

Continence requires effective functioning of the lower urinary tract, adequate cognitive and physical functioning, motivation, and an appropriate environment (Table 8-2). Thus, the pathophysiology of geriatric incontinence can relate to the anatomy and physiology of the lower urinary tract as well as to functional, psychological, and environmental factors. Several anatomic components participate in normal urination (Fig. 8-2). At the most basic level, urination is governed by reflexes centered in the sacral micturition center. Afferent pathways (via somatic and autonomic nerves) carry information on bladder volume to the spinal cord as the bladder fills. Motor output is adjusted accordingly (Fig. 8-3). Thus, as the bladder fills, sympathetic tone closes the bladder neck, relaxes the dome of the bladder, and inhibits parasympathetic tone; somatic innervation maintains tone in the pelvic floor musculature (including striated muscle around the urethra).

TABLE 8-2   REQUIREMENTS FOR CONTINENCE

Effective lower urinary tract function
  Storage
    Accommodation by bladder of increasing volumes of urine under low
    pressure
      Closed bladder outlet
      Appropriate sensation of bladder fullness
      Absence of involuntary bladder contractions
  Emptying
    Bladder capable of contraction
    Lack of anatomic obstruction to urine flow
    Coordinated lowering of outlet resistance with bladder contractions
Adequate mobility and dexterity to use toilet or toilet substitute and to
  manage clothing
Adequate cognitive function to recognize toileting needs and to find a toilet
  or toilet substitute
Motivation to be continent
Absence of environmental and iatrogenic barriers such as inaccessible toilets
  or toilet substitutes, unavailable caregivers, or drug side effects

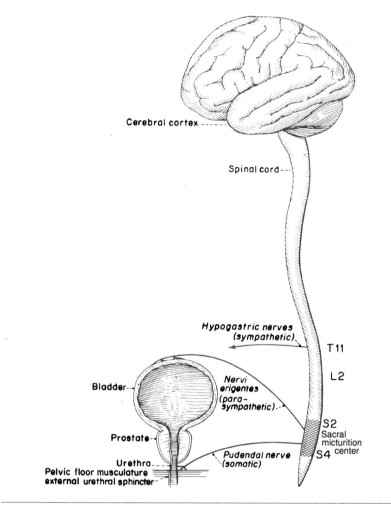

Cerebral cortex

Spinal cord

Hypogastric nerves
(sympathetic)

T 11

L 2

Bladder

Nervi
erigentes
(para-
sympathetic)

S 2
Sacral
micturition
center
S 4

Prostate

Urethra
Pelvic floor musculature
external urethral sphincter

Pudendal nerve
(somatic)

— FIGURE 8-2 — Structural components of normal micturition.

When urination occurs, sympathetic and somatic tones diminish, and parasympathetic cholinergically mediated impulses cause the bladder to contract. All these processes are under the influence of higher centers in the brain stem, cerebral cortex, and cerebellum. This is a simplified description of a very complex process, and the neurophysiology of urination remains incompletely understood. The cerebral cortex exerts a predominantly inhibitory influence and the brain stem facilitates urination. Thus, loss of the central cortical inhibiting influences over the sacral micturition center from diseases such as dementia, stroke, and parkinsonism can produce incontinence in elderly patients. Disorders of the

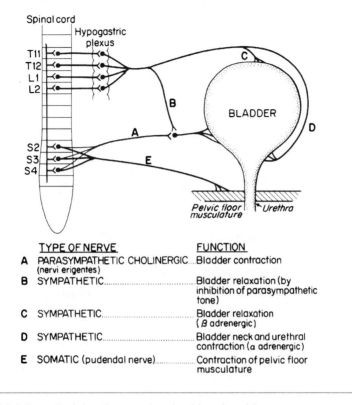

Spinal cord

Hypogastric plexus

T11
T12
L1
L2

B

C

BLADDER

A

D

S2
S3
S4

E

Pelvic floor musculature   Urethra

	TYPE OF NERVE	FUNCTION
A	PARASYMPATHETIC CHOLINERGIC (nervi erigentes)	Bladder contraction
B	SYMPATHETIC	Bladder relaxation (by inhibition of parasympathetic tone)
C	SYMPATHETIC	Bladder relaxation (β adrenergic)
D	SYMPATHETIC	Bladder neck and urethral contraction (a adrenergic)
E	SOMATIC (pudendal nerve)	Contraction of pelvic floor musculature

— FIGURE 8-3 — Peripheral nerves involved in micturition.

brain stem and suprasacral spinal cord can interfere with the coordination of bladder contractions and lowering of urethral resistance, and interruptions of the sacral innervation can cause impaired bladder contraction and problems with continence.

Normal urination is a dynamic process, requiring the coordination of several physiological processes. Figure 8-4 depicts a simplified schematic diagram of the pressure–volume relationships in the lower urinary tract, similar to measurements made in urodynamic studies. Under normal circumstances, as the bladder fills, bladder pressure remains low (eg, <15 cm H_2O). The first urge to void is variable but generally occurs between 150 and 300 mL, and normal bladder capacity is 300 to 600 mL. When normal urination is initiated, true detrusor pressure (bladder pressure minus intra-abdominal pressure) increases, urethral resistance decreases, and urine flow occurs when detrusor pressure exceeds urethral resistance. If at any time during bladder filling total intravesicular pressure (which includes intra-abdominal pressure) exceeds outlet resistance, urinary leakage will occur. This will happen if, for example, intra-abdominal pressure rises without a

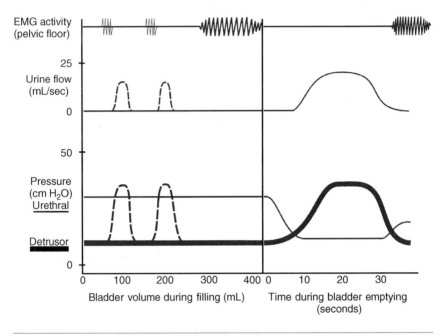

— FIGURE 8-4 —   Simplified schematic of the dynamic function of the lower urinary tract during bladder filling (left) and emptying (right). As the bladder fills, true detrusor pressure (thick line at bottom) remains low (<15 cm H_2O) and does not exceed urethral resistance pressure (thin line at bottom). As the bladder fills to capacity (generally 300-600 mL), pelvic floor and sphincter activity increase as measured by electromyography (EMG). Involuntary detrusor contractions (illustrated by dashed lines) occur commonly among incontinent geriatric patients (see text). They may be accompanied by increased EMG activity in attempts to prevent leakage (dashed lines at top). If detrusor pressure exceeds urethral pressure during an involuntary contraction, as shown, urine will flow. During bladder emptying, detrusor pressure rises, urethral pressure falls, and EMG activity ceases in order for normal urine flow to occur (right side of figure).

rise in true detrusor pressure when someone with low outlet or urethral sphincter weakness coughs or sneezes. This would be defined as genuine stress incontinence in urodynamic terminology. Alternatively, the bladder can contract involuntarily and cause urinary leakage. Involuntary detrusor contractions have been defined as detrusor hyperreflexia in patients with neurological disorders. Increasing attention is being paid to the role of sensory afferent innervation in the pathogenesis of detrusor overactivity. Sensory afferent innervation may therefore become a target for therapeutic intervention in the future.

CAUSES AND TYPES OF INCONTINENCE

Basic Causes

There are four basic categories of causes for geriatric urinary incontinence (Fig. 8-5). Determining the cause(s) is essential to proper management.

It is important to distinguish between urological and neurological disorders that cause incontinence and other problems (such as diminished mobility and/or mental function, inaccessible toilets, and psychological problems) which can cause or contribute to the condition. As is the case for a number of other common geriatric problems discussed in this text, multiple disorders often interact to cause urinary incontinence, as depicted in Fig. 8-5.

Aging alone does not cause urinary incontinence. Several age-related changes can, however, contribute to its development.

In general, with age, bladder capacity declines, residual urine increases, and involuntary bladder contractions become more common. These contractions are found in up to 80% of older incontinent patients, as well as in 5% to 10% of older women and in 33% or more of older men with no or minimal urinary symptoms. Combined with impaired mobility, these contractions account for a substantial proportion of incontinence in frail geriatric patients.

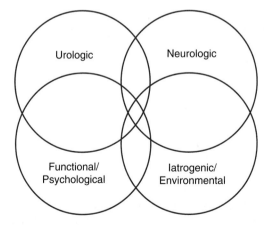

— FIGURE 8-5 —   Basic underlying causes of geriatric urinary incontinence.

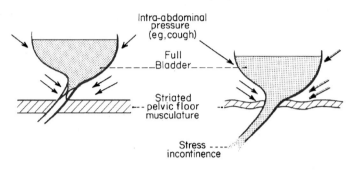

— FIGURE 8-6 — Simplified schematic depicting age-associated changes in pelvic floor muscle, bladder, and urethra–vesicle position, predisposing to stress incontinence. Normally (left), the bladder and outlet remain anatomically inside the intra-abdominal cavity, and rises in pressure contribute to bladder outlet closure. Age-associated changes (eg, estrogen deficiency, surgeries, childbirth) can weaken the structures maintaining bladder position (right); in this situation, increases in intra-abdominal pressure can cause urine loss (stress incontinence).

Aging is associated with a decline in bladder outlet and urethral resistance pressure in women. This decline which is related to diminished estrogen influence and laxity of pelvic structures associated with prior childbirths, surgeries, and deconditioned muscles predisposes to the development of stress incontinence (Fig. 8-6). Decreased estrogen can also cause atrophic vaginitis and urethritis, which can, in turn, cause symptoms of dysuria and urgency and predispose to the development of urinary infection and urge incontinence. In men, prostatic enlargement is associated with decreased urine flow rates and detrusor overactivity and can lead to urge and/or overflow types of incontinence (see below). Aging is also associated with abnormalities of arginine vasopressin (AVP) and atrial natriuretic peptide (ANP) levels. Lack of the normal diurnal rhythm of AVP secretion and increased levels of ANP may contribute to nocturnal polyuria and predispose many older people to nighttime incontinence.

Reversible Factors Causing or Contributing to Incontinence

Numerous potentially reversible conditions and medications may cause or contribute to geriatric incontinence (Tables 8-3 and 8-4).

TABLE 8-3   REVERSIBLE CONDITIONS THAT CAUSE OR CONTRIBUTE TO GERIATRIC URINARY INCONTINENCE

CONDITION	MANAGEMENT
Conditions affecting the lower urinary tract	
Urinary tract infection (symptomatic with frequency, urgency, dysuria, etc)	Antimicrobial therapy
Atrophic vaginitis/urethritis	Topical estrogen
Stool impaction	Disimpaction; appropriate use of stool softeners, bulk-forming agents, and laxatives if necessary; implement high fiber intake, adequate mobility, and fluid intake (see Table 8-21)
Drug side effect (see Table 8-4)	Discontinue or change therapy if clinically appropriate. Dosage reduction or modification (eg, flexible scheduling of rapid-acting diuretics) may also help
Increased urine production	
Metabolic (hyperglycemia, hypercalcemia)	Better control of diabetes mellitus. Therapy for hypercalcemia depends on underlying cause
Excess fluid intake	Reduction in intake of diuretic fluids (eg, caffeinated beverages)
Volume overload	
Venous insufficiency with edema	Support stockings Leg elevation Sodium restriction Diuretic therapy
Congestive heart failure	Medical therapy
Impaired ability or willingness to reach a toilet	
Delirium	Diagnosis and treatment of underlying cause(s)

TABLE 8-3   REVERSIBLE CONDITIONS THAT CAUSE OR CONTRIBUTE
TO GERIATRIC URINARY INCONTINENCE (*Continued*)

CONDITION	MANAGEMENT
Chronic illness, injury, or restraint that interferes with mobility	Regular toileting Use of toilet substitutes Environmental alterations (eg, bedside commode, urinal) Remove restraints if possible
Psychological	Appropriate nonpharmacologic and/or pharmacologic treatment

Reproduced with permission from Fantl et al., 1996.

TABLE 8-4   MEDICATIONS THAT CAN CAUSE INCONTINENCE

TYPE OF MEDICATION	POTENTIAL EFFECTS ON INCONTINENCE
Diuretics	Polyuria, frequency, urgency
Anticholinergics	Urinary retention, overflow incontinence, stool impaction
Psychotropics Tricyclic Antidepressants	Anticholinergic actions, sedation
Antipsychotics	Anticholinergic actions, sedation, immobility
Sedative-hypnotics	Sedation, delirium, immobility, muscle relaxation
Narcotic analgesics	Urinary retention, fecal impaction, sedation, delirium
α-Adrenergic blockers	Urethral relaxation
α-Adrenergic agonists	Urinary retention
Cholinesterase inhibitors	Urinary frequency, urgency
Angiotensin-converting enzyme inhibitors	Cough precipitating stress incontinence

TABLE 8-4   MEDICATIONS THAT CAN CAUSE INCONTINENCE
             (*Continued*)

Type of Medication	Potential Effects on Incontinence
β-Adrenergic agonists	Urinary retention
Calcium channel blockers	Urinary retention, edema (nocturia)
Gabapentin, pregabalin, glitazones	Edema (nocturia)
Alcohol	Polyuria, frequency, urgency, sedation, delirium, immobility
Caffeine	Polyuria, bladder irritation

The term acute incontinence refers to those situations in which the incontinence is of sudden onset, usually related to an acute illness or an iatrogenic problem, and subsides once the illness or medication problem has been resolved (this has also been termed transient incontinence). Persistent incontinence refers to incontinence that is unrelated to an acute illness and persists over time.

Potentially reversible conditions can play a role in both acute and persistent incontinence. A search for these factors should be undertaken in all incontinent geriatric patients.

The causes of acute and reversible forms of urinary incontinence can be remembered by the mnemonic DRIP (Table 8-5).

TABLE 8-5   ACRONYM FOR POTENTIALLY REVERSIBLE CONDITIONS

D	Delirium
R	Restricted mobility, retention
I	Infection, inflammation, impaction
P	Polyuria, pharmaceuticals

* See Tables 8-3 and 8-4.

Many older persons, because of urinary frequency and urgency, especially when they are limited in mobility, carefully arrange their schedules (and may even limit social activities) in order to be close to a toilet. Thus, an acute illness (eg, pneumonia, cardiac decompensation, stroke, lower extremity, or vertebral fracture) can precipitate incontinence by disrupting this delicate balance. Hospitalization with its attendant environmental barriers (such as bed rails, poorly lit rooms) and the immobility that often accompanies acute illnesses can precipitate acute incontinence. Acute incontinence in these situations is likely to resolve with resolution of the underlying acute illness. Unless an indwelling or external catheter is necessary during an acute illness to record urine output accurately, this type of incontinence should be managed by environmental manipulations, scheduled toiletings, appropriate use of toilet substitutes (eg, urinals, bedside commodes, and pads), and careful attention to skin care. In a substantial proportion of patients, incontinence may persist for several weeks after hospitalization and should be evaluated as for persistent incontinence (see below).

Fecal impaction is a common problem in both acutely and chronically ill geriatric patients. Large impactions may cause mechanical obstruction of the bladder outlet in women and may stimulate involuntary bladder contractions induced by sensory input related to rectal distention. Whatever the underlying mechanism, relief of fecal impaction can lead to improvement and sometimes resolution of the urinary incontinence.

Urinary retention with overflow incontinence should be considered in any patient who suddenly develops urinary incontinence. Immobility, anticholinergic and narcotic drugs, and fecal impaction can all precipitate urinary retention and overflow incontinence in geriatric patients. In addition, this condition may be a manifestation of an underlying process causing spinal cord compression and presenting acutely.

Any acute inflammatory condition in the lower urinary tract that causes frequency and urgency can precipitate incontinence. Treatment of an acute cystitis, atrophic vaginitis, or urethritis can restore continence.

Conditions that cause polyuria, including hyperglycemia and hypercalcemia, as well as diuretics (especially the rapid-acting loop diuretics), can precipitate acute incontinence. Some older people drink excessive amounts of fluids, and others ingest a large amount of caffeine without understanding the prominent effects it can have on the bladder. Patients with volume-expanded states, such as congestive heart failure and lower extremity venous insufficiency, may have polyuria at night, which can contribute to nocturia and nocturnal incontinence.

As in the case of many other conditions discussed throughout this text, a wide variety of medications can play a role in the development of incontinence in elderly patients via several different mechanisms (see Table 8-4). Whether the incontinence is acute or persistent, the potential role of these medications in causing or contributing to the patients' incontinence should be considered. Whenever feasible, stopping the medication, switching to an alternative, or modifying the dosage schedule can be an important component (and possibly the only one necessary) of the treatment for incontinence.

Persistent Incontinence

Persistent forms of incontinence can be classified clinically into four basic types. As depicted in Fig. 8-7, these types can overlap. Thus, an individual patient may have more than one type simultaneously. While this classification does not include all the neurophysiological abnormalities associated with incontinence, it is helpful in approaching the clinical assessment and treatment of incontinence in the geriatric population.

Three of these types—stress, urge, and overflow—result from one or a combination of the two basic abnormalities in lower genitourinary tract function: (1) failure to store urine, caused by a hyperactive or poorly compliant bladder or by diminished outflow resistance; (2) failure to empty bladder, caused by a poorly contractile bladder or by increased outflow resistance. Table 8-6 shows the clinical definitions and common causes of persistent urinary incontinence.

Stress incontinence is common in older women, especially in ambulatory clinic settings. It may be infrequent and involve very small amounts of urine and need no specific treatment in women who are not bothered by it. On the other hand, it may be so severe and bothersome that it necessitates surgical correction. It is most often associated with weakened supporting tissues and consequent hypermobility of the bladder outlet and urethra caused by lack of estrogen and/or

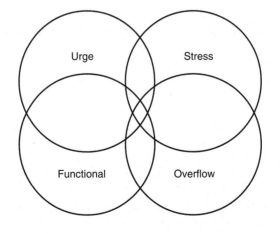

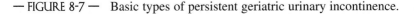

— FIGURE 8-7 — Basic types of persistent geriatric urinary incontinence.

TABLE 8-6 BASIC TYPES AND CAUSES OF PERSISTENT URINARY
INCONTINENCE

Types	Definition	Common Causes
Stress	Involuntary loss of urine (usually small amounts) with increases in intra-abdominal pressure (eg, cough, laugh, exercise)	Weakness of pelvic floor musculature and urethral hypermobility Bladder outlet or urethral sphincter weakness
Urge	Leakage of urine (variable but often larger volumes) because of inability to delay voiding after sensation of bladder fullness is perceived	Detrusor overactivity, isolated or associated with one or more of the following: Local genitourinary condition such as tumors, stones, diverticula, or outflow obstruction Central nervous system disorders such as stroke, dementia, parkinsonism, spinal cord injury
Overflow (incontinence associated with incomplete bladder emptying)	Symptoms are variable and nonspecific. Classic "overflow" incontinence involves leakage of urine (usually small amounts) resulting from mechanical forces on an overdistended bladder	Anatomic obstruction by prostate, stricture, cystocele Acontractile bladder associated with diabetes mellitus or spinal cord injury Neurogenic (detrusor-sphincter dyssynergy), associated with multiple sclerosis and other suprasacral spinal cord lesions
Functional	Urinary incontinence associated with inability to toilet because of impairment of cognitive and/or physical functioning, psychological unwillingness, or environmental barriers	Severe dementia and other neurological disorders Psychological factors such as depression and hostility

previous vaginal deliveries or surgery (see Fig. 8-6). Obesity and chronic coughing can exacerbate this condition. Women who have had previous vaginal repair and/or surgical bladder neck suspension may develop a weak urethra (intrinsic sphincter deficiency [ISD]). These women generally present with severe incontinence and symptoms of constant wetting with any activity. This condition should be suspected during office evaluation if a woman loses urine involuntarily with coughing in the supine position during a pelvic examination when her bladder is relatively empty. In general, women with ISD are less responsive to nonsurgical treatment but may benefit from periurethral injections or a surgical sling procedure (see below). Stress incontinence is unusual in men but can occur after transurethral surgery and/or radiation therapy for lower urinary tract malignancy when the anatomic sphincters are damaged.

Urge incontinence can be caused by a variety of lower genitourinary and neurological disorders (see Table 8-6). Patients with urge incontinence typically present with irritative symptoms of an overactive bladder, including frequency (voiding more than every 2 h), urgency, and nocturia (two or more voids during usual sleeping hours). Urge incontinence is most often, but not always, associated with detrusor motor instability or detrusor hyperreflexia (see Fig. 8-4). Some patients have a poorly compliant bladder without involuntary contractions (eg, as a result of radiation or interstitial cystitis, both relatively unusual conditions).

Other patients have symptoms of an overactive bladder but do not exhibit detrusor motor instability on urodynamic testing. Some patients with neurological disorders have detrusor hyperreflexia on urodynamic testing but do not have urgency and are incontinent without any warning symptoms ("unconscious incontinence"). The above-described patients are generally treated as if they had urge incontinence if they empty their bladders and do not have other correctable genitourinary pathology. A subgroup of older incontinent patients with detrusor motor instability also have impaired bladder contractility—emptying less than one-third of their bladder volume with involuntary contractions on urodynamic testing (Resnick and Yalla, 1987; Elbadawi et al., 1993). This condition has been termed detrusor hyperactivity with impaired contractility (DHIC). Patients with DHIC may present with symptoms that are not typical of urge incontinence and may strain to complete voiding. These patients may be difficult to manage because of their urinary retention.

Some older patients suffer from an overactive bladder, but are not incontinent. The hallmark symptom of overactive bladder is urinary urgency. Patients with overactive bladder usually also complain of urinary frequency (>8 voids in 24 h) and nocturia (awakening from sleep to void). Overactive bladder symptoms are common in the elderly; approximately 30% of women and 40% of men age 75 and older admit to these symptoms, most of whom also have urge incontinence. The conditions that contribute to symptoms of overactive bladder as well as the diagnostic evaluation and management of this symptom complex are the same as for urge incontinence (Ouslander, 2004).

Overflow incontinence, or incontinence associated with incomplete bladder emptying, can result from anatomic or neurogenic outflow obstruction, a hypotonic or acontractile bladder, or both. The most common causes include prostatic enlargement, diabetic neuropathic bladder, and urethral stricture. Low spinal cord injury and anatomic obstruction in females (caused by pelvic prolapse and urethral distortion) are less common causes of overflow incontinence. Several types of drugs can also contribute to this type of persistent incontinence (see Table 8-4). Some patients with suprasacral spinal cord lesions (eg, multiple sclerosis) develop detrusor-sphincter dyssynergy and consequent urinary retention, which must be treated in a similar manner as overflow incontinence; in some instances a sphincterotomy is necessary. The symptoms of overflow incontinence are nonspecific and urinary retention is easily missed on physical examination. Thus, a postvoid residual determination must be performed to exclude this condition.

The term functional incontinence refers to incontinence associated with the inability or lack of motivation to reach a toilet on time. Factors that contribute to functional incontinence (such as inaccessible toilets and psychological disorders) can also exacerbate other types of persistent incontinence. Patients with incontinence that appears to be predominantly related to functional factors may also have abnormalities of the lower genitourinary tract. In some patients, it can be very difficult to determine whether the functional factors or the genitourinary factors predominate without a trial of specific types of treatment. However, no matter what specific treatments are prescribed, patients with functional incontinence require systematic toileting assistance as a component of their management plan.

These basic types of incontinence may occur in combination, as depicted by the overlap in Fig. 8-7. Older women commonly have a combination of stress and urge incontinence (generally referred to as mixed incontinence). Frail geriatric patients often have urge incontinence with detrusor instability as well as functional disabilities that contribute to their incontinence.

EVALUATION

Basic Evaluation

The first step in evaluating incontinent patients is to identify the incontinence by direct observation or the screening questions discussed earlier. In patients with the sudden onset of incontinence (especially when associated with an acute medical condition and hospitalization), the reversible factors that can cause acute incontinence (see Tables 8-3, 8-4, and 8-5) can be ruled out by a brief history, physical examination, postvoid residual determination, and basic laboratory studies (urinalysis, culture, serum glucose, and calcium). Table 8-7 shows the

TABLE 8-7   COMPONENTS OF THE DIAGNOSTIC EVALUATION OF PERSISTENT URINARY INCONTINENCE

All patients
  History, including bladder record
  Physical examination
  Urinalysis
  Postvoid residual determination*

Selected patients[†]
  Laboratory studies
    Urine culture
    Urine cytology
    Blood glucose, calcium
    Renal function tests
    Renal ultrasonography
  Gynecologic evaluation
  Urological evaluation
  Cystourethroscopy
  Urodynamic tests
    Simple
      Observation of voiding
      Cough test for stress incontinence
    Complex
      Urine flowmetry[‡]
      Multichannel cystometrogram
      Pressure-flow study
      Leak-point pressure
      Urethral pressure profilometry
      Sphincter electromyography
      Videourodynamics

*Postvoid residual determination may not be necessary in carefully selected patients (see text).
[†]See text and Table 8-9.
[‡]Urine flowmetry is a useful screening test in older men (see text).

basic components of the evaluation of persistent urinary incontinence. Practice guidelines suggest that the basic evaluation should include a focused history, targeted physical examination, urinalysis, and postvoiding residual (PVR) determination (Fantl et al. 1996; American Medical Directors Association, 2006; Fung et al., 2007). The history should focus on the characteristics of the incontinence, current medical problems and medications, the most bothersome symptom(s), and the impact of the incontinence on the patient and caregivers (Table 8-8). Bladder

TABLE 8-8   KEY ASPECTS OF AN INCONTINENT PATIENT'S HISTORY

Active medical conditions, especially neurologic disorders, diabetes
  mellitus, congestive heart failure, venous insufficiency

Medications (see Table 8-4)

Fluid intake pattern
  Type and amount of fluid (especially caffeine and fluids before bedtime)

Past genitourinary history, especially childbirth, surgery, dilatations, urinary
  retention, recurrent urinary tract infections

Symptoms of incontinence
  Onset and duration
  Type—stress vs. urge vs. mixed vs. other
  Frequency, timing, and amount of incontinence episodes and of continent
    voids (see Figs. 8-8 and 8-9)

Other lower urinary tract symptoms
  Irritative—dysuria, frequency, urgency, nocturia
  Voiding difficulty—hesitancy, slow or interrupted stream, straining,
    incomplete emptying
  Other—hematuria, suprapubic discomfort

Other symptoms
  Neurological (indicative of stroke, dementia, parkinsonism, normal-
    pressure hydrocephalus, spinal cord compression, multiple
    sclerosis)
  Psychological (depression)
  Bowel (constipation, stool incontinence)
  Symptoms suggestive of volume-expanded state (eg, lower extremity
    edema, shortness of breath while horizontal or with exertion)

Environmental factors
  Location and structure of bathroom
  Availability of toilet substitutes

Perceptions of incontinence
  Patient's concerns or ideas about underlying cause(s)
  Most bothersome symptom(s)
  Interference with daily life
  Severity (eg, is it enough of a problem for you to consider surgery?)

BLADDER RECORD

Day:_____   Date:_____/_____.

                                              month   day

1NSTRUCTIONS:

(1) In the 1st column make a mark every time during the 2-hour period you urinate into the toilet

(2) Use the 2nd column to record the amount you urinate (if you are measuring amounts)

(3) In the 3rd or 4th column, make a mark every time you accidentally leak urine

Time interval	Urinated in toilet	Amount	Leaking accident	or	Large accident	Reason for accident *
6–8 AM						
8–10 AM						
2–4 PM						
4–6 PM						
6–8 PM						
8–10 PM						
10–12 PM						
Overnight						

Number of pads used today:_____

* For example, if you coughed and have a leaking accident, write "cough".
  If you had a large accident after a strong urge to urinate, write "urge".

— FIGURE 8-8 — Example of a bladder record for ambulatory care settings.

records or voiding diaries such as those shown in Fig. 8-8 (for outpatients) and Fig. 8-9 (for institutionalized patients) can be helpful in initially characterizing symptoms as well as in following the response to treatment.

Physical examination should focus on abdominal, rectal, and genital examinations and an evaluation of lumbosacral innervation (Table 8-9). During the history and physical examination, special attention should be given to factors such as mobility, mental status, medications, and accessibility of toilets that may either be causing the incontinence or interacting with urological and neurological disorders to worsen the condition. The pelvic examination in women should include careful inspections of the labia and vagina for signs of inflammation suggestive of atrophic vaginitis and for pelvic prolapse. Most older women have

INCONTINENCE MONITORING RECORD

INSTRUCTIONS: EACH TIME THE PATIENT IS CHECKED:
1) Mark *one* of the circles in the BLADDER section at the hour closest to the time the patient is checked.
2) Make an X in the BOWEL section if the patient has had an incontinent or normal bowel movement.

| 🍩 = Incontinent, small amount | ∅ = Dry | X = Incontinent BOWEL |
| 🍩 = Incontinent, large amount | ⩘ = Voided correctly | X = Normal BOWEL |

PATIENT NAME _____ ROOM # _____ DATE _____

| | BLADDER | | | BOWEL | | | |
	INCONTINENT OF URINE	DRY	VOIDED CORRECTLY	INCONTINENT X	NORMAL X	INITIALS	COMMENTS
12 AM	● ●	○	△ cc ___				
1	● ●	○	△ cc ___				
2	● ●	○	△ cc ___				
3	● ●	○	△ cc ___				
4	● ●	○	△ cc ___				
5	● ●	○	△ cc ___				
6	● ●	○	△ cc ___				
7	● ●	○	△ cc ___				
8	● ●	○	△ cc ___				
9	● ●	○	△ cc ___				
10	● ●	○	△ cc ___				
11	● ●	○	△ cc ___				
12 PM	● ●	○	△ cc ___				
1	● ●	○	△ cc ___				
2	● ●	○	△ cc ___				
3	● ●	○	△ cc ___				
4	● ●	○	△ cc ___				
5	● ●	○	△ cc ___				
6	● ●	○	△ cc ___				
7	● ●	○	△ cc ___				
8	● ●	○	△ cc ___				
9	● ●	○	△ cc ___				
10	● ●	○	△ cc ___				
11	● ●	○	△ cc ___				
TOTALS:							

— FIGURE 8-9 — Example of a record to monitor bladder and bowel functions in institutional settings. This type of record is especially useful for implementing and following the results of various training procedures and other treatment protocols. Reproduced with permission from Ouslander et al., 1986a.

TABLE 8-9   KEY ASPECTS OF AN INCONTINENT PATIENT'S PHYSICAL
EXAMINATION

Mobility and dexterity
   Functional status compatible with ability to self-toilet
   Gait disturbance (parkinsonism, normal-pressure hydrocephalus)
Mental status
   Cognitive function compatible with ability to self-toilet
   Motivation
   Mood and effect
Neurological
   Focal signs (especially in lower extremities)
   Signs of parkinsonism
   Sacral arc reflexes
Abdominal
   Bladder distension
   Suprapubic tenderness
   Lower abdominal mass
Rectal
   Perianal sensation
   Sphincter tone (resting and active)
   Impaction
   Masses
   Size and contour of prostate
Pelvic
   Perineal skin condition
   Perineal sensation
   Atrophic vaginitis (friability, inflammation, bleeding)
   Pelvic prolapse (ie, cystocele, rectocele; see Fig. 8-10)
   Pelvic mass
   Other anatomic abnormality
Other
   Lower extremity edema or signs of congestive heart failure (if nocturia is
   a prominent complaint)

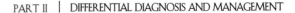

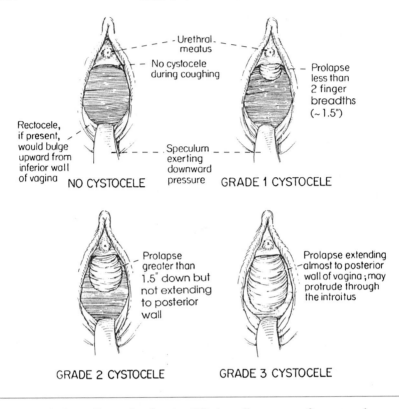

- - Urethral - - - -
meatus

– No cystocele
during coughing

– Prolapse
less than
2 finger
breadths
(~1.5")

Rectocele,
if present,
would bulge
upward from
inferior wall
of vagina   NO CYSTOCELE

.Speculum _ _ _ _ _
exerting
downward
pressure   GRADE 1 CYSTOCELE

Prolapse
greater than
1.5" down but
not extending
to posterior
wall

Prolapse extending
almost to posterior
wall of vagina; may
protrude through
the introitus

GRADE 2 CYSTOCELE   GRADE 3 CYSTOCELE

— FIGURE 8-10 — Example of a simplified grading system for cystoceles.

some degree of pelvic prolapse (eg, grade 1 or 2 cystocele as depicted in Fig. 8-10). Not all incontinent older women with these degrees of prolapse need gynecological evaluation (see below).

A clean urine sample should be collected for urinalysis. For men who are frequently incontinent, making a "clean-catch" specimen difficult to obtain, a clean specimen can be obtained using a condom catheter after cleaning the penis. For cognitively and functionally impaired women, a clean specimen can be obtained by cleaning the urethral and perineal area and having the patient void into a disinfected bedpan as an alternative to in-and-out catheterization. Persistent microscopic hematuria (>5 red blood cells per high-power field) in the absence of infection is an indication for further evaluation to exclude a tumor or other urinary tract pathology.

Because the prevalence of "asymptomatic bacteriuria" roughly parallels the prevalence of incontinence, incontinent geriatric patients commonly have significant bacteriuria. In the initial evaluation of incontinent noninstitutionalized patients, especially those in whom the incontinence is new or worsening, otherwise asymptomatic bacteriuria should be treated before further evaluation is undertaken. In the nursing home population, eradicating bacteriuria does not affect the severity of chronic, stable incontinence (Ouslander et al., 1995a). However, the new onset of incontinence, worsening incontinence, unexplained fever, and declines in mental and/or functional status may be the manifestations of a urinary tract infection in this population.

A PVR determination can be done either by catheterization or ultrasonogram to detect urinary retention, which cannot always be detected by physical examination. A portable ultrasonographic device that can detect significant residual urine is available (Verathon, Bothell, WA). Although the symptoms of incontinence associated with urinary retention can be nonspecific, and significant residual urine can be easily missed on physical examination, some elderly incontinent patients may not need a PVR before a trial of treatment. Examples of such patients include those with pure symptoms of stress incontinence, urge incontinence, or overactive bladder who have no symptoms of voiding difficulty and no risk factors or urinary retention (eg, diabetes, spinal cord disease).

Patients with residual volumes of more than 200 mL should be considered for further evaluation. The need for further evaluation in patients with lesser degrees of retention should be determined on an individual basis, considering the patient's symptoms and the degree to which they complain of straining or are observed to strain with voiding.

In older men, a noninvasive flow rate determination can be very helpful in screening for impaired bladder contractility or obstruction. Very low peak urinary flow rates (eg, < 10 m/s) after an adequate void (eg, > 150 mL) are suggestive of one of these conditions. Uroflowmeters are relatively inexpensive, but are rare in physicians' offices (except for urologists).

Further Evaluation

The need for further evaluation and the specific diagnostic procedures listed in Table 8-7 should be determined on an individual basis. Clinical practice guidelines state that not all incontinent geriatric patients require further evaluation. Patients who have unexplained polyuria should have their blood glucose and calcium levels determined. Patients with significant urinary retention should have renal function tests and be considered for renal ultrasound and urodynamic testing to determine whether obstruction, impaired bladder contractility, or both are present. Persistent microscopic hematuria in the absence of infection is an indication for urine cytology and urological evaluation, including cystoscopy. Even in the absence of hematuria, patients with the recent and sudden onset of irritative urinary symptoms who have risk factors for bladder cancer (heavy smoking, industrial exposure to aniline dyes) should be considered for these evaluations.

Women with marked pelvic prolapse (see Fig. 8-10) should be referred for gynecological evaluation.

Complex urodynamic testing is helpful in guiding treatment in selected patients, and is essential to determine the cause(s) of urinary retention and for any older patient for whom surgical intervention is being considered. Table 8-10 summarizes criteria for referral for further evaluation and Fig. 8-11 summarizes the overall approach to the evaluation of geriatric urinary incontinence.

TABLE 8-10   CRITERIA FOR CONSIDERING REFERRAL OF INCONTINENT PATIENTS FOR UROLOGICAL, GYNECOLOGICAL, OR URODYNAMIC EVALUATION

CRITERIA	DEFINITION	RATIONALE
History		
Recent history of lower urinary tract or pelvic surgery or irradiation	Surgery or irradiation involving the pelvic area or lower urinary tract within the past 6 months.	A structural abnormality relating to the recent procedure should be sought.
Recurrent symptomatic urinary tract infections	Two or more symptomatic episodes in a 12-month period.	A structural abnormality or or pathological condition in the urinary tract predisposing to infection should be excluded.
Risk factors for bladder cancer	Recent or sudden onset of irritative symptoms, history of heavy smoking, or exposure to aniline dyes.	Urine for cytology and cystoscopy to exclude bladder cancer should be considered.
Physical examination		
Marked pelvic prolapse	A prominent cystocele that descends the entire height of the vaginal vault with coughing during speculum examination.	Anatomic abnormality may underlie the pathophysiology of the incontinence, and selected patients may benefit from a pessary or surgical repair.

TABLE 8-10   CRITERIA FOR CONSIDERING REFERRAL OF INCONTINENT
             PATIENTS FOR UROLOGICAL, GYNECOLOGICAL, OR
             URODYNAMIC EVALUATION (*Continued*)

CRITERIA	DEFINITION	RATIONALE
Marked prostatic enlargement and/ or suspicion of cancer	Gross enlargement of the prostate on digital examination; prominent induration or asymmetry of the lobes.	An evaluation to exclude prostate cancer may be appropriate and have therapeutic implications.
Postvoid residual Difficulty passing a 14-F straight catheter	Impossible catheter passage, or passage requiring considerable force, or a larger, more rigid catheter.	Anatomic blockage of the urethra or bladder neck may be present.
Postvoid residual volume >200	Volume of urine remaining in the bladder within a few minutes after the patient voids spontaneously in as normal a fashion as possible.	Anatomic or neurogenic obstruction or poor bladder contractility may be present.
Urinalysis Hematuria	>5 red blood cells per high-power field on repeated microscopic examinations in the absence of infection.	A pathological condition in the urinary tract should be excluded.
Therapeutic trial Failure to respond	Persistent symptoms that are bothersome to the patient after adequate trials of behavioral and/or drug therapy.	Urodynamic evaluation may help guide specific therapy

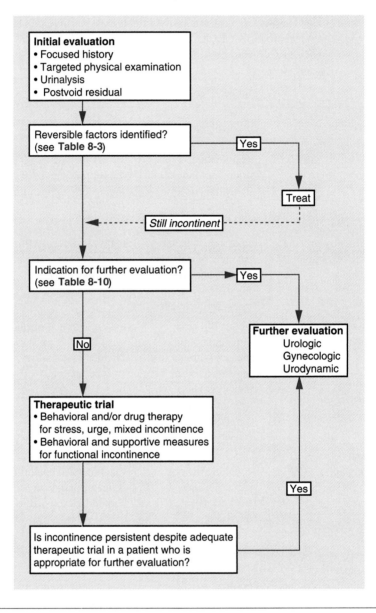

— FIGURE 8-11 — Algorithm protocol for evaluating incontinence.

MANAGEMENT

General Principles

Several evidenced-based reviews are available that can help clinicians manage incontinence in geriatric patients. Readers who are particularly interested in the evidence base are referred to these reviews for in-depth coverage of the issues (Fung et al., 2007; Shamliyan et al., 2008; Fonda et al., 2005; Holroyd-Leduc and Straus, 2006).

Several therapeutic modalities can be used in managing incontinent geriatric patients (Table 8-11). Treatment can be especially helpful if specific diagnoses are made and attention is paid to all factors that may be contributing to the incontinence in a given patient. Even when cure is not possible, the comfort and satisfaction of both patients and caregivers can almost always be enhanced.

Special attention should be given to the management of acute incontinence which is most common among older patients in acute care hospitals. Acute incontinence may be transient if managed appropriately; on the other hand, inappropriate management may lead to a permanent problem. The most common approach to incontinent geriatric patients in acute care hospitals is indwelling catheterization. In some instances, this is justified by the necessity for accurate measurement of urine output during the acute phase of an illness. In many instances, however, it is unnecessary and poses a substantial and unwarranted risk of catheter-induced infection. Although it may be more difficult and time consuming, making toilets and toilet substitutes accessible and combining this with some form of scheduled toileting is probably a more appropriate approach in patients who do not require indwelling catheterization. Launderable or disposable and highly absorbent bed pads and undergarments may also be helpful in managing these patients. These products may be more costly than catheters but probably result in less morbidity (and, therefore, overall cost) in the long run.

All of the potential reversible factors that can cause or contribute to incontinence (see Tables 8-3, 8-4, and 8-5) should be attended to in order to maximize the potential for regaining continence.

Supportive measures are critical in managing all forms of incontinence and should be used in conjunction with other, more specific treatment modalities. A positive attitude, education, environmental manipulations, appropriate use of toilet substitutes, avoidance of iatrogenic contributions to incontinence, modifications of diuretic and fluid intake patterns, and good skin care are all important.

TABLE 8-11   TREATMENT OPTIONS FOR GERIATRIC URINARY INCONTINENCE

Nonspecific supportive measures
    Education
    Modifications of fluid (eg, caffeine) and medication intake
    Use of toilet substitutes
    Environmental manipulations
    Garments and pads

Behavioral interventions (see Table 8-13)
    Patient dependent
        Pelvic muscle exercises
        Bladder training
        Bladder retraining (see Table 8-14)
    Caregiver dependent
        Scheduled toileting
        Habit training
        Prompted voiding (see Table 8-15)

Drugs (see Table 8-16)
    Bladder relaxants
    α-Antagonists
    α-Agonists
    Estrogen

Periurethral injections

Surgery
    Bladder neck suspension or sling
    Removal of obstruction or pathological lesion

Mechanical devices
    Penile clamps
    Artificial sphincters
    Sacral nerve stimulators

Catheters
    External
    Intermittent
    Indwelling

Specially designed incontinence undergarments and pads can be very helpful in many patients but must be used appropriately. They are marketed on television and are readily available in stores. Although they can be effective, several caveats should be noted:

1. Garments and pads are a nonspecific treatment. They should not be used as the first response to incontinence or before some type of diagnostic evaluation is done.
2. Many patients are curable if treated with specific therapies, and some have potentially serious factors underlying their incontinence that must be diagnosed and treated.
3. Underpants and pads can interfere with attempts at behavioral intervention and thereby foster dependency.
4. Many disposable products are relatively expensive and are not covered by Medicare or other insurance.

TABLE 8-12 PRIMARY TREATMENTS FOR DIFFERENT TYPES OF GERIATRIC URINARY INCONTINENCE

Type of Incontinence	Primary Treatments
Stress	Pelvic muscle (Kegel) exercises Other behavioral interventions (see Table 8-13) α-Adrenergic agonists Topical estrogen Periurethral injections Surgical bladder neck suspension or sling
Urge	Bladder relaxants Topical estrogen (if atrophic vaginitis present) Bladder training (including pelvic muscle exercises)
Overflow	Surgical removal of obstruction Bladder retraining (see Table 8-14) Intermittent catheterization Indwelling catheterization
Functional	Behavioral interventions (caregiver dependent; see Tables 8-13 and 8-15) Environmental manipulations Incontinence undergarments and pads

To a large extent the optimal treatment of persistent incontinence depends on identifying the type(s). Table 8-12 outlines the primary treatments for the basic types of persistent incontinence in the geriatric population. Each treatment modality is briefly discussed below. Behavioral interventions have been well studied in the geriatric population. These interventions are generally recommended by guidelines as an initial approach to therapy in many patients because they are generally noninvasive and nonspecific (ie, patients with stress and/or urge incontinence respond equally well).

Behavioral Interventions

Many types of behavioral interventions have been described for the management of urinary incontinence. The term bladder training has been used to encompass a wide variety of techniques. It is, however, important to distinguish between procedures that are patient dependent (ie, necessitate adequate function, learning capability, and motivation of the patient), in which the goal is to restore a normal pattern of voiding and continence, and procedures that are caregiver dependent that can be used for functionally disabled patients, in which the goal is to keep the patient and environment dry. Table 8-13 summarizes behavioral interventions. All of the patient-dependent procedures generally involve the patient's continuous self-monitoring, using a record such as the one depicted in Fig. 8-8; the caregiver-dependent procedures usually involve a record such as the one shown in Fig. 8-9.

Pelvic muscle (Kegel) exercises are an essential component of patient-dependent behavioral interventions. They have been shown to produce the greatest benefit in treating urinary incontinence (Shamliyan, 2008) These exercises consist of repetitive contractions and relaxations of the pelvic floor muscles. The exercises may be taught by having the patient interrupt voiding to get a sense of the muscles being used or by having women squeeze the examiner's fingers during a vaginal examination (without doing a Valsalva maneuver, which is the opposite of the intended effect). A randomized trial has documented that many young-old women (mean age in the mid to upper sixties) can be taught these exercises during an in-office examination and derive significant reductions in incontinence (Burgio et al., 2002). Many women, however, especially those older than age 75, require biofeedback to help them identify the muscles and practice the exercises. One full exercise is a 10-second squeeze and a 10-second relaxation. Most older women will have to build endurance gradually to this level. Once learned, the exercises should be practiced many times throughout the day (up to 40 exercises per day) and, importantly, should be used in everyday life during situations (eg, coughing, standing up, hearing running water) that might precipitate incontinence. Vaginal cones (weights) may be useful adjuncts to pelvic muscle exercises in some patients. Electrical stimulation may also be used to help identify and train pelvic muscles. This technique (using a different frequency of

TABLE 8-13   EXAMPLES OF BEHAVIORAL INTERVENTIONS FOR URINARY INCONTINENCE

PROCEDURE	DEFINITION	TYPES OF INCONTINENCE	COMMENTS
Patient dependent			
Pelvic muscle (Kegel) exercises	Repetitive contraction and relaxation of pelvic floor muscles	Stress and urge	Requires adequate function and motivation Biofeedback often helpful in teaching the exercise
Bladder training	Use of education, bladder records, pelvic muscle, and other behavioral techniques	Stress and urge	Requires trained therapist, adequate cognitive and physical functioning, and motivation
Bladder retraining	Progressive lengthening or shortening of intervoiding interval, with intermittent catheterization used in patients recovering from overdistention injuries with persistent retention (see Table 8-14)	Acute (eg, postcatheterization with urge or overflow, poststroke)	Goal is to restore normal pattern of voiding and continence Requires adequate cognitive and physical function and motivation

TABLE 8-13   EXAMPLES OF BEHAVIORAL INTERVENTIONS FOR URINARY INCONTINENCE (*Continued*)

PROCEDURE	DEFINITION	TYPES OF INCONTINENCE	COMMENTS
Caregiver dependent			
Scheduled toileting	Routine toileting at regular intervals (scheduled toileting)	Urge and functional	Goal is to prevent wetting episodes Can be used in patients with impaired cognitive or physical functioning Requires staff or caregiver's availability and motivation
Habit training	Variable toileting schedule based on patient's voiding patterns	Urge and functional	Goal is to prevent wetting episodes Can be used in patients with impaired cognitive or physical functioning Requires staff or caregiver's availability and motivation
Prompted voiding	Offer opportunity to toilet every 2 h during the day; toilet only on request; social reinforcement; routine offering of fluids (see Table 8-15)	Urge, stress, mixed, functional	Same as above 25%–40% of nursing home residents respond well during the day and can be identified during a 3-day trial (see text and Table 8-15)

stimulation) may also be useful in suppressing the involuntary bladder contractions associated with urge incontinence. Many older patients are reluctant to purchase the devices for a therapeutic trial.

Biofeedback can be very effective for teaching pelvic muscle exercises. It generally involves the use of vaginal (or rectal) pressure or electromyography (EMG) and abdominal muscle EMG recordings to train patients to contract pelvic floor muscles and relax the abdomen. Studies show that these techniques improve management of both stress and urge incontinence in the geriatric population. Numerous software packages are now available to assist with biofeedback training.

Other forms of patient-dependent interventions include bladder training and bladder retraining. Bladder training involves education, pelvic muscle exercises (with or without biofeedback), strategies to manage urgency, and the regular use of bladder records (see Fig. 8-8). Bladder training is highly effective in selected community-dwelling patients, especially those who are motivated and functional.

Table 8-14 provides an example of a bladder retraining protocol. This protocol is applicable to patients who have had indwelling catheterization for monitoring of urinary output during a period of acute illness or for treatment of urinary retention with overflow incontinence. Such catheters should be removed as soon as possible, and this type of bladder retraining protocol should enable most indwelling catheters to be removed from patients in acute care hospitals as well as some in long-term care settings. A patient who continues to have difficulty voiding after 1 to 2 weeks of bladder retraining should be examined for other potentially reversible causes of voiding difficulties, such as those mentioned in the preceding discussion of acute incontinence. When difficulties persist, a urological referral should be considered in order to rule out correctable lower genitourinary pathology.

The goal of caregiver-dependent interventions is to prevent incontinence episodes rather than to restore normal patterns of voiding and complete continence. Such procedures are effective in reducing incontinence in selected nursing home residents (Ouslander et al., 1995b; Ouslander et al., 2005). In its simplest form, scheduled toileting involves toileting the patient at regular intervals, usually every 2 hours during the day and every 4 hours during the evening and night. Habit training involves a schedule of toiletings or prompted voidings that is modified according to the patient's pattern of continent voids and incontinence episodes as demonstrated by a monitoring record such as that shown in Fig. 8-9. Adjunctive techniques to prompt voiding (eg, running tap water, stroking the inner thigh, or suprapubic tapping) and to facilitate complete emptying of the bladder (eg, bending forward after completion of voiding) may be helpful in some patients. Prompted voiding has been the best studied of these procedures. Table 8-15 provides an example of a prompted voiding protocol. Up to 40% of incontinent nursing home residents may be essentially dry during the day with a consistent prompted voiding program (Ouslander et al., 1995b). The success of these interventions is largely dependent on the knowledge and motivation of the caregivers who are implementing them, rather than on the physical functional and

TABLE 8-14   EXAMPLE OF A BLADDER RETRAINING PROTOCOL

Objective: To restore a normal pattern of voiding and continence after the removal of an indwelling catheter

1. Remove the indwelling catheter (clamping the catheter before removal is not necessary)

2. Treat urinary tract infection if present

3. Initiate a toileting schedule. Begin by toileting the patient:
   a. Upon awakening
   b. Every 2 h during the day and evening
   c. Before getting into bed
   d. Every 4 h at night

4. Monitor the patient's voiding and continence pattern with a record that allows for the recording of:
   a. Frequency, timing, and amount of continent voids
   b. Frequency, timing, and amount of incontinence episodes
   c. Fluid intake pattern
   d. Postvoid catheter volume

5. If the patient is having difficulty voiding (complete urinary retention or very low urine outputs, eg, 240 mL in an 8-h period while fluid intake is adequate):
   a. Perform in-and-out catheterization, recording volume obtained, every 6-8 h until residual values are 200 mL
   b. Instruct the patient on techniques to trigger voiding (eg, running water, stroking inner thigh, suprapubic tapping) and to help completely empty bladder (eg, bending forward, suprapubic pressure, double voiding)
   c. If the patient continues to have high residual volumes after 1-2 weeks, consider urodynamic evaluation

6. If the patient is voiding frequently (ie, more often than every 2 h):
   a. Perform postvoid residual determination to ensure the patient is completely emptying the bladder
   b. Encourage the patient to delay voiding as long as possible and instruct them to use techniques to help completely empty bladder
   c. If the patient continues to have frequency and nocturia with or without urgency and incontinence:
      1. Rule out other reversible causes (eg, urinary tract infection medication effects, hyperglycemia, and congestive heart failure)
      2. Consider further evaluation to rule out other pathology

TABLE 8-15   EXAMPLE OF A PROMPTED VOIDING PROTOCOL FOR A NURSING HOME

Assessment period (3-5 days)

1. Contact resident every hour from 7 AM to 7 PM for 2-3 days, then every 2 h for 2-3 days
2. Focus attention on voiding by asking them whether they are wet or dry
3. Check residents for wetness, record results on bladder record, and give feedback on whether response was correct or incorrect
4. Whether wet or dry, ask residents if they would like to use the toilet or urinal. If they say yes:
   • Offer assistance
   • Record results on bladder record
   • Give positive reinforcement by spending extra time talking with them

   If they say no:
   • Repeat the question once or twice
   • Inform them that you will be back in 1 h and request that they try to delay voiding until then
   • If there has been no attempt to void in the last 2-3 h, repeat the request to use the toilet at least twice more before leaving
5. Offer fluids

Targeting

1. Prompted voiding is more effective in some residents than others
2. The best candidates are residents who show the following characteristics during the assessment period:
   • Void in the toilet, commode, or urinal (as opposed to being incontinent in a pad or garment) more than two-thirds of the time
   • Wet on ≤ 20% of checks
   • Show substantial reduction in incontinence frequency on 2-hour prompts
3. Residents who do not show any of these characteristics may be candidates for either:
   • Further evaluation to determine the specific type of incontinence if they attempt to toilet but remain frequently wet
   • Supportive management by padding and adult diapers, and a checking-and-changing protocol if they do not cooperate with prompting

Prompted voiding (ongoing protocol)

1. Contact the resident every 2 h from 7 AM to 7 PM
2. Use same procedures as for the assessment period
3. For nighttime management, use either modified prompted voiding schedule or padding, depending on resident's sleep pattern and preferences
4. If a resident who has been responding well has an increase in incontinence frequency despite adequate staff implementation of the protocol, the resident should be evaluated for reversible factors

mental status of the incontinent patient. Targeting of prompted voiding to selected patients after a 3-day trial (see Table 8-15) may enhance its cost-effectiveness.

Toileting at night should be individualized, because prompted voiding and other similar interventions can disrupt sleep. Many frail patients are managed supportively at night with pads and adults diapers. This type of supportive management is appropriate for incontinent patients whose sleep is not disrupted and whose skin is not irritated. Quality improvement methods, based on principles of industrial statistical quality control, have been shown to be helpful in maintaining the effectiveness of prompted voiding in nursing homes (Ouslander, 2007). However, unless adequate staffing, training, and administrative support for the program persist, the effectiveness of prompted voiding will not be maintained in an institutional setting.

Drug Treatment

Table 8-16 lists the drugs used to treat various types of incontinence.

Several clinical trials show that the efficacy of drug treatment in the geriatric population is similar to that in younger populations. Drug treatment can be prescribed in conjunction with various behavioral interventions (Burgio et al., 1998; Ouslander et al., 1995c). Treatment decisions should be individualized and will depend in large part on the characteristics and preferences of the patient (including risks and costs) and the preference of the health-care professional.

For urge incontinence, antimuscarinic drugs with anticholinergic and relaxant effects on the bladder smooth muscle are used. All of them have proven efficacy in older patients, but they can have bothersome systemic anticholinergic side effects, especially dry mouth and constipation. Dry mouth can be relieved by small sips of water, hard candy, or over-the-counter oral lubricants. Constipation can be managed proactively (see section at end of chapter). Patients should be warned about exacerbation of gastroesophageal reflux and glaucoma. Although open-angle glaucoma is not an absolute contraindication, patients being treated for glaucoma should be instructed to consult their ophthalmologist before initiating treatment.

All antimuscarinic drugs have anticholinergic properties and can theoretically cause problems with memory and other central nervous system side effects. Many older incontinent patients with urge incontinence or overactive bladder have memory loss or early dementia and are already on cholinesterase inhibitors. In these patients, the decision to add an antimuscarinic for the bladder must be based on careful weighing of the bother of the symptoms versus the potential risks of the drugs (Kay et al., 2005).

The maximum effect of antimuscarinic drugs may not be achieved for up to 1 to 2 months. Patients should therefore be educated so that they do not have unrealistic expectations about a quick cure and complete dryness. In order to maximize adherence, they should be told that many patients benefit from these drugs,

TABLE 8-16 DRUG TREATMENT FOR URINARY INCONTINENCE AND OVERACTIVE BLADDER

DRUGS	DOSAGES	MECHANISMS OF ACTION	TYPE OF INCONTINENCE	POTENTIAL COMMON ADVERSE EFFECTS
Antimuscarinic				
Darifenacin	7.5-15 mg daily	Increase bladder capacity and diminish involuntary bladder contractions	Urge or mixed with urge predominant	Dry mouth, constipation, blurry vision, elevated intraocular pressure, cognitive impairment, delirium
			Overactive bladder with incontinence	
Oxybutynin				
Short-acting	2.5-5 mg tid			
Long-acting	5-30 mg daily			
Transdermal	3.9 mg patch changed after each 3 days			
Solifenacin	5-10 mg daily			
Tolterodine				
Short-acting	2 mg bid			
Long-acting	4 mg daily			
Trospium				
Short-acting	20 mg bid			
Long-acting	60 mg daily			

TABLE 8-16   DRUG TREATMENT FOR URINARY INCONTINENCE AND OVERACTIVE BLADDER (*Continued*)

DRUGS	DOSAGES	MECHANISMS OF ACTION	TYPE OF INCONTINENCE	POTENTIAL COMMON ADVERSE EFFECTS
α-Adrenergic agonists		Relax smooth muscle of urethra and prostatic capsule	Urge incontinence and related irritative symptoms associated with benign prostatic enlargement	Postural hypotension
Alfuzosin	10 mg qd		May be more effective in combination with an antimuscarinic drug	
Doxazosin	1-8 mg qd			
Tamsulosin	0.4 mg qd			
Terazosin	1-10 mg qhs			
α-Adrenergic antagonists*				
Pseudoephedrine	30-60 mg tid or 60-120 mg, long acting	Stimulates contraction of urethral smooth muscle	Stress	Headache, tachycardia, elevation of blood pressure
Duloxetine	20-40 mg daily	Increases α-adrenergic tone to the urethra		Nausea

Topical estrogen†				
Topical cream	0.5-1.0 g/day for 2 weeks, then twice weekly	Strengthen periurethral tissues	Urge associated with severe vaginal atrophy or atrophic vaginitis	Local irritation
Vaginal estradiol ring	One ring every 3 months	Increase periurethral blood flow	Stress	
Vaginal tablets	One 25 µg tablet per day for 2 weeks, then twice weekly			
Arginine vasopressin‡				
DDAVP oral	0.1-0.4 mg at night	Prevents water loss from the kidney	Nocturia that is bothersome and does not respond to other treatments	Hyponatremia (serum sodium must be monitored closely at the onset of treatment)
Nasal spray	10-20 µg of nasal spray in each nostril at night			Flushing, nausea, rhinitis

TABLE 8-16 DRUG TREATMENT FOR URINARY INCONTINENCE AND OVERACTIVE BLADDER (*Continued*)

DRUGS	DOSAGES	MECHANISMS OF ACTION	TYPE OF INCONTINENCE	POTENTIAL COMMON ADVERSE EFFECTS
Cholinergic agonist[§]				
Bethanechol	10-30 mg tid	Stimulate bladder contraction	Acute incontinence associated with incomplete bladder emptying in the absence of obstruction	Bradycardia, hypotension, bronchoconstriction, gastric acid secretion, diarrhea

* α-Adrenergic agonists are not approved by the US Food and Drug Administration for this indication.
† Topical estrogen alone is not effective in relieving symptoms and should be considered an adjunctive treatment. There is also evidence that estrogen (given orally) may worsen incontinence in some women (Hendrix et al., 2005).
‡ DDAVP is not approved by the US Food and Drug Administration for this indication.
§ Bethanechol may be helpful in selected patients after an episode of acute urinary retention; there is no evidence that it is useful on a chronic basis.

some are cured, and that it may take a couple of months to achieve the desired effect. As with many other therapeutic agents, some patients respond to one drug better than others in the same class, so patients who are bothered and not responsive to one drug could be given a trial of another.

Among older men, symptoms of overactive bladder, including urge incontinence, overlap with the irritative symptoms of benign prostate hyperplasia (BPH). Men with large prostate glands (eg, > 40 g) may benefit from a 5-α reductase inhibitor. α-Adrenergic blockers (listed in Table 8-16) are effective for many older men for lower urinary tract symptoms associated with BPH, but must be used carefully because of their potential to cause postural hypotension, especially among men already on cardiovascular medications. Alfuzosin and tamsulosin may have less effect on blood pressure than other α-blockers, but still must be used carefully in the elderly. There is now good evidence that combining an α-blocker with an antimuscarinic drug is more efficacious than either alone, and that the incidence of significant urinary retention with combination is very low (Kaplan et al., 2006).

Carefully selected patients with bothersome nocturia and/or nocturnal incontinence may benefit from a careful trial of intranasal arginine vasopressin (DDAVP) (Table 8-16). However, the incidence of hyponatremia with this agent is very high in the elderly, and treated patients must be carefully monitored for its development. Currently this would be an off-label use of this drug.

For stress incontinence, there are no drug treatments approved by the US Food and Drug Administration (FDA). If drug treatment is considered, it usually involves a combination of an α-agonist and estrogen. Drug treatment is appropriate for motivated patients who have mild to moderate degrees of stress incontinence, do not have a major anatomic abnormality (eg, grade 3 cystocele or ISD), and do not have any contraindications to these drugs. Pseudoephedrine is contraindicated in elderly patients with hypertension. Duloxetine, a selective serotonin uptake inhibitor (SSRI) antidepressant, increases α-adrenergic tone to the lower urinary tract through a spinal cord mechanism. It is approved in some countries for the treatment of stress incontinence. Neither pseudoephedrine nor duloxetine is FDA approved for stress incontinence and would be used off label for this indication. Patients with stress incontinence may also respond to concomitant behavioral interventions, as described above.

For stress incontinence, estrogen alone is not as effective as it is in combination with an α-agonist. Estrogen is also used for the treatment of irritative voiding symptoms and urge incontinence in women with atrophic vaginitis and urethritis. Oral estrogen is not as effective as topical estrogen for these symptoms. Vaginal estrogen can be prescribed five nights per week for 1 to 2 months initially and then reduced to a maintenance dose of one to three times per week. A vaginal ring that slowly releases estradiol and vaginal tables is also available. Recent data suggest that oral (not topical) estrogen may actually worsen incontinence in some women (Henderix et al., 2005).

Drug treatment for chronic overflow incontinence using a cholinergic agonist or an α-adrenergic antagonist is rarely efficacious. Bethanechol may be helpful when given for a brief period subcutaneously in patients with persistent bladder contractility problems after an overdistention injury, but it is seldom effective when given over the long term orally. α-Adrenergic blockers may be helpful in relieving symptoms associated with outflow obstruction in some patients but are probably not efficacious for long-term treatment of overflow incontinence.

Surgery

Surgery should be considered for older women with stress incontinence that continues to be bothersome after attempts at nonsurgical treatment and in women with a significant degree of pelvic prolapse or ISD. As with many other surgical procedures, patient selection and the experience of the surgeon are critical to success. All women being considered for surgical therapy should have a thorough evaluation, including urodynamic tests, before undergoing the procedure.

Women with mixed stress incontinence and detrusor motor instability may also benefit from surgery, especially if the clinical history and urodynamic findings suggest that stress incontinence is the predominant problem. Many modified techniques of bladder neck suspension can be done with minimal risk and are successful in achieving continence over about a 5-year period. Urinary retention can occur after surgery, but it is usually transient and can be managed by a brief period of suprapubic catheterization. Recent data suggest that a fascial sling is more efficacious than a Burch culposuspension, but it is also associated with more postoperative complications (Albo et al., 2007). Periurethral injection of collagen and other materials is now available and may offer patients with ISD an alternative to surgery.

Surgery may be indicated in men in whom incontinence is associated with anatomically and/or urodynamically documented outflow obstruction. Men who have experienced an episode of complete urinary retention without any clear precipitant are likely to have another episode within a short period of time and should have a prostatic resection, as should men with incontinence associated with a sufficient amount of residual urine to be causing recurrent symptomatic infections or hydronephrosis. The decision about surgery in men who do not meet these criteria must be an individual one, weighing carefully the degree to which the symptoms bother the patient, the potential benefits of surgery (obstructive symptoms often respond better than irritative symptoms), and the risks of surgery, which may be minimal with newer prostate resection techniques. A small number of older patients, especially men who have stress incontinence related to sphincter damage caused by previous transurethral surgery, may benefit from the surgical implantation of an artificial urinary sphincter.

Catheters and Catheter Care

Catheters should be avoided in managing incontinence, unless specific indications are present. Three basic types of catheters and catheterization procedures are used for the management of urinary incontinence: external catheters, intermittent straight catheterization, and chronic indwelling catheterization.

External catheters generally consist of some type of condom connected to a drainage system. Improvements in design and observance of proper procedure and skin care when applying the catheter will decrease the risk of skin irritation as well as the frequency with which the catheter falls off. Patients with external catheters are at increased risk of developing symptomatic infection. External catheters should be used only to manage intractable incontinence in male patients who do not have urinary retention and who are extremely physically dependent. As with incontinence undergarments and padding, these devices should not be used as a matter of convenience, since they may foster dependency.

Intermittent catheterization can help in the management of patients with urinary retention and overflow incontinence because of an acontractile bladder or DHIC. The procedure can be carried out by either the patient or a caregiver and involves straight catheterization two to four times daily, depending on catheter urine volumes and patient tolerance. In general, bladder volume should be kept to less than 400 mL. In the home setting, the catheter should be kept clean (but not necessarily sterile).

Intermittent catheterization may be useful for certain patients in acute care hospitals and nursing homes, for example, following removal of an indwelling catheter in a bladder retraining protocol (see Table 8-14). Nursing home residents, however, may be difficult to catheterize, and the anatomic abnormalities commonly found in older patients' lower urinary tracts may increase the risk of infection as a consequence of repeated straight catheterizations. In addition, using this technique in an institutional setting (which may have an abundance of organisms that are relatively resistant to many commonly used antimicrobial agents) may yield an unacceptable risk of nosocomial infections, and using sterile catheter trays for these procedures would be very expensive; thus, it may be extremely difficult to implement such a program in a typical nursing home setting.

Indwelling catheterization is overused in acute hospital settings and increases the incidence of a number of complications, including chronic bacteriuria, bladder stones, periurethral abscesses, and even bladder cancer with long-term use. Nursing home residents, especially men, managed by chronic catheterization are at relatively high risk of developing symptomatic infections. Given these risks, it seems appropriate to recommend that the use of chronic indwelling catheters be limited to certain specific situations (Table 8-17). When indwelling catheterization is used, certain principles of catheter care should be observed in order to attempt to minimize complications (Table 8-18).

TABLE 8-17   INDICATIONS FOR CHRONIC INDWELLING CATHETER USE

Urinary retention that
  Is causing persistent overflow incontinence, symptomatic infections, or renal dysfunction
  Cannot be corrected surgically or medically
  Cannot be managed practically with intermittent catheterization

Skin wounds, pressure ulcers, or irritations that are being contaminated by incontinent urine

Care of terminally ill or severely impaired patients for whom bed and clothing changes are uncomfortable or disruptive

Preference of patient when toileting or changing cause excessive discomfort

TABLE 8-18   KEY PRINCIPLES OF CHRONIC INDWELLING CATHETER CARE

1. Maintain sterile, closed gravity-drainage system
2. Avoid breaking the closed system
3. Use clean techniques in emptying and changing the drainage system; wash hands between patients in institutionalized setting
4. Secure the catheter to the upper thigh or lower abdomen to avoid perineal contamination and urethral irritation because of movement of the catheter
5. Avoid frequent and vigorous cleaning of the catheter entry site; washing with soapy water once per day is sufficient
6. Do not routinely irrigate
7. If bypassing occurs in the absence of obstruction, consider the possibility of a bladder spasm which can be treated with a bladder relaxant
8. If catheter obstruction occurs frequently, increase the patient's fluid intake and acidify the urine with dilute acetic acid irrigations
9. Do not routinely use prophylactic or suppressive urinary antiseptics or antimicrobials
10. Do not do surveillance cultures to guide management of individual patients because all chronically catheterized patients have bacteriuria (which is often polymicrobial) and the organisms change frequently
11. Do not treat infection unless the patient develops symptoms; symptoms may be nonspecific and other possible sources of infection should be carefully excluded before attributing symptoms to the urinary tract
12. If a patient develops frequent symptomatic urinary tract infections, a genitourinary evaluation should be considered to rule out pathology such as stones, periurethral or prostatic abscesses, and chronic pyelonephritis

FECAL INCONTINENCE

Fecal incontinence is less common than urinary incontinence. Its occurrence is relatively unusual in older patients who are continent with regard to urine; however, a large proportion (30%-50%) of geriatric patients with frequent urinary incontinence also have episodes of fecal incontinence, especially in the nursing home population. This coexistence suggests common pathophysiological mechanisms. Several evidence-based reviews are now available on this topic (Shamliyan et al., 2008; Wald, 2007; Fonda et al., 2005).

Defecation, like urination, is a physiological process that involves smooth and striated muscles, central and peripheral innervation, coordination of reflex responses, mental awareness, and physical ability to get to a toilet. Disruption of any of these factors can lead to fecal incontinence. The most common causes of fecal incontinence are problems with constipation and laxative use, unrecognized lactose intolerance, neurological disorders, and colorectal disorders (Table 8-19). Constipation is extremely common in the geriatric population and, when chronic, can lead to fecal impaction and incontinence. The hard stool (or scybalum) of fecal impaction irritates the rectum and results in the production of mucus and fluid. This fluid leaks around the mass of impacted stool and precipitates incontinence. Constipation is difficult to define; technically it indicates less than three bowel movements per week, although many patients use the term to describe difficult passage of hard stools or a feeling of incomplete evacuation (Lembo and Camilleri, 2003). Poor dietary and toilet habits, immobility,

TABLE 8-19   CAUSES OF FECAL INCONTINENCE

Fecal impaction

Laxative overuse or abuse

Neurological disorders
  Dementia
  Stroke
  Spinal cord disease/injury

Colorectal disorders
  Diarrheal illnesses
  Lactose intolerance
  Diabetic autonomic neuropathy
  Rectal sphincter damage

TABLE 8-20   CAUSES OF CONSTIPATION

Diet low in bulk and fluid

Poor toilet habits

Immobility

Laxative abuse

Colorectal disorders
     Colonic tumor, stricture, volvulus
     Painful anal and rectal conditions (hemorrhoids, fissures)

Depression

Drugs
     Anticholinergic
     Narcotic

Diabetic autonomic neuropathy

Endocrine or metabolic
     Hypothyroidism
     Hypercalcemia
     Hypokalemia

and chronic laxative abuse are the most common causes of constipation in geriatric patients (Table 8-20).

Appropriate management of constipation will prevent fecal impaction and resultant fecal incontinence. The first step in managing constipation is the identification of all possible contributory factors. If the constipation is a new complaint and represents a recent change in bowel habit, then colonic disease, endocrine or metabolic disorders, depression, or drug side effects should be considered (see Table 8-19).

Proper diet, including adequate fluid intake and bulk, is important in preventing constipation. Crude fiber in amounts of 4 to 6 g/day (equivalent to three or four tablespoons of bran) is generally recommended. Improving mobility, positioning of body during toileting, and the timing and setting of toileting are all important in managing constipation.

Defecation should optimally take place in a private, unrushed atmosphere and should take advantage of the gastrocolic reflex, which occurs a few minutes after eating. These factors are often overlooked, especially in nursing home settings.

TABLE 8-21   DRUGS USED TO TREAT CONSTIPATION

Type	Examples	Mechanism of Action
Stool softeners and lubricants	Dioctyl sodium succinate Mineral oil	Soften and lubricate fecal mass
Bulk-forming agents	Bran Psyllium mucilloid	Increase fecal bulk and retain fluid in bowel lumen
Osmotic cathartics	Milk of magnesia Magnesium sulfate/ citrate Lactulose Sorbitol	Poorly absorbed and retain fluid in bowel lumen; increase net secretions of fluid in small intestine
Stimulants and irritants	Cascara Senna Bisacodyl Phyenolphthalein	Alter intestinal mucosal permeability; stimulate muscle activity and fluid secretions
Enemas	Tap water Saline Sodium phosphate Oil	Induce reflex evacuations
Suppositories	Glycerin Bisacodyl	Cause mucosal irritation

A variety of drugs can be used to treat constipation (Table 8-21). These drugs are often overused; in fact, their overuse may cause an atonic colon and contribute to chronic constipation ("cathartic colon").

Laxative drugs can also contribute to fecal incontinence. Rational use of these drugs necessitates knowing the nature of the constipation and quality of the stool. For example, stool softeners will not help a patient with a large mass of already soft stool in the rectum. These patients would benefit from glycerin or irritant suppositories. The use of osmotic and irritant laxatives should be limited to no more than three or four times a week.

Fecal incontinence from neurological disorders is sometimes amenable to pelvic floor muscle training, although most severely demented patients are unable to cooperate. For those patients with end-stage dementia who fail to respond to a regular toileting program and suppositories, a program of alternating constipating agents (if necessary) and laxatives on a routine schedule (such as giving laxatives or enemas three times a week) is often effective in controlling defecation.

Experience suggests that these measures should permit management of even severely demented patients. As a last resort, specially designed incontinence undergarments are sometimes helpful in managing fecal incontinence and preventing complications. Frequent changing is essential, because fecal material, especially in the presence of incontinent urine, can cause skin irritation and predispose to pressure ulcers.

EVIDENCE SUMMARY

Do's

- Assess for correctable underlying causes of overactive bladder and incontinence by history and targeted physical examination.
- Manage constipation.
- Utilize education and simple behavioral interventions for all incontinent patients.
- Follow symptomatic response and satisfaction with treatment after a 4- to 6-week period to determine the need to adjust the treatment plan.

Don'ts

- Send all patients for specialist consultation or urodynamics.
- Automatically prescribe medication for all older patients with symptoms of overactive bladder and incontinence.
- Prescribe oral estrogen.

Consider

- Referring selected patients for further urologic, gynecologic, and/or urodynamic evaluation.
- A trial of pharmacologic therapy for older patients with overactive bladder and urge incontinence.
- Antimuscarinic agent for women.

References

Albo ME, Richter HE, Brubaker L, et al. Burch colposuspension versus fascial sling to reduce urinary stress incontinence. *N Engl J Med.* 2007;356:2143-2155.

American Medical Directors Association. *Urinary Incontinence: Clinical Practice Guideline.* Columbia, MD: AMDA; 2006.

Appell RA. Clinical efficacy and safety of tolterodine in the treatment of overactive bladder: a pooled analysis. *Urology.* 1997;50(suppl 6A):90-96.

Burgio KL, Locher JL, Goode PS, et al. Behavioral vs. drug treatment for urge urinary incontinence in older women. *JAMA.* 1998;280(23):1995-2000.

Burgio KL, Goode PS, Locher JL, et al. Behavioral training with and without biofeedback in the treatment of urge incontinence in older women. *JAMA.* 2002;288(18):2293-2299.

Elbadawi A, Yalla SV, Resnick N. Structural basis of geriatric voiding dysfunction: I. Methods of a prospective ultrastructural/urodynamic study and an overview of the findings. *J Urol.* 1993;150:1650-1656.

Fantl JA, Newman DK, Colling J, et al. *Urinary Incontinence in Adults: Acute and Chronic Management.* Clinical Practice Guideline No. 2, 1996, Update (AHCPR Publication No. 96-0682). Rockville, MD: US Department of Health and Human Services, Public Health Service, Agency for Health Care Policy and Research; 1996.

Fonda D, DuBeau CE, Harari MD, et al. Incontinence in the frail elderly. In: Abrams P, Cardozo L, Khoury S, et al, eds. *Incontinence.* Paris, France: Health Publications Ltd; 2005;1165-1239.

Fung CH, Spencer B, Eslami M, et al. Quality indicators for the screening and care of urinary incontinence in vulnerable elders. *J Am Geriatr Soc.* 2007;55:S443-S449.

Hendrix SL, Cochrane BB, Nygaar IE, et al. Effects of estrogen with and without progestin on urinary incontinence. *JAMA.* 2005;293:935-948.

Holroyd-Leduc JM, Straus SE. Management of urinary incontinence in women. *JAMA.* 2004;291:986-995.

Kaplan SA, Roehrborn CG, Rovner ES, et al. Tolterodine and tamsulosin for treatment of men with lower urinary tract symptoms and overactive bladder. *JAMA.* 2006;296: 2319-2328.

Kay GG, Abou-Donia MB, Messer WS, et al. Antimuscarinic drugs for overactive bladder and their potential effects on cognitive function in older patients. *J Am Geriatr Soc.* 2005;53:2195-2201.

Lembo A, Camilleri M. Chronic constipation. *N Engl J Med.* 2003;349:1360-1368.

Ouslander JG, Uman GC, Urman HN. Development and testing of an incontinence monitoring record. *J Am Geriatr Soc.* 1986a;34:83-90.

Ouslander JG, Schapira M, Schnelle J, et al. Does eradicating bacteriuria affect the severity of chronic urinary incontinence among nursing home residents? *Ann Intern Med.* 1995a;122:749-754.

Ouslander JG, Schnelle JF, Uman G, et al. Predictors of successful prompted voiding among incontinent nursing home residents. *JAMA.* 1995a;273:1366-1370.

Ouslander JG, Schnelle JF, Uman G, et al. Does oxybutynin add to the effectiveness of prompted voiding for urinary incontinence among nursing home residents? A placebo-controlled trial. *J Am Geriatr Soc.* 1995c;43:610-617.

Ouslander JG. Management of overactive bladder. *N Engl J Med.* 2004;350:786-799.

Ouslander JG, Griffiths PC, McConnell E, et al. Functional incidental training: a randomized, controlled, crossover trial in Veterans Affairs nursing homes. *J Am Geriatr Soc.* 2005; 53:1091-1100.

Ouslander JG. Quality improvement initiatives for urinary incontinence in nursing homes. *J Am Med Dir Assoc.* 2007;8:S6-S11.

Resnick NM, Yalla SV. Detrusor hyperactivity with impaired contractile function: an unrecognized but common cause of incontinence in elderly patients. *JAMA.* 1987;257:3076-3081.

Shamliyan T, Wyman J, Bliss DZ, et al. *Prevention of Fecal and Urinary Incontinence in Adults.* Evidence Report/Technology Assessment. AHRQ Publication No. 08-8003. Rockville, MD: Agency for Healthcare Research and Quality; December, 2007.

Wald A. Fecal incontinence in adults. *N Engl J Med.* 2007;356:1648-1655.

Suggested Readings

Andersson KE. LUTS treatment: future treatment options. *Neurourol Urodyn.* 2007; 26:934-947.

Barry MJ. A 73-year-old man with symptomatic benign prostatic hyperplasia. *JAMA.* 1997;287(24):2178-2184.

Brown JS, Vittinghoff E, Wyman JF, et al. Urinary incontinence: does it increase risk for falls and fractures? *J Am Geriatr Soc.* 2000;48:721-725.

Gibbs CF, Johnson TM II, Ouslander JG. Office management of geriatric urinary incontinence. *Am J Med.* 2007;120:211-220.

Ouslander JG, ed. Aging and the lower urinary tract. *Am J Med Sci.* 1997;314(4):214-218.

Ouslander JG, Maloney C, Grasela TH, et al. Implementation of a nursing home urinary incontinence management program with and without tolterodine. *J Am Med Dir Assoc.* 2001;2:207-214.

Ouslander JG, Schnelle JF. Incontinence in the nursing home. *Ann Intern Med.* 1995; 122:438-449.

Pfisterer MHD, Griffiths DJ, Schaefer W, et al. The effect of age on lower urinary tract function: a study in women. *J Am Geriatr Soc.* 2006;54:405-412.

Saigal CS. Quality indicators for benign prostatic hyperplasia in vulnerable elders. *J Am Geriatr Soc.* 2007;55:S2-S257.

Skelly J, Flint AJ. Urinary incontinence associated with dementia. *J Am Geriatr Soc.* 1995;42:286-294.

Taylor III JA, Kuchel GA. Detrusor underactivity: clinical features and pathogenesis of an underdiagnosed geriatric condition. *J Am Geriatr Soc.* 2006;54:1920-1932.

Yoshimura N, Chancellor MB. Current and future pharmacological treatment for overactive bladder. *J Urol.* 2002;168:1897-1913.

Selected Web Sites (Accessed on March 16, 2008)

http://www.nafc.org/
http://www.simonfoundation.org/

http://www.urinary-incontinence.org/
http://www.healthinaging.org/agingintheknow/chapters_ch_trial.asp?ch=20
α-Blocker with or without an antimuscarinic for men
Tools
Assessment—General
http://www.ofmq.com/Websites/ofmq/Images/INCONTINENCE_ASSESSMENT.pdf.
   (Accessed on April 12, 2008)
http://www.woundcarestrategies.com/shop/forms/UIAT%20SAMPLE.pdf
(Accessed on April 12, 2008)
Assessment for Women
http://www.stressui.org/clinical_tools.htm (Accessed on April 12, 2008)
Assessment for Men
http://www.bphtreatment.org/auasymptomindex.html (Accessed on April 12, 2008)

CHAPTER 9

FALLS

Falls are among the major cause of morbidity in the geriatric population. Close to one-third of those aged 65 years and older living at home suffer a fall each year. Among nursing homes residents, as many as half suffer a fall each year; 10% to 25% cause serious injuries. Accidents are the fifth leading cause of death in persons older than age 65, and falls account for two-thirds of these accidental deaths. Of deaths from falls in the United States, more than 70% occur in the population older than age 65. Fear of falling can adversely affect older persons' functional status and overall quality of life. Repeated falls and consequent injuries can be important factors in the decision to institutionalize an elderly person.

Table 9-1 lists potential complications of falls. Fractures of the hip, femur, humerus, wrist, and ribs and painful soft tissue injuries are the most frequent physical complications. Many of these injuries will result in hospitalization, with the attendant risks of immobilization and iatrogenic illnesses (see Chap. 10). Fractures of the hip and lower extremities often lead to prolonged disability because of impaired mobility. A less common, but important, injury is subdural hematoma. Neurological symptoms and signs that develop days to weeks after a fall should prompt consideration of this treatable problem.

Even when the fall does not result in serious injury, substantial disability may result from fear of falling, loss of self-confidence, and restricted ambulation (either self-imposed or imposed by caregivers).

A growing body of studies suggests that at least some falls can be prevented (see below). Moreover, it is possible to prevent the untoward consequences of falls (ie, fractures) by changing the way old people fall. The potential for prevention together with the use of falling as an indicator of underlying frailty combine to make an understanding of the causes of falls and a practical approach to the evaluation and management of patients with instability and falls important components of geriatric care. Similar to many other conditions in the geriatric population, factors that can contribute to or cause falls are multiple, and very often more than one of these factors plays an important role (Fig. 9-1).

Falling may be an indicator of frailty in general. Persons with a history of falling have higher levels of subsequent health-care use and poor functional status. Inability to get up after a fall can also indicate a poor prognosis. Assessing fallers thoroughly assessed for the intrinsic and extrinsic causes of falls illustrated in Fig. 9-1 may improve functional outcomes over those who were not, even when the precise cause of the fall cannot be determined or treated.

TABLE 9-1   COMPLICATIONS OF FALLS IN ELDERLY PATIENTS

Injuries
    Painful soft tissue injuries
    Fractures
    Hip
    Femur
    Humerus
    Wrist
    Ribs

Subdural hematoma

Hospitalization
    Complications of immobilization (see Chap. 10)
    Risk of iatrogenic illnesses (see Chap. 5)

Disability
    Impaired mobility because of physical injury
    Impaired mobility from fear, loss of self-confidence, and restriction of
    ambulation

Increased risk of institutionalization

Increased risk of death

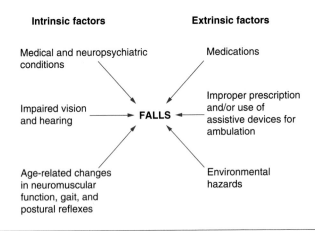

— FIGURE 9-1 —   Multifactorial causes and potential contributors to falls in older
persons.

AGING AND INSTABILITY

Several age-related factors contribute to instability and falls (Table 9-2). Most "accidental" falls are caused by one or a combination of these factors interacting with environmental hazards.

TABLE 9-2   AGE-RELATED FACTORS CONTRIBUTING TO INSTABILITY AND FALLS

Changes in postural control and blood pressure
   Decreased proprioception
   Slower righting reflexes
   Decreased muscle tone
   Increased postural sway
   Orthostatic hypotension
   Postprandial hypotension

Changes in gait
   Feet not picked up as high
   Men develop flexed posture and wide-based, short-stepped gait
   Women develop narrow-based, waddling gait

Increased prevalence of pathologic conditions predisposing to instability
   Degenerative joint disease
   Fractures of hip and femur
   Stroke with residual deficits
   Muscle weakness from disuse and deconditioning
   Peripheral neuropathy
   Diseases or deformities of the feet
   Impaired vision
   Impaired hearing
   Impaired cognition and judgment
   Other specific disease processes (eg, cardiovascular disease, parkinsonism—
      see Table 9-3)

Increased prevalence of conditions causing nocturia (eg, congestive heart
   failure, venous insufficiency)

Increased prevalence of dementia

Aging changes in postural control and gait probably play a major role in many falls among older persons. Increasing age is associated with diminished proprioceptive input; slower righting reflexes; diminished strength of muscles, important in maintaining posture; and increased postural sway. All these changes can contribute to falling—especially the ability to avoid a fall after encountering an environmental hazard or an unexpected trip. Changes in gait also occur with increasing age. Although these changes may not be sufficiently prominent to be labeled truly pathological, they can increase susceptibility to falls. In general, elderly people do not pick their feet up as high, thus increasing the tendency to trip. Elderly men tend to develop wide-based, short-stepped gaits; elderly women often walk with a narrow-based, waddling gait. These gait changes have been associated with white matter changes in the brain on magnetic resonance imaging (MRI) and with subsequent development of cognitive impairment.

Orthostatic hypotension (defined as a drop in systolic blood pressure of 20 mm Hg or more when moving from a lying to a standing position) occurs in approximately 20% of older persons. Although not all elderly individuals with orthostatic hypotension are symptomatic, this impaired physiological response could play a role in causing instability and precipitating falls in a substantial proportion of patients. Older people have been shown to experience a postprandial fall in blood pressure as well. People with orthostatic and/or postprandial hypotension are at particular risk for near syncope and falls when treated with diuretics and antihypertensive drugs.

Several pathological conditions that increase in prevalence with increasing age can contribute to instability and falling. Degenerative joint disease (especially of the neck, the lumbosacral spine, and the lower extremities) can cause pain, unstable joints, muscle weakness, and neurological disturbances. Healed fractures of the hip and femur can cause an abnormal and less steady gait. Residual muscle weakness or sensory deficits from a recent or remote stroke can also cause instability.

Muscle weakness as a result of disuse and deconditioning (caused by pain and/or lack of exercise) can contribute to an unsteady gait and impair the ability to right oneself after a loss of balance. Diminished sensory input, such as in diabetes and other peripheral neuropathies, visual disturbances, and impaired hearing diminish cues from the environment that normally contribute to stability and thus predispose one to falls. Impaired cognitive function may result in the creation of, or wandering into, unsafe environments and may lead to falls. Podiatric problems (bunions, calluses, nail disease, joint deformities, etc) that cause pain, deformities, and alterations in gait are common, correctable causes of instability. Other specific disease processes common in older people (such as Parkinson disease and cardiovascular disorders) can cause instability and falls and are discussed later in the chapter.

CAUSES OF FALLS IN OLDER PERSONS

Table 9-3 outlines the multiple and often interacting causes of falls among older persons. More than half of all falls are related to medically diagnosed conditions, emphasizing the importance of a careful medical assessment for patients who fall (see below). Several studies have examined risk factors for falls among older persons and have found a variety of these factors—including cognitive impairment, impaired lower extremity strength or function, gait and balance abnormalities, nocturia, and the number and nature of medications being taken—as important risk factors. Frequently overlooked, environmental factors can increase susceptibility to falls and other accidents. Homes of elderly people are often full of environmental hazards (Table 9-4). Unstable furniture, rickety stairs with inadequate railings, throw rugs and frayed carpets, and poor lighting should be specifically looked for on-home visits. Several factors are associated with falls among older nursing home residents (Table 9-5). Awareness of these factors can help prevent morbidity and mortality in these settings. Attention to these environmental hazards is important in individual people; however, the impact on morbidity of addressing environmental hazards in general has not been demonstrated in older people.

Several factors can hinder precise identification of the specific causes for falls. These factors include lack of witnesses, inability of the elderly person to recall the circumstances surrounding the event, the transient nature of several causes (eg, arrhythmia, transient ischemic attack [TIA], postural hypotension), and the fact that the majority of elderly people who fall do not seek medical attention. Somewhat more detailed information is available on the circumstances surrounding falls in nursing homes (see Table 9-5), but these individuals represent a relatively low proportion and a highly select group among the total senior population.

Close to half of all falls can be classified as accidental. Usually an accidental trip or a slip can be precipitated by an environmental hazard, often in conjunction with factors listed in Table 9-2. Addressing the environmental hazards begins with a careful assessment of the environment. Some older persons have developed a strong attachment to their cluttered surroundings and may need active encouragement to make the necessary changes, but many may simply take such environmental risks for granted until they are specifically identified.

Syncope, "drop attacks," and "dizziness" are commonly cited causes of falls in elderly persons. If there is a clear history of loss of consciousness, a cause for true syncope should be sought. Although the complete differential diagnosis of syncope is beyond the scope of this chapter, some of the more common causes of syncope in older people include vasovagal responses, carotid sinus hypersensitivity, cardiovascular disorders (such as bradycardia and tachyarrhythmias and aortic stenosis), acute neurological events (such as TIA, stroke, and seizure), pulmonary embolus, and metabolic disturbances (eg, hypoxia, hypoglycemia).

TABLE 9-3   CAUSES OF FALLS

Accidents
    True accidents (trips, slips, etc)
    Interactions between environmental hazards and factors increasing
    susceptibility (see Table 9-2)

Syncope (sudden loss of consciousness)

Drop attacks (sudden leg weaknesses without loss of consciousness)

Dizziness and/or vertigo
    Vestibular disease
    Central nervous system disease

Orthostatic hypotension
    Hypovolemia or low cardiac output
    Autonomic dysfunction
    Impaired venous return
    Prolonged bed rest
    Drug-induced hypotension
    Postprandial hypotension

Drug-related causes
    Antihypertensives
    Antidepressants
    Antiparkinsonian
    Diuretics
    Sedatives
    Antipsychotics
    Hypoglycemics
    Alcohol

Specific disease processes
    Acute illness of any kind ("premonitory fall")
    Cardiovascular
        Arrhythmias
        Valvular heart disease (aortic stenosis)
        Carotid sinus hypersensitivity
    Neurological causes
        TIA
        Stroke (acute)
        Seizure disorder
        Parkinson disease

TABLE 9-3   CAUSES OF FALLS (*Continued*)

Cervical or lumbar spondylosis (with spinal cord or nerve root compression)
Cerebellar disease
Normal-pressure hydrocephalus (gait disorder)
Central nervous system lesions (eg, tumor, subdural hematoma)
Urinary
  Overactive bladder
  Urge incontinence
  Nocturia

TIA, transient ischemic attack.

Cardiovascular causes for syncope are more common in the elderly than in younger populations. A precise cause for syncope may remain unidentified in 40% to 60% of elderly patients.

Drop attacks, described as sudden leg weakness causing a fall without loss of consciousness, may be overdiagnosed in elderly people who fall. They are often attributed to vertebrobasilar insufficiency, frequently precipitated by a change in head position. Although a small proportion of older people who fall have truly

TABLE 9-4   COMMON ENVIRONMENTAL HAZARDS

Old, unstable, and low-lying furniture

Beds and toilets of inappropriate height

Unavailability of grab bars

Uneven or poorly demarcated stairs and inadequate railing

Throw rugs, frayed carpets, cords, wires

Slippery floors and bathtubs

Inadequate lighting, glare

Cracked and uneven sidewalks

Pets that get under foot

TABLE 9-5   FACTORS ASSOCIATED WITH FALLS AMONG OLDER
NURSING HOME RESIDENTS

Recent admission

Dementia

Hip flexor muscle weakness

Certain activities (toileting, getting out of bed)

Psychotropic drugs causing daytime sedation

Cardiovascular medications (vasodilators, antihypertensives, diuretics)

Polypharmacy

Low staff-patient ratio

Unsupervised activities

Unsafe furniture

Slippery floors

had a drop attack, the underlying pathophysiology is poorly understood, and care should be taken to rule out other causes.

Dizziness and unsteadiness are common complaints among elderly people who fall (as well as those who do not). A feeling of light-headedness can be associated with several different disorders, but is a nonspecific symptom and should be interpreted with caution. Patients complaining of light-headedness should be carefully evaluated for postural hypotension and intravascular volume depletion.

Vertigo (a sensation of rotational movement), on the other hand, is a more specific symptom and is probably an uncommon precipitant of falls in the elderly. It is most commonly associated with disorders of the inner ear, such as acute labyrinthitis, Ménière disease, and benign positional vertigo. Vertebrobasilar ischemia and infarction and cerebellar infarction can also cause vertigo. Patients with vertigo caused by organic disorders often have nystagmus, which can be observed by having the patient quickly lie down and turning the patient's head to the side in one motion. Many older patients with symptoms of dizziness and unsteadiness are anxious, depressed, and chronically afraid of falling, and the evaluation of their symptoms is quite difficult. Some patients, especially those with symptoms suggestive of vertigo, will benefit from a thorough otological examination including auditory testing, which may help clarify the symptoms and differentiate inner ear from central nervous system (CNS) involvement.

Orthostatic hypotension is best detected by taking the blood pressure and pulse rate in supine position, after 1 minute in the sitting position, and after 1 and

3 minutes in the standing position. A drop of more than 20 mm Hg in systolic blood pressure is generally considered to represent significant orthostatic hypotension. In many instances, this condition is asymptomatic; however, several conditions can cause orthostatic hypotension or worsen it to a severity sufficient to precipitate a fall. These conditions include low cardiac output from heart failure or hypovolemia, autonomic dysfunction (which can result from diabetes or Parkinson disease), impaired venous return (eg, venous insufficiency), prolonged bed rest with deconditioning of muscles and reflexes, and several different drugs. Simply eating a full meal can precipitate a reduction in blood pressure in an older person that may be worsened when the person stands up and lead to a fall.

Drugs that should be suspected of playing a role in falls include diuretics (hypovolemia), antihypertensives (hypotension), antidepressants (postural hypotension), sedatives (excessive sedation), antipsychotics (sedation, muscle rigidity, postural hypotension), hypoglycemics (acute hypoglycemia), and alcohol (intoxication). Combinations of these drug types may greatly increase the risk of a fall. Many older patients are on a diuretic and one or two other antihypertensives with consequent hypotension or postural hypotension precipitate a fall. Psychotropic drugs are commonly prescribed and appear to substantially increase the risk of falls and hip fractures, especially in patients concomitantly prescribed antidepressants.

Many disease processes, especially of the cardiovascular and neurological systems, can be associated with falls. Cardiac arrhythmias are common in ambulatory elderly persons and may be difficult to associate directly with a fall or syncope. In general, cardiac monitoring should document a temporal association between a specific arrhythmia and symptoms (or a fall) before the arrhythmia is diagnosed (and treated) as the cause of falls.

Syncope can be a symptom of aortic stenosis and is an indication of the need to evaluate a patient suspected of having significant aortic stenosis for valve replacement. Aortic stenosis is difficult to diagnose by physical examination alone, and all patients suspected of having this condition should have an echocardiogram.

Some elderly individuals have sensitive carotid baroreceptors and are susceptible to syncope resulting from reflex increase in vagal tone (caused by cough, straining at stool, micturition, etc), which leads to bradycardia and hypotension. Carotid sinus sensitivity can be detected by bedside maneuvers (see below).

Cerebrovascular disease is often implicated as a cause or contributing factor for falls in older patients. Although cerebral blood flow and cerebrovascular autoregulation may be diminished, these aging changes alone are not enough to cause unsteadiness or falls. They may, however, render the elderly person more susceptible to stresses such as diminished cardiac output which will more easily precipitate symptoms. Acute strokes (caused by thrombosis, hemorrhage, or embolus) can cause and may initially manifest themselves in falls. TIAs of both the anterior and posterior circulations frequently last only minutes and are often poorly described. Thus, care must be taken in making these diagnoses. Anterior circulation TIAs may cause unilateral weakness and thus precipitate a fall. Vertebrobasilar (posterior circulation) TIAs may cause vertigo, but a history of transient vertigo alone is not a sufficient basis for the diagnosis of TIA. The diagnosis of posterior circulation TIA necessitates that one or more other symptoms (visual field cuts, dysarthria, ataxia, or limb weakness—which can be bilateral) be associated with vertigo. Vertebrobasilar insufficiency, as mentioned above, is often cited as a cause of drop attacks; in addition, mechanical compression of the vertebral arteries by osteophytes of the cervical spine when the head is turned has also been proposed as a cause of unsteadiness and falling. Both of these conditions are poorly documented, are probably overdiagnosed, and should not be used as causes of a fall simply because nothing else can be found.

Other diseases of the brain and CNS can also cause falls. Parkinson disease and normal-pressure hydrocephalus can cause disturbances of gait, which lead to instability and falls. Cerebellar disorders, intracranial tumors, and subdural hematomas can cause unsteadiness, with a tendency to fall. A slowly progressive gait disability with a tendency to fall, especially in the presence of spasticity or hyperactive reflexes in the lower extremities, should prompt consideration of cervical spondylosis and spinal cord compression. It is especially important to consider these diagnoses because treatment may improve the condition before permanent disability ensues.

Urinary tract disorders including overactive bladder, urge incontinence, and nocturia are also associated with falling. Urinary urgency may cause a distraction, similar to the "dual-tasking" studies mentioned above, and thereby predispose to falls. Awakening at night to void, especially among people who have taken hypnotics or other psychotropic drugs, may substantially increase the risk of falls.

Despite this long list, the precise causes of many falls will remain unknown—even after a thorough evaluation. The ultimate test of the etiology for falls is its reversibility. As noted earlier, we are better at finding putative causes than in correcting them.

EVIDENCE ON FALLS PREVENTION

Updated quality indicators for the identification, evaluation, and management of vulnerable elderly people with falls and mobility problems have recently been published as a component of the Assessing Care for the Vulnerable Elderly (ACOVE) project (Chang and Ganz, 2007). These quality indicators (a series of "If...Then," "Because" statements) are based on research data and expert opinion. Recommendations in this chapter are consistent with these ACOVE quality indicators. In terms of intervention, meta-analysis concluded that there was evidence that interventions could prevent the rate of falls, but the cost-effectiveness of falls prevention still remains unclear (RAND, 2002). Table 9-6 presents selected findings from some of these studies. In general, they suggest that it is possible to reduce the rate of falling, but not the rate of injurious falls. Relatively few interventions were effective in controlled trials. Despite this mixed message, there is growing enthusiasm for undertaking preventive efforts. Moreover, good clinical sense still dictates active efforts to identify remediable risk factors in individual older people. A meta-analysis of the several studies conducted under the auspices of the Frailty and Injuries: Cooperative Studies of Intervention Techniques (FICSIT) trials showed only modest results. In only two cases did an intervention lead to a significant reduction in falls; exercise and balance training were associated with fewer falls, but not with injurious falls. Tai chi training was shown to increase the time to a fall but not to a serious fall compared with an educational control group. When a specific fall prevention program was compared with a more general chronic disease prevention program, the fall program achieved lower rates of falls and serious falls at the end of the first year, but by year 2, the differences disappeared. A fact to remember when interpreting the effect of exercise on falls prevention is that exercise needs to be sustained, probably for at least 6 months. The dropout rate for many of these exercise programs is quite high (approximately one-third to one-half of participants), suggesting that at least part of the problem in demonstrating an effect may lie in maintaining the intervention.

Although many caregivers, especially in nursing home settings, think of physical restraints as a means of preventing falls, the evidence points in the opposite direction. Physical restraints should therefore not generally be used as an intervention to decrease falls. Rates of restraint use have, in fact, dropped substantially in US nursing homes as a result of a national emphasis on restraint reduction through Medicare's quality improvement initiatives. Whenever feasible, cognitively impaired patients, who are at special risk of falling, should be kept in environments that reduce the risk of making bad choices and falling as a result.

EVALUATING THE ELDERLY PATIENT WHO FALLS

Older patients who report a fall (or recurrent falls) that is not clearly the result of an accidental trip or slip should be carefully evaluated, even if the falls have not resulted in serious physical injury. A jointly developed set of recommendations for assessing people who fall has been issued by the American Geriatrics Society, The British Geriatrics Society, and the American Academy of Orthopaedic Surgeons (American Geriatrics Society et al., 2001). Table 9-7 lists the hallmarks of these recommendations. An example of an assessment from for older patients who fall is included in the appendix. A thorough fall evaluation consists of a focused history, targeted physical examination, gait and balance assessment, and, in certain instances, selected laboratory studies.

The history should focus on the general medical history and medications, the patient's thoughts about what caused the fall, the circumstances surrounding it

TABLE 9-6   SUMMARY OF SELECTED COMMUNITY-BASED FALLS INTERVENTION STUDIES

INTERVENTION	FINDINGS	REFERENCE
Combination of medication adjustment, behavioral instructions, exercise program	At 1 year RR for falls 0.69; no significant effect on injurious falls	Tinetti et al., 1994
Removing safety hazards, behavior program, strength, range of motion, and proprioception exercises	At 2 years' RR for falling 0.85; no significant effect on injurious falls	Hornbrook et al., 1994
Nurse home assessment with and without specific attention to falls risks	Both intervention groups have lower rates of falls and injurious falls after 1 year, but not at 2 years	Wagner et al., 1994
Various exercise programs	RR for falls among general exercise group 0.90, including balance 0.83; no significant effect on injurious falls	FICSIT (Province et al., 1995)
Tai chi	Relative hazard for falling 0.51	Wolf et al., 1996
Strength and endurance training	Relative hazard for falls 0.53	Buchner et al., 1997
Weight-bearing exercise	Number of falls over 2 years not significant but difference in rate for months 12-18 was significant	McMurdo et al., 1997
Home-based physical therapy exercise program	Hazard ratio for the first fall was not significant, but for fall with injury it was 0.61	Campbell et al., 1997

Medical and occupational therapy assessment and referrals	RR for falls at 12 months 0.39, for recurrent falls 0.33; RR for hospital admission 0.61	PROFET (Close et al., 1999)
Home-based strength and balance exercise program	RR for falls at 2 years' 0.69; RR for moderate/severe injury 0.63	Campbell et al., 1999
Home visit by occupational therapist for environmental assessment and modification	Decrease in number of persons falling; among prior fallers, RR of fall was 0.64	Cumming et al., 1999
Falls prevention strategies in nursing homes	Only two-thirds completed 6 months intervention; no difference in fall rates	McMurdo, Millar, and Daly, 2000
Additive model: education, exercise, home safety advice, clinical assessment	Compared to education group, significant reduction in slips and trips, but not falls	Steinberg et al., 2000
Home hazard assessment, information on hazard reduction, installation of safety devices	No significant difference in rate of falls in the home	Stevens et al., 2001
Nurse-delivered home exercise program	Significant decrease in numbers of falls and serious injurious falls	Robertson et al., 2001
Multiple strategies in residential care facilities (education, environmental modifications, reviewing drug regimens, etc)	Adjusted OR for falls 0.49; adjusted incidence rate for falls 0.60	Jensen et al., 2002

TABLE 9-6 SUMMARY OF SELECTED COMMUNITY-BASED FALLS INTERVENTION STUDIES (*Continued*)

Intervention	Findings	Reference
CGA with home visit and interventions and modifications	Intervention group had fewer falls compared to CGA alone. Incident rate ratio 0.69 (0.51-0.97)	Nikolaus et al., 2003
Multifactorial intervention in residential care, including 3 months of gait/balance training, medication review, podiatry, optometry	Lower fall rate in intervention group, but not significant after accounting for clustering effects 2.2 vs. 4.0 falls per resident year ($p = 0.2$)	Dyer et al., 2004
Individualized fall risk assessment and interventions in a residential care setting	Higher proportion of intervention groups fell over 2 months (56% vs. 43% [$p < 0.018$])	Kerse et al., 2004
Home safety assessment and modifications by an occupational therapist among people with severe visual impairment	Intervention reduced falls compared to control group (incident rate ratio 0.59 [0.42-0.83])	Campbell et al., 2005
Vitamin D 1000 IU daily for 2 years and 600 mg of calcium	No effect of exercise and vitamin D but adherence was poor Incidence of falls reduced compared to placebo (incident rate ratio 0.73 [0.57-0.95]); ratio lower in those who adhered to treatment (0.63 [0.48-0.82])	Flicker et al., 2005

Intervention	Result	Reference
Individualized exercise and strategies for maximizing vision and sensation	Reduced fall risk factors No reduction in falls over 6 months compared to a group that get advice and a control group	Lord et al., 2005
Tai chi for 48 weeks	Reduction in fear of falling compared to a wellness education control group	Sattin et al., 2005
Tai chi for 1 year	Nonsignification reduction in injurious falls No change in fear of falling compared to an education control group	Lin et al., 2006
Two in-home visits by a nurse or physical therapist, recommendations, referrals for therapy, monthly phone calls, and balance exercises	No difference in falls compared to control group who got a home safety assessment (incident rate ration 0.81 [$p = 0.27$])	Mahoney et al., 2007
Tai chi: 1-h classes for 16 months	Time to first fall longer Fewer falls No difference in proportion who fell one or more times compared to controls	Voukelatos et al., 2007

CGA, comprehensive geriatric assessment; FICSIT, Frailty and Injuries: Cooperative Studies of Intervention Techniques; OR, odds ratio; PROFET, Prevention of Falls in the Elderly Trial; RR, relative risk.

TABLE 9-7   RECOMMENDATIONS FOR FALLS ASSESSMENT

1. All older people should be asked about falls in the prior year
2. Those with a single prior fall should have a "get up and go" test or its equivalent (rising from a chair without using their arms and walking at a normal pace and turning 360° and then sitting back down). Those who can do this normally and have no history of falling need no further assessment
3. Those with two or more falls should be given a full falls assessment
4. Fall assessment consists of
   • History of fall circumstances, medications, acute or chronic medical problems, that may contribute (Table 9-3)
   • Examination of vision, gait and balance, and lower extremity joint function
   • Basic neurological examination (mental status, muscle strength, lower extremity sensation, reflexes, tests of cortical, extrapyramidal and cerebellar function)
   • Basic cardiovascular assessment (heart rate and rhythm, postural pulse and blood pressure, and possibly carotid sinus stimulation test)

American Geriatrics Society et al., 2001.

including ingestion of a meal and/or medication, any premonitory or associated symptoms (such as palpitations caused by a transient arrhythmia or focal neurological symptoms caused by a TIA), and whether there was loss of consciousness (Table 9-8). Information of the history of loss of consciousness after the fall (which is often difficult to document) is important and should raise the suspicion of a cardiac event (transient arrhythmia or heart block) or a seizure (especially if there has been incontinence). Falls are often unwitnessed, and elderly patients may not recall any details of the circumstances surrounding the event. Detailed questioning can sometimes lead to identification of environmental factors that may have played a role in the fall and to symptoms that may lead to a specific diagnosis. Many elderly patients will not be able to give details about an unwitnessed fall and will simply report, "I just fell down, I don't know what happened." The skin, extremities, and painful soft tissue areas should be assessed to detect any injury that may have resulted from a fall.

Several other aspects of the physical examination can be helpful in determining the cause(s) (Table 9-9). Because a fall can herald the onset of a variety of acute illnesses (premonitory falls), careful attention should be given to vital signs.

TABLE 9-8   EVALUATING THE ELDERLY PATIENT WHO FALLS: KEY
POINTS IN THE HISTORY

General medical history

History of previous falls

Medications (especially antihypertensive and psychotropic agents)

Patient's thoughts on the cause of the fall
  Was patient aware of impending fall?
  Was it totally unexpected?
  Did patient trip or slip?

Circumstances surrounding the fall
  Location and time of day
  Activity
  Situation: alone or not alone at the time of the fall
  Witnesses
  Relationship to changes in posture, turning of head, cough, urination, a
    meal, medication intake

Premonitory or associated symptoms
  Light-headedness, dizziness, vertigo
  Palpitations, chest pain, shortness of breath
  Sudden focal neurologic symptoms (weakness, sensory disturbance,
    dysarthria, ataxia, confusion, aphasia)
  Aura
  Incontinence of urine or stool

Loss of consciousness
  What is remembered immediately after the fall?
  Could the patient get up and, if so, how long did it take?
  Can loss of consciousness be verified by a witness?

Fever, tachypnea, tachycardia, and hypotension should prompt a search for an
acute illness (such as pneumonia or sepsis, myocardial infarction, pulmonary
embolus, or gastrointestinal bleeding). Postural blood pressure and pulse
determinations taken supine, sitting, and standing (after 1 and 3 min) are critical
in the diagnosis and management of falls in older patients. As noted earlier,
postural hypotension (generally defined as a drop of 20 mm Hg or more upon
change in posture) occurs in a substantial number of healthy, asymptomatic
elderly persons as well as in those who are deconditioned from immobility or

TABLE 9-9   EVALUATING THE ELDERLY PATIENT WHO FALLS: KEY ASPECTS OF THE PHYSICAL EXAMINATION

Vital signs
   Fever, hypothermia
   Respiratory rate
   Pulse and blood pressure (lying, sitting, standing)

Skin
   Turgor (over the chest; other areas unreliable)
   Pallor
   Trauma

Eyes
   Visual acuity

Cardiovascular
   Arrhythmias
   Carotid bruits
   Signs of aortic stenosis
   Carotid sinus sensitivity

Extremities
   Degenerative joint disease
   Range of motion
   Deformities
   Fractures
   Podiatric problems (calluses; bunions; ulcerations; poorly fitted,
      inappropriate, or worn-out shoes)

Neurological
   Mental status
   Focal signs
   Muscles (weakness, rigidity, spasticity)
   Peripheral innervation (especially position sense)
   Cerebellar (especially heel-to-shin testing)
   Resting tremor, bradykinesia, other involuntary movements
   Observation of gait and balance
      Get up and go test (Table 9-10)

Evaluation of assistive devices for hazards, such as missing tips on canes
   and walkers, impaired locking devices, or broken footrests on wheelchairs

---

have venous insufficiency. This finding can also be a sign of dehydration, acute blood loss (occult gastrointestinal bleeding), or a drug side effect (especially with cardiovascular medications and antidepressants). Visual acuity should be assessed for any possible contribution to instability and falls. The cardiovascular examination should focus on the presence of arrhythmias (many of which are easily missed during a brief examination) and signs of aortic stenosis. Because both of these conditions are potentially serious and treatable, yet difficult to diagnose by physical examination, the patient should be referred for continuous monitoring and echocardiography if they are suspected. If the history suggests carotid sinus sensitivity, the carotid can be gently massaged for 5 seconds to observe whether this precipitates a profound bradycardia (50% reduction in heart rate) or a long pause (2 s). The extremities should be examined for evidence of deformities, limits to range of motion, or active inflammation that might underlie instability and cause a fall.

Special attention should be given to the feet because deformities; painful lesions (calluses, bunions, ulcers); and poorly fitted, inappropriate, or worn-out shoes are common and can contribute to instability and falls.

Neurological examination is also an important aspect of this physical assessment. Mental status should be assessed (see Chap. 6), with a careful search for focal neurological signs. Evidence of muscle weakness, rigidity, or spasticity should be noted, and signs of peripheral neuropathy (especially posterior column signs such as loss of position or vibratory sensation) should be ruled out. Abnormalities in cerebellar function (especially heel-to-shin testing and heel tapping) and signs of Parkinson disease (such as resting tremor, muscle rigidity, and bradykinesia) should be sought.

Gait and balance assessments are a critical component of the examination and are probably more useful in identifying remediable problems than is the standard neuromuscular examination. Although sophisticated techniques have been developed to assess gait and balance, careful observation of a series of maneuvers is the most practical and useful assessment technique. The "get up and go" test and other practical performance-based balance and gait assessments have been developed (Table 9-10). While timing of this test has been used in research, timing in clinical practice is not necessary and may distract the observer from careful assessment of gait and balance. Abnormalities on this assessment may be helpful in identifying patients who are likely to fall again and potentially remediable problems that might prevent future falls.

There is no specific laboratory workup for an elderly patient who falls. Laboratory studies should be ordered based on information gleaned from the history and physical examination. If the cause of the fall is obvious (such as a slip or a trip) and no suspicious symptoms or signs are detected, laboratory studies are unwarranted. If the history or physical examination (especially vital signs) suggests an acute illness, appropriate laboratory studies (such as complete blood count, electrolytes, blood urea nitrogen, chest film, electrocardiogram) should

TABLE 9-10   EXAMPLE OF A PERFORMANCE BASED-ASSESSMENT OF GAIT AND BALANCE (GET UP AND GO)

Maneuver	Normal	Adaptive	Abnormal
Sitting balance	Steady, stable	Holds onto chair to keep upright	Leans, slides down in chair
Arising from chair	Able to arise in a single movement without using arms	Uses arms (on chair or walking aid) to pull or push up and/or moves forward in chair before attempting to rise	Multiple attempts required or unable without human assistance
Immediate standing balance (first 3–5 s)	Steady without holding onto walking aid or other object for support	Steady, but uses walking aid or support grabbing objects for support	Any sign of unsteadiness (eg, other object for staggering, more than minimal trunk sway)
Standing balance	Steady, able to stand with feet together without holding onto an object for support	Steady, but cannot put feet together	
Balance with eyes closed (Romberg test)	Steady without holding onto any object with feet together	Steady with feet apart	Any sign of unsteadiness or needs to hold onto an object

Maneuver			
Nudge on sternum (patient standing with eyes closed; examiner pushes with light, even pressure over sternum three times; reflects ability to withstand displacement)	Steady, able to withstand pressure	Needs to move feet, but able to maintain balance	Begins to fall, or examiner has to help maintain balance
Walking (usual pace with assistive device if used)	Stable, smooth gait	Use of cane, walker, holding onto furniture	Decreased step height and/or step length; unsteadiness or staggering gait
Turning balance (360°)	No grabbing or staggering; no need to hold onto any objects; steps are continuous (turn is a flowing movement)	Steps are discontinuous (patient puts one foot completely on floor before raising other foot)	Any sign of unsteadiness or holds onto an object; more than four steps to turn 360°
Neck turning (patient asked to turn head side to side and look up while standing with feet as close together as possible)	Able to turn head at least halfway side to side and able to bend head back to look at ceiling; no staggering, grabbing, or symptoms of light-headedness, unsteadiness, or pain	Decreased ability to turn side to side or extend neck, but no staggering, grabbing, or symptoms of light-headedness, unsteadiness, or pain	Any sign of unsteadiness or symptoms when turning head or extending neck

TABLE 9-10 EXAMPLE OF A PERFORMANCE BASED-ASSESSMENT OF GAIT AND BALANCE (GET UP AND GO) (*Continued*)

Maneuver	Normal	Adaptive	Abnormal
Back extension (ask patient to lean back as far as possible, without holding onto object if possible)	Good extension without holding object or staggering	Tries to extend, but range of motion is decreased or needs to hold object to attempt extension	Will not attempt, no extension seen, or staggers
Reaching up (have patient attempt to remove an object from a shelf high enough to necessitate stretching or standing on toes)	Able to take down object without needing to hold onto other object for support and without becoming unsteady	Able to get object but needs to steady self by holding onto something for support	Unable or unsteady
Bending down (patient is asked to pick up small objects, such as pen, from the floor)	Able to bend down and pick up the object and able to get up easily in single attempt without needing to pull self up with arms	Able to get object and get upright in single attempt but needs to pull self up with arms or hold onto something for support	Unable to bend down or unable to get upright after bending down or takes multiple attempts to upright self
Sitting down	Able to sit down in one smooth movement	Needs to use arms to guide self into chair or not a smooth movement	Falls into chair, misjudges distances (lands off center)

be ordered. Because increasing evidence suggests that vitamin D may be helpful in preventing falls (Bischoff-Ferrari et al., 2004; Table 9-6), evaluating patients who fall recurrently for vitamin D deficiency is appropriate. If a transient arrhythmia or heart block is suspected, ambulatory electrocardiographic monitoring should be done. Although the sensitivity and specificity of this procedure for determining the cause of falls in the elderly is unknown, and many elderly people have asymptomatic ectopy, cardiac abnormalities detected on continuous monitoring that are clearly related to symptoms should be treated.

Because it is difficult to diagnose aortic stenosis on physical examination, echocardiography should be considered in all patients with suggestive histories and a systolic heart murmur or those who have a delay in the carotid upstroke. If the history suggests anterior circulation TIA, noninvasive vascular studies should be considered to rule out treatable vascular lesions. Computed tomography (CT) scans or MRI scans should be reserved for those patients in whom there is a high suspicion of an intracranial lesion or seizure disorder.

MANAGEMENT

Table 9-11 outlines the basic principles of managing elderly patients with instability and a history of falls. Assessment and treatment of physical injury should not be overlooked because it may be helpful in preventing recurrent falls.

When specific conditions are identified by history, physical examination, and laboratory studies, they should be treated in order to minimize the risk of subsequent falls, morbidity, and mortality. Table 9-12 lists examples of treatments for some of the more common conditions. This table is meant only as a general outline; most of these topics are discussed in detail in general textbooks of medicine.

Physical therapy and patient education are important aspects of the management. Gait training, muscle strengthening, the use of assistive devices, and adaptive behaviors (such as rising slowly, using rails or furniture for balance, and techniques of getting up after a fall) are all helpful in preventing subsequent morbidity from instability and falls.

Environmental manipulations can be critical in preventing further falls in individual patients. The environments of the elderly are often unsafe (see Table 9-4) and appropriate interventions can often be instituted to improve safety (see Table 9-12). Physical restraints (vests, belts, mittens, geri-chairs, etc) are used in institutional settings for those felt to be at high risk of falling. Federal nursing home regulations and quality improvement initiatives reflect increasing recognition that physical restraints probably do not decrease and may in fact

TABLE 9-11   PRINCIPLES OF MANAGEMENT FOR ELDERLY PATIENTS
WITH COMPLAINTS OF INSTABILITY AND/OR FALLS

Assess and treat physical injury

Treat underlying conditions (Table 9-12)

Prevent future falls

Provide physical therapy and education
  Gait and balance retraining
  Muscle strengthening
  Aids to ambulation
  Properly fitted shoes
  Adaptive behaviors

Alter the environment
  Safe and proper-size furniture
  Elimination of obstacles (loose rugs, etc)
  Proper lighting
  Rails (stairs, bathroom)

increase falls and injuries (Tinetti, Liu, and Ginter, 1992; Neufeld et al., 1999), have led to the reduced and more appropriate use of these devices in many institutional settings. Multifaceted interventions for fall prevention in long-term care settings have been designed and tested, but the results of these trials have been mixed (Ray et al., 1997; Taylor, 2002; Ray et al., 2005; Rask et al., 2007).

For elderly patients who are at high risk for falls and hip fractures, the use of hip protectors should be considered. Despite numerous clinical trials as well as meta-analyses (Kannus et al., 2000; Parker, Gillespie, and Gillespie, 2001; Honkanen et al., 2006; Kiel et al., 2007; Sawka et al., 2007; van Schoor et al., 2007), there is no definitive evidence that hip protectors reduce morbidity in a population of fallers. However, in individual high-risk patients who will wear them, hip protectors may be a simple and relatively inexpensive preventive intervention to consider.

Table 9-13 summarizes the American Geriatrics Society recommendations on fall prevention. While the scientific strength of these recommendations is limited, they are based on the best available evidence and expert opinion available at the time they were published.

TABLE 9-12   EXAMPLES OF TREATMENT FOR UNDERLYING CAUSES OF FALLS

Condition and Cause	Potential Treatment
CARDIOVASCULAR	
Tachyarrhythmias	Antiarrhythmics*
Bradyarrhythmias	Pacemaker*
Aortic stenosis	Valve surgery (for syncope)
Postural hypotension	
Drug-related	Elimination of drugs(s) that may contribute
Intravascular volume depletion	Rehydrate as appropriate Evaluate for blood loss if indicated
With venous insufficiency	Support stockings Leg elevation Adaptive behaviors
Autonomic dysfunction or idiopathic	Support stockings Mineralocorticoids Midodrine hydrochloride Adaptive behaviors (eg, pausing and getting up slowly)
TIA	Aspirin and/or surgery[†]
Cervical spondylosis (with spinal cord compression)	Physical therapy Neck brace Surgery
Parkinson disease	Antiparkinsonian drugs
Visual impairment	Ophthalmological evaluation and specific treatment
Seizure disorder	Anticonvulsants
Normal-pressure hydrocephalus	Surgery (shunt)[†]
Dementia	Supervised activities Hazard-free environment
Benign positional vertigo	Habituation exercises Antivertiginous medication

TABLE 9-12 EXAMPLES OF TREATMENT FOR UNDERLYING CAUSES OF FALLS (*Continued*)

CONDITION AND CAUSE	POTENTIAL TREATMENT
OTHERS	
Foot disorders	Podiatric evaluation and treatment
Gait and balance disorders (miscellaneous)	Properly fitted shoes Physical therapy Exercise with balance training (eg, tai chi)
Muscle weakness, deconditioning	Lower extremity strength training
Drug overuse (eg, sedatives, alcohol, other psychotropic drugs, antihypertensives)	Elimination of drug(s)
Vitamin D deficiency	Vitamin D supplementation
Recurrent falls in high-risk patients	Consider hip protectors

*These treatments may be indicated only if the cardiac disturbance is clearly related to symptoms.
†Risk-benefit ratio must be carefully assessed.
TIA, transient ischemic attack.

TABLE 9-13 RECOMMENDED INTERVENTIONS TO PREVENT FALLS

1. Among community-dwelling older persons
   - Gait training and advice on appropriate assistive devices
   - Review and modify medications, especially antihypertensives and psychotropics
   - Exercise programs that include balance training (eg, tai chi)
   - Treat postural hypertension
   - Modify environmental hazards
   - Treat cardiovascular disorders, including arrhythmias
2. In long-term care and assisted-living settings
   - Education and quality improvement programs
   - Gait and balance training and advice on appropriate assistive devices
   - Review and modify medication, especially antihypertensives and psychotropics

Adapted from American Geriatrics Society et al., 2001.

EVIDENCE SUMMARY

Do's

■ Distinguish between falls, syncope, and seizure.
■ Distinguish between "dizziness" and true vertigo.
■ Assess for correctable underlying causes of falls by history and targeted physical examination.
■ Pay particular attention to:
   ■ Uncorrected vision impairment
   ■ Postural vital signs
   ■ Psychotropic medications
   ■ Gait and balance abnormalities
   ■ Inappropriate footwear
   ■ Incorrect use of canes and other assistive devices
   ■ Environmental hazards
   ■ A simple "get up and go" test on all patients who have fallen.
■ Ensure safety in recurrent fallers by urgent intervention(s) to prevent injury.
■ Refer patients to rehabilitation therapists (physical and occupational) whenever appropriate for detailed environmental and safety assessments, strengthening, and proper prescription and use of assistive devices.

Don'ts

■ Send all patients for extensive diagnostic studies or cardiac monitoring.

Consider

■ Referring selected patients for tai chi if they have balance problems and classes are available
■ Prescribing vitamin D
■ Recommending hip protectors in carefully selected patients who are at high risk for fracture and who are recurrently falling

References

American Geriatrics Society, British Geriatrics Society, American Academy of Orthopaedic Surgeons Panel on Falls Prevention. Guideline for the prevention of falls in older persons. *J Am Geriatr Soc.* 2001;49:664-672.

Bischoff-Ferrari HA, Dawson-Hughes B, Willett WC, et al. Effect of vitamin D on falls: a meta-analysis. *JAMA.* 2004;291:1999-2006.

Buchner DM, Cress ME, deLateur BJ, et al. The effect of strength and endurance training on gait, balance, fall risk and health services use in community-living older adults. *J Gerontol A Biol Sci Med Sci.* 1997;52A:M218-M224.

Campbell AJ, Robertson MC, Gardener MM, et al. Randomised controlled trial of a general practice programme of home-based exercise to prevent falls in elderly women. *BMJ.* 1997;315:1065-1069.

Campbell AJ, Robertson MC, Gardner MM, et al. Falls prevention over 2 years: a randomised controlled trial in women 80 years and older. *Age Ageing.* 1999;28:513-518.

Campbell AJ, Robertson MC, LaGrow SJ, et al. Randomised controlled trial of prevention of falls in people aged > or = 75 with severe visual impairment: the VIP trial. *BMJ.* 2005;331:817.

Chang JT, Morton SC, Rubenstein LZ, et al. Interventions for the prevention of falls in older adults: systematic review and meta-analysis of randomised clinical trials. *BMJ.* 2004;328:680.

Chang JT, Ganz D. Quality indicators for falls and mobility problems in vulnerable elders. *J Am Geriatr Soc.* 2007;55:S327-S334.

Close J, Ellis M, Hooper R, et al. Prevention of Falls in the Elderly Trial (PROFET): a randomized controlled trial. *Lancet.* 1999;353:93-97.

Cumming RG, Thomas M, Szonyi G, et al. Home visits by an occupational therapist for assessment and modification of environmental hazards: a randomized trial of falls prevention. *J Am Geriatr Soc.* 1999;47:1397-1402.

Dyer CA, Taylor GJ, Reed M, et al. Falls prevention in residential care homes: a randomized control trial. *Age Ageing.* 2004;33:596-602.

Fiatarone MA, O'Neill EF, Ryan ND, et al. Exercise training and nutritional supplementation for physical frailty in very elderly people. *N Engl J Med.* 1994;330:1769-1775.

Flicker L, Macinnis RJ, Stein MS, et al. Should older people in residential care receive vitamin D to prevent falls? Results of a randomized trial. *J Am Geriatr Soc.* 2005;53:1881-1888.

Honkanen LA, Mushlin AI, Lachs M, et al. Can hip protector use cost-effectively prevent fractures in community-dwelling geriatric populations? *J Am Geriatr Soc.* 2006;54:1658-1665.

Hornbrook MC, Stevens VJ, Wingfield DJ, et al. Preventing falls among community-dwelling older persons: results from a randomized trial. *Gerontologist.* 1994;34:16-23.

Jensen J, Lundin-Olsson L, Nyberg L, et al. Fall and injury prevention in older people living in residential care facilities: a cluster randomized trial. *Ann Intern Med.* 2002;136:733-741.

Kannus P, Parkkari J, Niemi S, et al. Prevention of hip fracture in elderly people with use of a hip protector. *N Engl J Med.* 2000;343:1506-1513.

Kerse N, Butler M, Robinson E, et al. Fall prevention in residential care: a cluster, randomized, controlled trial. *J Am Geriatr Soc.* 2004;52:524-531.

Kiel DP, Magaziner J, Zimmerman S, et al. Efficacy of a hip protector to prevent hip fracture in nursing home residents: the HIP PRO randomized controlled trial. *JAMA.* 2007;298:413-422.

Lauritzen JB, Petersen MM, Lund B. Effect of external hip protectors on hip fractures. *Lancet.* 1993;341:11-13.

Lin MR, Hwang HF, Wang YW, et al. Community-based Tai Chi and its effects on injurious falls, balance, gait and fear of falling in older people. *Phys Ther.* 2006;86:1189-1201.

Lord SR, Tiedemann A, Chapman K, et al. The effect of an individualized fall prevention program on fall risk and falls in older people: a randomized, controlled trial. *J Am Geriatr Soc.* 2005;53:1296-1304.

Mahoney JE, Shea TA, Przybelski R, et al. Kenosha County falls prevention study: a randomized, controlled trial of an intermediate-intensity, community-based multifactorial falls intervention. *J Am Geriatr Soc.* 2007;55:489-498.

Mathias SN, Nayak USL, Isaacs B. Balance in elderly patients: the "get up and go" test. *Arch Phys Med Rehabil.* 1986;67:387-389.

McMurdo MET, Mole PA, Paterson CR. Controlled trial of weight-bearing exercise in older women in relation to bone density and falls. *BMJ.* 1997;314:569.

McMurdo ME, Millar AM, Daly F. A randomized controlled trial of fall prevention strategies in old peoples' homes. *Gerontology.* 2000;46(2):83-87.

Neufeld RR, Libow LS, Foley WJ, et al. Restraint reduction reduces serious injuries among nursing home residents. *J Am Geriatr Soc.* 1999;47:1202-1207.

Nikolaus T, Bach M. Preventing falls in community-dwelling frail older people using a home intervention team (HIT): results from the randomized Falls-HIT trial. *J Am Geriatr Soc.* 2003;51:300-305.

Parker MJ, Gillespie LD, Gillespie WJ. Hip protectors for preventing hip fractures in the elderly (Cochrane Review): Oxford (update software.com): The Cochrane Library, 2001, Issue 2, 2001.

Province MA, Hadley EC, Hornbrook MC, et al. The effects of exercise on falls in elderly patients: a preplanned meta-analysis of the FICSIT trials. *JAMA.* 1995;273:1341-1347.

RAND. *Falls Prevention Interventions in the Medicare Population.* Santa Monica, CA: RAND; 2002; Contract No. 500–98–0281. Prepared for the Centers for Medicare and Medicaid Services.

Rask K, Parmelee P, Taylor JA, et al. Implementation and evaluation of a fall management program. *J Am Geriatr Soc.* 2007;55:342-349.

Ray WA, Taylor JA, Brown AK, et al. Prevention of fall-related injuries in long-term care: a randomized controlled trial of staff education. *Arch Intern Med.* 2005;165:2293-2298.

Ray WA, Taylor JA, Meador KG, et al. A randomized trial of a consultation service to reduce falls in nursing homes. *JAMA.* 1997;278:557-562.

Robertson MC, Devlin N, Gardner MM, et al. Effectiveness and economic evaluation of a nurse delivered home exercise programme to prevent falls. 1: randomized controlled trial. *BMJ.* 2001;322:697-701.

Rubenstein LZ, Robbins AS, Josephson KR, et al. The value of assessing falls in an elderly population. *Ann Intern Med.* 1990;113:308-316.

Sattin RW, Easley KA, Wolf SL, et al. Reduction in fear of falling through intense Tai Chi exercise training in older, transitionally frail adults. *J Am Geriatr Soc.* 2005;53: 11;68-1178.

Sawka AM, Boulos P, Beattie K, et al. Hip protectors decrease hip fracture risk in elderly nursing home residents: a Bayesian meta-analysis. *J Clin Epidemiol.* 2007;60:336-344.

Steinberg M, Cartwright C, Peel N, et al. A sustainable programme to prevent falls and near falls in community-dwelling older people: results of a randomized trial. *J Epidemiol Community Health.* 2000;54:227-232.

Stevens M, Holman CDJ, Bennett N, et al. Preventing falls in older people: outcome evaluation of a randomized controlled trial. *J Am Geriatr Soc.* 2001;49:1448-1455.

Taylor JA. The Vanderbilt fall prevention program for long-term care: eight years of field experience with nursing home staff. *J Am Med Dir Assoc.* 2002;3:180-185.

Tinetti M, Baker D, McAvay G, et al. A multifactorial intervention to reduce the risk of falling among elderly people living in the community. *N Engl J Med.* 1994;331: 821-827.

Tinetti ME, Liu W, Ginter SF. Mechanical restraint use and fall-related injuries among residents of skilled nursing facilities. *Ann Intern Med.* 1992;116:369-374.

Van Schoor NM, Smit JH, Bouter LM, et al. Maximum potential preventive effect of hip protectors. *J Am Geriatr Soc.* 2007;55:507-510.

Voukelatos A, Cumming RG, Lord SR, et al. A randomized, controlled trial of Tai Chi for the prevention of falls: a Central Sydney Tai Chi trial. *J Am Geriatr Soc.* 2007;55:1185-1191.

Wagner EH, LaCroix AZ, Grothaus L, et al. Preventing disability and falls in older adults: a population-based randomized trial. *Am J Public Health.* 1994;84:1800-1806.

Wolf SL, Barnhart HX, Kutner NG, et al. Reducing frailty and falls in older persons: an investigation of Tai Chi and computerized balance training. *J Am Geriatr Soc.* 1996;44: 489-497.

Suggested Readings

Agostini JV, Baker DI, Bogardus STJ. *Prevention of Falls in Hospitalized and Institutionalized Older People: Making Health Care Safer: A Critical Analysis of Patient Safety Practices.* Rockville, MD: Agency for Healthcare Research and Quality; 2001.

Alexander N. Gait disorders in older adults. *J Am Geriatr Soc.* 1996;44:434-451.

Connell B. Role of the environment in falls prevention. *Clin Geriatr Med.* 1996;12: 859-880.

Coussement J, De Paepe L, Schwendimann R, et al. Interventions for preventing falls in acute- and chronic-care hospitals: a systematic review and meta-analysis. *J Am Geriatr Soc.* 2007;56:29-36.

Gillespie LD, Gillespie WJ, Robertson MC, et al. Interventions for preventing falls in elderly people. *Cochrane Database Syst Rev.* 2001;3:CD000340.

King MB, Tinetti ME. Falls in community-dwelling older persons. *J Am Geriatr Soc.* 1995;43:1146-1154.

National Council on Aging. *Falls Free™ National Action Plan: A Progress Report.* Washington, DC: 20036; 2007.

Tinetti ME, Williams CS, Gill TM. Dizziness among older adults: a possible geriatric syndrome. *Ann Intern Med.* 2000;132:337-344.

Tinetti ME. Preventing falls in elderly persons. *N Engl J Med.* 2003;348:42-49.

Selected Web Sites (Accessed on March 16, 2008)

http://www.cdc.gov/ncipc/factsheets/adultfalls.htm

http://www.fallsprevention.org.au/resources.htm

http://www.guideline.gov/summary/summary.aspx?ss=15&doc_id=6118&nbr=3968

http://www.healthinaging.org/agingintheknow/chapters_ch_trial.asp?ch=21

Tools

http://www.medicine.emory.edu/ger/edu_resources/compAsses.cfm (Accessed on April 12, 2008)

Click on Consider Full Fall Assessment under Fall Risk.

CHAPTER 10

IMMOBILITY

Immobility refers to any disease or disability that requires complete bed rest or extremely limits an individual's ability to move. Patients who have had a stroke resulting in partial or complete hemiparesis/paralysis, spinal cord injury resulting in paraplegia or quadriplegia, fracture or musculoskeletal disorder limiting function, or prolonged bed rest after surgery or acute illness are considered immobilized. Immobility is a common pathway by which a series of subsequent diseases and problems can occur in older individuals which produces further pain, disability, and impaired quality of life. Optimizing mobility should be the goal of all members of the health-care team working with older adults. Small improvements in mobility can decrease the incidence and severity of complications, improve the patient's well-being, and decrease the cost and burden of caregiving.

This chapter outlines the common causes and complications of immobility and reviews the principles of management for some of the more common conditions associated with immobility in the older population.

CAUSES

The causes of immobility can be divided into intrapersonal factors including psychological factors (eg, depression, fear, motivation), physical changes (cardiovascular, neurological, and musculoskeletal disorders, and associated pain), and environmental causes. Examples of these physical, psychological, and environmental factors include inappropriate caregiving, paralysis, lack of access to appropriate assistive devices, and environmental barriers such as lack of handrails on stairs or grab bars around a commode (Table 10-1).

The incidence of degenerative joint disease (DJD) is particularly high in older adults, although symptoms of disease may not manifest in all individuals who have radiographic changes (Andrianakos et al., 2006; Jordan et al., 2007). The pain and musculoskeletal changes associated with DJD can result in contractures and progressive immobility if not appropriately treated. In addition, podiatric problems associated with degenerative changes in the feet (eg, bunions and hammertoes) can likewise cause pain and contractures. These changes can result in painful ambulation and a subsequent decrease in the older individual's willingness and ability to ambulate (Keysor et al., 2005).

TABLE 10-1   COMMON CAUSES OF IMMOBILITY IN OLDER ADULTS

Musculoskeletal disorders
  Arthritides
  Osteoporosis
  Fractures (especially hip and femur)
  Podiatric problems
  Other (eg, Paget disease)

Neurological disorders
  Stroke
  Parkinson disease
  Neuropathies
  Normal-pressure hydrocephalus
  Dementias
  Other (cerebellar dysfunction, neuropathies)

Cardiovascular disease
  Congestive heart failure (severe)
  Coronary artery disease (frequent angina)
  Peripheral vascular disease (frequent claudication)

Pulmonary disease
  Chronic obstructive lung disease (severe)

Sensory factors
  Impairment of vision
  Decreased kinesthetic sense
  Decreased peripheral sensation

Environmental causes
  Forced immobility (in hospitals and nursing homes)
  Inadequate aids for mobility
  Acute and chronic pain

Other
  Deconditioning (after prolonged bed rest from acute illness)
  Malnutrition
  Severe systemic illness (eg, widespread malignancy)
  Depression
  Drug side effects (eg, antipsychotic-induced rigidity)
  Fear of falling
  Apathy and lack of motivation

Over the last decade, the number of stroke survivors has increased 30%, and worldwide we currently have the largest cohort of persons surviving stroke. The incidence of stroke doubles with each decade beyond 60 years of age, putting older adults particularly at risk (Zorowitz, Gross, and Polinski, 2002). About half of the individuals who suffer a stroke have residual deficits for which they require assistance, and often these deficits result in immobility. Parkinson disease (PD), another common neurological disorder found in older adults, can cause severe limitations in mobility. PD is a progressive neurological disorder that affects approximately 1.5 million people in the United States (Dorsey et al., 2007). As the disease progresses, it has a major impact on the individual's function caused by the associated bradykinesia (slow movement) or akinesia (absence of movement), resting tremor, and muscle rigidity, as well as cognitive changes.

Severe congestive heart failure, coronary artery disease with frequent angina, peripheral vascular disease with frequent claudication, orthostatic hypotension, and severe chronic lung disease can restrict activity and mobility in many elderly patients because of lack of cardiovascular endurance. Peripheral vascular disease, especially in older diabetics, can cause claudication, peripheral neuropathy, and altered balance, all of which limit ambulation.

The psychological and environmental factors that influence immobility are as important as the physical changes noted. Depression, lack of motivation, apathy, fear of falling, and health beliefs (ie, a belief that rest and immobility are beneficial to recovery) can all influence mobility in older adults. The environment, both the social and physical environment, can have a major impact on mobility. Well-meaning formal and informal caregivers may provide care for older individuals rather than help the individual optimize their underlying function. Inappropriate use of wheelchairs, bathing, and dressing of individuals who have the underlying capability to engage in these activities results in deconditioning and immobility. Lack of mobility aids (eg, canes, walkers, and appropriately placed railings), cluttered environments, uneven surfaces, and the shape of and positioning of chairs and beds can further lead to immobility. Negotiating stairs can be a special challenge.

Drug side effects in the management of acute and chronic illness may also contribute to immobility. Sedatives and hypnotics can result in drowsiness, dizziness, delirium, and ataxia, and can impair mobility. Antipsychotic drugs (especially the phenothiazine-like agents) have prominent extrapyramidal effects and can cause muscle rigidity and diminished mobility (see Chap. 14). The treatment of hypertension can result in orthostatic hypotension or bradycardia such that the individual experiences dizziness and is unable to ambulate independently.

COMPLICATIONS

Immobility can lead to complications in almost every major organ system (Table 10-2). Prolonged inactivity or bed rest has adverse physical and psychological consequences. Metabolic effects include a negative nitrogen and calcium balance

TABLE 10-2   COMPLICATIONS OF IMMOBILITY

Skin
   Pressure ulcers

Musculoskeletal
   Muscular deconditioning and atrophy

Contractures
   Bone loss (osteoporosis)
   Cardiovascular
   Deconditioning
   Orthostatic hypotension
   Venous thrombosis, embolism

Pulmonary
   Decreased ventilation
   Atelectasis
   Aspiration pneumonia

Gastrointestinal
   Anorexia
   Constipation
   Fecal impaction, incontinence

Genitourinary
   Urinary infection
   Urinary retention
   Bladder calculi
   Incontinence

Metabolic
   Altered body composition (eg, decreased plasma volume)
   Negative nitrogen balance
   Impaired glucose tolerance
   Altered drug pharmacokinetics

Psychological
   Sensory deprivation
   Delirium
   Depression

and impaired glucose tolerance. The older individual can also experience diminished plasma volume and subsequent changes in drug pharmacokinetics. Immobilized older patients often become depressed, are deprived of environmental stimulation, and, in some instances, become delirious. Deconditioning can occur rapidly, especially among older individuals who have little physiological reserve.

Musculoskeletal complications associated with immobility include loss of muscle strength and endurance; reduced skeletal muscle fiber size, diameter, and capillarity; contractures, disuse osteoporosis, and DJD. The severity of muscle atrophy is related to the duration and magnitude of activity limitation. If left unchecked, this muscle wasting can lead to long-term sequelae, including impaired functional capacity and permanent muscle damage. Moreover, immobility exacerbates bone turnover (Chen et al., 2005). The impact of immobility on skin can also be devastating. Varying degrees of immobility and decreased serum albumin significantly increase the risk for pressure ulcer development (Sharp and McLaws, 2006). Prolonged immobility results in cardiovascular deconditioning; the combination of deconditioned cardiovascular reflexes and diminished plasma volume can lead to postural hypotension. Postural hypotension may not only impair rehabilitative efforts but also predispose to falls and serious cardiovascular events such as stroke and myocardial infarction. Likewise, deep venous thrombosis and pulmonary embolism are well-known complications (Steier et al., 2006). Immobility, especially bed rest, also impairs pulmonary function. Tidal volume is diminished; atelectasis may occur, which, when combined with the supine position, predisposes to developing aspiration pneumonia.

Gastrointestinal and genitourinary problems are likewise influenced by immobility. Constipation and fecal impaction may occur because of decreased mobility and inappropriate positioning to optimize defecation. Urinary retention can result from inability to void lying down and/or rectal impaction impairing the flow of urine. These conditions and their management are discussed in Chap. 8.

ASSESSING IMMOBILE PATIENTS

Several aspects of the history and physical examination are important in assessing immobile patients (Table 10-3). Focused histories should address the intrapersonal aspect as well the environmental issues associated with immobility. It is important to explore the underlying cause, or perceived cause, of the immobility on the part of the patient and caregiver. Specific contributing factors to explore include medical conditions, treatments (eg, medications, associated treatments such as intravenous lines), pain, psychological (eg, mood and fear) and

TABLE 10-3   ASSESSMENT OF IMMOBILE OLDER PATIENTS

History
   Nature and duration of disabilities causing immobility
   Medical conditions contributing to immobility
   Pain
   Drugs that can affect mobility
   Motivation and other psychological factors
   Environment

Physical examination
   Skin
   Cardiopulmonary status

Musculoskeletal assessment
   Muscle tone and strength (see Table 10-4)
   Joint range of motion
   Foot deformities and lesions

Neurological deficits
   Focal weakness
   Sensory and perceptual evaluation

Levels of mobility
   Bed mobility
   Ability to transfer (bed to chair)
   Wheelchair mobility
   Standing balance
   Gait (see Chap. 9)
   Pain with movement

motivational factors. Nutrition status, particularly protein levels and evaluation of 25-hydroxy vitamin D is particularly useful to consider when evaluating the older patient as these have been associated with muscle weakness, poor physical performance, balance problems, and falls (Campbell and Allain, 2006; Dhesi et al., 2002; Hedstrom et al., 2002; Houston et al., 2007; Joseph, 2005; Morely et al., 2001; Mosekilde L, 2005; Trivedi, Doll, and Khaw, 2003). An assessment of the environment is critical and should include both the patient's physical and social environment (particularly caregiving interactions). Any and all of these factors can decrease the individual's willingness to engage in activities. While a comprehensive assessment is therefore critical, other members of the health-care team (eg, social work, physical therapy) can facilitate these evaluations and provide at least an aspect of that assessment.

In addition to the potential causes of immobility, the impact of immobility in older adults must always be considered. A comprehensive skin assessment should be done with a particular focus on bony prominences and areas of pressure against the bed, chair, splint, shoe, or any type of immobilizing device. Cardiopulmonary status, especially intravascular volume, and postural changes in blood pressure and pulse are important to consider, particularly as these may further limit mobility. A detailed musculoskeletal examination—including evaluation of muscle tone and strength, evaluation of joint range of motion, and assessment of podiatric problems that may cause pain should be performed. Standardized and repeated measures of muscle strength can be helpful in gauging a patient's progress (Table 10-4). The neurological examination should identify focal weakness as well as cognitive, sensory, and perceptual problems that can impair mobility and influence rehabilitative efforts.

TABLE 10-4   EXAMPLE OF HOW TO GRADE MUSCLE STRENGTH IN IMMOBILE OLDER PATIENTS

---

0 = Flaccid

1 = Trace/Slight contractility but no movement

2 = Weak with movement possible when gravity is eliminated

3 = Fair movement against gravity but not against resistance

4 = Good with movement against gravity with some resistance

5 = Normal with movement against gravity and some resistance

Upper extremity:
Shoulder extension: Have the individual hold up their arm at 90°. Place your hand on the individual's upper arm between elbow and shoulder and tell the individual not to let you push down their arm.
Elbow flexion: Have the individual bend their elbow fully and attempt to straighten the arm out while telling the individual not to let you pull the arm down.
Elbow extension: While the individual still has the elbow flexed, tell them to try and straighten out the arm while you resist.
Lower extremity:
Hip flexion: Place your hand on the individual's anterior thigh and ask them to raise the leg against your resisting hand (say to individual: don't let me push your leg down).
Knee extension: Have the individual bend their leg on the bed and place one of your hands just below the individual's knee and tell to try and straighten out the leg as you resist.
Ankle plantar flexion: Have the individual extend their foot against your hand.
Ankle dorsiflexion: Have the individual pull their foot up against your hand.

Most importantly, the patient's function and mobility should be assessed and reevaluated on an ongoing basis. Assessments should include bed mobility; transfers, including toilet transfers; and ambulation and stair climbing (see Table 10-3). Pain, fear, resistance to activity, and endurance should simultaneously be considered during these evaluations. As previously noted, other members of the healthcare team (eg, physical therapy, occupational therapy, and nursing) are skilled in completion of these assessments and are critical to the comprehensive evaluation of the patient.

MANAGEMENT OF IMMOBILITY

The goal in the management of any older adult is to optimize function and mobility to the individual's highest level. Medical management is central to assuring this goal as optimal management of underlying acute and chronic disease must be addressed to assure success. It is beyond the scope of this text to detail the management of all conditions associated with immobility in older adults; however important general principles of the management of the most common of these conditions are reviewed. Brief sections at the end of the chapter provide an overview of key principles in the management of pain and the rehabilitation of geriatric patients.

Arthritis

Arthritis includes a heterogeneous group of related joint disorders that have a variety of causes such as metabolism, joint malformation, joint trauma, or joint damage. The pathology of osteoarthritis (OA) is characterized by cartilage destruction with subsequent joint space loss, osteophyte formation, and subchondral sclerosis. OA is the most common joint disease among older adults and is the major cause of knee, hip, and back pain. OA is not, by definition, inflammatory, though hypertrophy of synovium and accumulation of joint effusions are typical. It is currently believed that the pathogenesis of OA progression revolves around a complex interplay of numerous factors: chondrocyte regulation of the extracellular matrix, genetic influences, local mechanical factors, and inflammation (Sun, Wu, and Kalunian, 2007).

Plain film radiography has been the main diagnostic modality for assessing the severity and progression of OA. Magnetic resonance imaging (MRI) and ultrasound, however, have been noted to be more accurate and comprehensive measures of joint changes. Once diagnosed, a wide variety of modalities can be used to treat OA as well as other painful musculoskeletal conditions. Treatment can be separated into three different categories: nonpharmacological, pharmacological, and surgical. Nonpharmacological includes weight loss, physical therapy to strengthen related musculature, and use of exercise programs to maintain strength and function. Braces and neoprene sleeves have also been shown to reduce pain and improve function (Brouwer et al., 2006).

Pharmacological management is targeted toward symptomatic relieve and includes use of analgesics (discussed further below), nonsteroidal anti-inflammatory drugs (NSAIDs), intraocular steroid injections, and viscosupplementation. In addition, colchicine, topical nonsteroidals, arthroscopic irrigation, acupuncture and nutraceuticals, which are a combination of pharmaceutical and nutritional supplements, have also been used. The most common nutraceuticals include glucosamine and chondroitin and there is some support for their effectiveness in pain management and reducing joint space narrowing at dosages of 1500 mg/day of glucosamine and 800 mg/day of chondroitin (Clegg, 2006; Herrero-Beaumont et al., 2007). Arthroscopic interventions are mainly recommended for situations in which there is known inflammation and when other non-invasive interventions have failed. Likewise, joint replacement should be reserved for individuals with severe symptomatic disease who do not respond to more conservative interventions. Optimal management often involves the use of multiple treatment modalities, and the best combination of treatments will vary from patient to patient.

Treating arthritis optimally requires a differential diagnosis as there are multiple different types of arthritic conditions and treatments may vary. For example, polymyalgia rheumatica is a common musculoskeletal problem for older women with symptoms that include weight loss; fever; muscle pain; aching of the neck, shoulder, and hip; and morning stiffness. Treatment involves use of steroids, such as prednisone, although alternative treatments with drugs such as infliximab have also been shown to be effective (Salvarani et al., 2007). Because of the close association between polymyalgia rheumatica and temporal arteritis, any symptoms suggestive of involvement of the temporal artery—headache, jaw claudication, recent changes in vision—especially when the sedimentation rate is very high (> 75 mm/h) should prompt consideration of temporal artery biopsy (Unwin, 2006). Acute treatment of temporal arteritis with high-dose steroids is needed to prevent blindness. The history and physical examination can be helpful in differentiating OA from inflammatory arthritis (Table 10-5); however, other procedures are often essential.

Gout, one of the oldest recognized forms of arthritis, is characterized by intra-articular monosodium urate crystals. Gout generally presents as acute affecting the first metatarsal phalangeal joint, mid foot, or ankle, although the knee, elbow, or wrist can also be involved. Tophi, which are subcutaneous urate deposits on extensor surfaces, can develop in later phases of the disease, and are sometimes confused with rheumatoid arthritis and associated nodules. Radiographs may reveal well-defined gouty erosions in or around joints. Some patients will have elevated uric acid levels (Wise, 2007). The definitive diagnosis of gout is established by observing the presence of needle-shaped crystals in the involved joint. The goal of treatment is to terminate the acute

TABLE 10-5   CLINICAL FEATURES OF OSTEOARTHRITIS VERSUS INFLAMMATORY ARTHRITIS

CLINICAL FEATURE	OSTEOARTHRITIS	INFLAMMATORY ARTHRITIS
Duration of stiffness	Minutes	Hours
Pain	Usually with activity	Occurs even at rest and at night
Fatigue	Unusual	Common
Swelling	Common but little synovial reaction	Very common, with synovial proliferation and thickening
Erythema and warmth	Unusual	Common

attack, and then prevent future attacks by considering underlying causes (eg, considering hypouricemic therapy). The acute phase of gout should be managed using short-term NSAIDs, colchicines, corticotrophin, and corticosteroids. Treatment choices should be based on patient comorbidities (eg, renal function, gastrointestinal disease). Treatment to decrease uric acid levels should not be initiated during the acute phase as drugs such as allopurinol or probenecid may exacerbate the acute attack. Owing to renal changes associated with aging, allopurinol is recommended over probenecid in older individuals. Colchicine can be used for acute management as well as for prophylaxis.

In addition to making specific diagnoses of rheumatological disorders whenever possible, careful physical examination can detect treatable nonarticular conditions such as tendinitis and bursitis. Bicipital tendinitis and olecranon and trochanteric bursitis are common in geriatric patients. Dramatic relief from pain and disability from these conditions can be achieved by local treatments such as the injection of steroids.

Carpal tunnel syndrome is another common musculoskeletal disorder among older adults and can be confused for gout, rheumatoid arthritis, or pseudogout. Carpal tunnel syndrome involves the entrapment of the median nerve where it passes through the carpal tunnel of the wrist and thereby causes nocturnal hand pain, numbness, and tingling affecting the median nerve distribution in the hand. Further atrophy of the thenar eminence can develop when there has been persistent nerve compression. Nerve conduction studies are needed to make the diagnosis and surgical intervention is often needed to relieve the nerve compression. For more conservative interventions, cock-up wrist splints, usually worn at night, isometric flexion exercises of metacarpal phalangeal joints, and steroid injections have been implemented.

Hip Fracture

In 2003, there were more than 309,500 hospital admissions for hip fractures and by the year 2030 more than 650,000 hip fractures will occur annually in older adults (Cummings and Melton, 2002). Recent evidence suggests, however, that there are fewer hospitalizations for hip fracture with the overall age-adjusted hospitalization rate for hip fractures from 1993 to 2003 showing a decrease of 15.5%, from 917.6 per 100,000 population to 775.7 ($P = 0.001$ test for trend) (Gehlbach, Avrunin, and Puleo, 2007). More specifically, the hospitalization rate for hip fracture in women declined 20.8% ($P < 0.01$), and trends over an 11-year interval have a peak of 248,000 fractures among women (National Center for Health Statistics, 2006). About 95% of the hospitalizations for hip fracture in older women occurred in those aged 65 and over and almost 80% occurred in those aged 75 and over. In the first year post hip fracture, approximately 30% of individuals die, 25% will have significant functional decline in activities of daily living such as bathing and dressing, 20% will need help with lower extremity dressing, and 90% will require help climbing the stairs (Di Monaco, 2006; Ryan, Enderby, and Rigby, 2006). Individuals who have had a hip fracture are noted to be impaired in their ability to independently rise from an armless chair or to step symmetrically, and approximately 38% to 50% need assistance to walk or are unable to walk at 12 months post hip fracture. The assessment and management of falls, the major cause of hip fracture, is discussed in Chap. 9.

The degree of immobility and disability caused by a hip fracture depends on several factors, including coexisting medical conditions, patient motivation, the nature of the fracture, and the techniques of management (Beloosesky et al., 2007). Many older patients with hip fracture already have impaired mobility, and there is a high incidence of medical illnesses that necessitate treatment (eg, infection, heart failure, anemia, dehydration) at the time of hip fracture. Patients with these underlying conditions and those with dementia are at especially high risk for poor functional recovery.

The location of the fracture is especially important in determining the most appropriate management plan (Fig. 10-1). Subcapital fractures (which are inside the joint capsule) disrupt the blood supply to the proximal femoral head, thus resulting in a higher probability of necrosis of the femoral head and nonunion of the fracture. Replacement of the femoral head is often warranted in these cases. Inter- and subtrochanteric fractures generally do not disrupt the blood supply to the femoral head and open reduction and pinning are usually successful. Generally, arthroplasty has been shown to be more clinically effective and probably

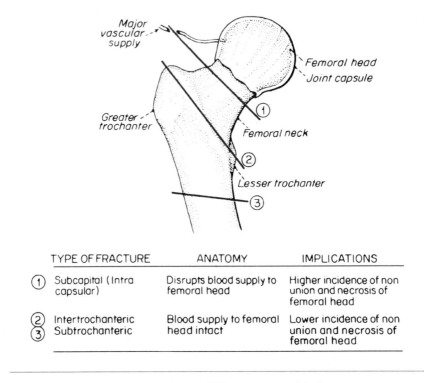

TYPE OF FRACTURE	ANATOMY	IMPLICATIONS
① Subcapital (Intra capsular)	Disrupts blood supply to femoral head	Higher incidence of non union and necrosis of femoral head
② Intertrochanteric ③ Subtrochanteric	Blood supply to femoral head intact	Lower incidence of non union and necrosis of femoral head

— FIGURE 10-1 —   Characteristics of different types of hip fractures.

less costly over a 2-year period post surgery when compared to open reduction and fixation, bipolar hemiarthroplasty and total arthroplasty (Blomfeldt et al., 2007; Keating et al., 2006).

Generally, the current trend in hip fracture management is to stabilize any associated comorbid or acute medical conditions; surgically repair the hip, ideally with spinal anesthesia; and encourage early ambulation and aggressive rehabilitation (Blomfeldt et al., 2007; Dillingham, 2007; Host et al., 2007). The current standard of care is for patients to receive prophylactic anticoagulation to prevent thromboembolic complications (Colwell, 2007). Subcutaneous injection of low-molecular-weight heparin is an effective method of prophylaxis in patients with hip fractures (Steier et al., 2006). Intermittent pneumatic compression is of value, but the equipment is costly and the need to apply and remove the device limits its usefulness. In addition to traditional interdisciplinary rehabilitation programs which are known to improve outcomes (Stenvall et al., 2007), participation in ongoing exercise activities is critical to recovery

(Mangione et al., 2005; Petrella and Jones, 2007). As with most older adults, motivational interventions are effective and should be implemented to increase time spent in exercise post hip fracture (Resnick et al., 2007).

Parkinson Disease

The first step in successful management of PD is to recognize its presence. Pathologically, PD is associated with a progressive loss of dopamine-producing cells, especially in the substantia nigra which sends dopamine to the corpus striatum. These structures, located in the basal ganglia, are stimulated by the neurotransmitter dopamine and are responsible for planning and controlling automatic movements of the body, such as walking, writing, or rising from a seated position. Once the level of dopamine loss has reached a threshold, individuals typically develop a triad of symptoms: bradykinesia (slow movement) or akinesia (absence of movement), resting tremor, and muscle rigidity. Many elderly patients, especially in long-term care institutions, have undiagnosed, treatable forms of parkinsonism. Some of these individuals have drug-induced parkinsonism resulting from the extrapyramidal side effects of antipsychotics (see Chap. 14). Nonmotor symptoms of PD are also common and include depression, psychosis, anxiety, sleep disturbances, dysautonomia, dementia, and others. Left untreated, parkinsonian patients eventually become immobile and can develop flexion contractures, pressure sores, malnutrition, and aspiration pneumonia.

Pharmacological treatment of PD is based on an attempt to increase the ratio of dopamine to acetylcholine in the central nervous system, specifically the nigrostriatal system. There are many drugs that are used in the treatment of the disease including amantadine, anticholinergic drugs, levodopa, monoamine oxidase inhibitors B (MAO-B), catechol O-methyltransferase (COMT), and dopamine agonists (Schapira, 2005). Surgical options are also gaining more attention and are a viable choice for a select group of individuals (Bronte-Stewart, 2003). Several drugs can be used, sometimes in combination (Table 10-6). Clinical response may take several weeks. Side effects are common and often limit pharmacological treatment. Wide variations in response can also occur, including morning akinesia, peak-dose dyskinesias, and freezing episodes (sometimes referred to as the "on–off phenomenon"). Excessive dopamine can also cause sleep disturbances, delirium, and psychosis. Surgical procedures such as deep brain stimulation (DBS) of the subthalamic nuclei (STN) or globus pallidum (GPi) are available for individuals with advanced PD (Rascol et al., 2006).

Exercise therapy has long been recommended for individuals with PD and is sometimes used as an adjunct to pharmacologic therapies (Suchowersky O, 2006). Aerobic exercise, specifically treadmill training, had significantly positive effects on perceived functional independence, motor function, and ADL as reported on the Unified Parkinson Disease Rating Scale (UPDRS) (Toole et al., 2005).

TABLE 10-6   DRUGS USED TO TREAT PARKINSON DISEASE

Drug (Brand Name)	Usual Dosages	Mechanism of Action	Potential Side Effects
Carbidopa, levodopa (Sinemet)	40/400-200/2000 mg/day in divided doses*	Increases dopamine availability and decreases peripheral dopamine metabolism	Nausea, vomiting, anorexia Dyskinesias Orthostatic hypotension Behavioral disturbances Vivid dreams and hallucinations
Amantadine (Symmetrel)	100-300 mg/day†	Increases dopamine release	Delirium and hallucinations
Bromocriptine (Parlodel)	1-1.5 mg tid or qid (initial); gradually increase to maximum of 30-40 mg in divided doses	Directly activates dopamin-ergic receptors	Behavioral changes Hypotension Nausea
Pramipexole (Mirapex)	0.5-1.5 mg tid	Dopamine agonist	Hallucinations Nausea Somnolence
Ropinirole (Requip)	3-8 mg tid	Dopamine agonist	Orthostatic hypotension Syncope Nausea Somnolence
Anticholinergic agents,‡ trihexyphenidyl (Artane, Tremin)	2-20 mg/day in divided doses	Decreases effects of acetyl-choline and helps to restore balance between cholinergic and dopaminergic systems	Dry mouth Constipation Urinary retention Blurred vision

Drug	Dosage	Mechanism	Side effects
Benztropine mesylate (Cogentin)	0.5–8.0 mg/day in divided doses		Exacerbation of glaucoma Tachycardia Confusion Behavioral changes
Selegiline (Eldepryl)	10 mg/day in one dose	MAO-B inhibitor	As above Nausea Confusion Agitation Insomnia Involuntary movements
Rasagiline (Azilect)	1 mg/day in one dose	Selective, irreversible MAO-B inhibitor	Balance difficulties Anorexia Vomiting Weight loss Depressive symptoms No dietary restrictions
Entacapone (Comtan)	200 mg with each dose of levodopa	Inhibits catechol methyltransferase	Nausea Dyskinesias Orthostatic hypotension Diarrhea
Tolcapone (Tasmar)	100–200 mg tid		Liver dysfunction§

*Top number represents carbidopa; bottom number, levodopa.
†Eliminated by kidney; dosages should be adjusted when renal function is diminished.
‡Several other anticholinergic agents are available.
MAO-B, monoamine oxidase type B.

Stroke

To prevent the progression of immobility moving toward disability and subsequent complications, patients with completed strokes should receive prompt and intensive rehabilitative therapy. In many elderly patients, coexisting medical conditions (eg, cardiovascular disease) limit the intensity of rehabilitation treatment that can be tolerated in order to qualify for Medicare coverage in an inpatient or skilled nursing facility. However, all patients should be evaluated and managed as actively as possible during the first several weeks after a stroke. Although all stroke patients deserve an assessment and consideration for intensive rehabilitation, the cost-effectiveness of various approaches to stroke rehabilitation is controversial. Whether the rehabilitative efforts occur in the acute care hospital, special rehabilitation unit, nursing home, or at home, these efforts should involve a multidisciplinary rehabilitation team, and the basic principles remain the same (see Rehabilitation later in this chapter).

Despite the lack of data from controlled trials, even some of the most severely affected stroke patients can achieve meaningful improvements in functional status by early rehabilitative efforts. Although complete functional recovery occurs in less than half of stroke patients, immobility and its attendant complications can almost always be prevented or minimized. Innovative interventions with motor training consisting of voluntary movements assisted by a robot device have recently been tested. Such interventions led to significant improvements in motor performance in stroke patients (Colombo et al., 2007). Similarly, treadmill training in stroke patients has been shown to have a positive effect on gait (Chen and Patten, 2006). In addition to innovative and intensive rehabilitation in the immediate poststroke period, ongoing exercise and physical activity is critical post stroke to maintain optimal function and prevent future strokes. The management of older patients with cerebrovascular disease is discussed further in Chap. 11.

Pressure Ulcers

A pressure ulcer is defined as damage caused to the skin and underlying soft tissue by unrelieved pressure when the tissue is compressed between a bony prominence and external surface over a period of time. Three main factors contribute to the development of pressure sores: pressure, shearing forces, and friction. The amount of pressure necessary to occlude blood supply to the skin (and thus predispose to irreversible tissue damage) depends on the quality of the tissue, blood flow to the area, and the amount of pressure applied. For example, a patient with peripheral artery disease heel pressure over a relatively short period of time may cause an ulceration to occur.

Shearing forces (such as those created when the head of a bed is elevated and the torso slides down and transmits pressure to the sacral area) contribute to the stretching and angulation of subcutaneous tissues. Friction, caused by the repeated movement of skin across surfaces such as bedsheets or clothing, increases the shearing force. This can eventually lead to thrombosis of small blood vessels, thus undermining and then destroying skin. Shearing forces and friction are worsened by loose, folded skin, which is common in the elderly because of loss of subcutaneous tissue and/or dehydration. Moisture from bathing, sweat, urine, and feces compounds the damage. Three out of nineteen risk factors are consistently included in screening tools: mobility, continence, and nutrition, although these risk factors have not been supported as causal (Sharp and McLaws, 2006). In light of the many risk factors and their variable influence, numerous scales have been developed to quantify a person's risk of developing pressure ulcers. The two most commonly used scales are the Braden scale (http://www.bradenscale.com/), and the Norton scale (http://www.ncbi.nlm. nih.gov/books/bv.fcgi?rid=hstat2.table.4948).

Pressure ulcers can be classified into four stages, depending on their clinical appearance and extent (Table 10-7). The area of damage below the pressure ulcer can be much larger than the ulcer itself. This is caused by the manner in which pressure and shearing forces are transmitted to subcutaneous tissues. More than 90% of pressure ulcers occur in the lower body—mainly in the sacral and coccygeal areas, at the ischial tuberosities, and in the greater trochanter area.

The cornerstone of management of the skin in immobile patients is prevention of pressure ulcers (Table 10-8), as outlined in the Agency for Health Care Research and Quality Pressure Ulcers in Adults: Prediction and Prevention (www.ahrq.gov/news/pubcat/c_clin.htm). Once a stage I or II pressure ulcer develops, all preventive measures listed in Table 10-8 should be used to avoid progression of the ulcer, and intensive local skin care must be instituted. Many techniques have been advocated for local skin care; none is more successful than the others. The most important factor in all these techniques is the attention that the skin gets, including relief from pressure. Almost any technique that involves removing pressure from the area and regularly cleansing and drying the skin will work. Alternating pressure mattresses and alternating pressure overlays are equally effective in terms of prevention and management of pressure ulcers (Nixon et al., 2006).

The management of stages III and IV pressure ulcers is more complicated. Debridement of necrotic tissue and frequent irrigation (two to three times daily), cleansing (with saline or peroxide), and dressing of the wound are essential. Eschars should be undermined and removed if they are suspected of hiding large amounts of necrotic and infected tissue. Chemical debriding agents can be helpful. The role of wound cultures and antimicrobials in the management of stage III pressure ulcers is controversial. Topical antimicrobials may be useful, especially when bacterial colony counts are high, but they are generally not recommended. Systemic antimicrobials should not be used because they do not reach sufficient concentrations in the area of the ulcer; topical therapy will be more effective

TABLE 10-7   CLINICAL CHARACTERISTICS OF PRESSURE SORES

CHARACTERISTICS	DIAGNOSTIC TIPS
Stage I	
Acute inflammatory response limited to epidermis	Pressure areas at stage I do not blanch when pressed
Presents as irregular area of erythema, induration, edema; may be firm or boggy	May be different with different skin pigments
	Redness with pressure persists after 30 min; in dark skin the color may be red, blue, or a purple hue
Often over a bony prominence	
Skin is unbroken	
Stage II	
Extension of acute inflammatory response through dermis to the junction of subcutaneous fat	May look like an abrasion or a blister
Appears as a blister, abrasion, or shallow ulcer with more distinct edges	
Early fibrosis and pigment changes occur	
Stage III	
Full-thickness skin ulcer extending through subcutaneous fat. This may extend down to but not through the underlying fascia	This presents like a crater and may have undermining of the adjacent tissue
The skin may have undermining	
Base of ulcer infected, often with necrotic, foul-smelling tissue	
Stage IV	
Extension of ulcer through deep fascia, so that bone is visible at base of ulcer	Undermining is even more common and there may be sinus tracts
Osteomyelitis and septic arthritis can be present	

TABLE 10-8   PRINCIPLES OF SKIN CARE IN IMMOBILE OLDER
PATIENTS

Preventive
Identify patients at risk
Decrease pressure, friction, and skin folding
Keep skin clean and dry
Avoid excessive bed rest: optimize and encourage function
Avoid oversedation
Provide adequate nutrition and hydration (30-35 kcal/kg) overall, protein
(1-1.5 g/kg), and fluid (1mL/kcal)

Stages I and II pressure sores
Clean wounds with warm, normal saline or water
Avoid pressure and moisture
Cover open wounds with an occlusive dressing: determined based on
ulcer condition (eg, presence of granulation, necrotic tissue), type and
amount of drainage, surrounding tissue, and evidence of infection
Prevent further injury and infection: use antibiotics very judiciously
Provide intensive local skin care[*]
Manage associated pain

Stage III pressure sores
Debride necrotic tissue: autolytic, chemical, mechanical, sharp, or
surgical options
Cleanse and dress wound as above[*]
Culture wound: treat only in cases of confirmed bacteremia, sepsis,
osteomyelitis, and cellulitis[†]
Manage associate pain

Stage IV pressure sores
Take tissue biopsy for culture
Use systemic antimicrobials as noted in stage III
Cleanse and dress wound as above
Have surgical consultation to consider surgical repair
Manage associated pain

[*]Many techniques are effective (see text).
[†]Cultures and topical antimicrobials should not be used routinely (see text).

unless cellulitis is present. Routine wound cultures are probably not warranted for stage III lesions because they almost always grow several different organisms and do not detect anaerobic bacteria, which are often pathogenic. Results of such cultures generally reflect colonization rather than infection. Once a lesion has progressed to stage IV, systemic antimicrobials are often necessary. Routine and anaerobic cultures of tissue or bone are most helpful in directing antimicrobial therapy. Patients with large pressure ulcers which become septic should be treated with broad-spectrum antimicrobials that will cover anaerobes, gram-negative organisms, and *Staphylococcus aureus*. In selected instances, consideration of plastic surgery for stage IV lesions is warranted.

Documentation of pressure sores is critical and should include the following components: (1) the type of ulcer, how long it has been present, and in what setting it occurred; (2) the size measured as length × width × depth in centimeters (area of the wound bed that is deepest, without a tract); (3) the color as percentage with red indicating amount of granulation tissue, yellow indicating the amount of slough present, and black being necrotic tissue or eschar; (4) exudate as serous, serosanguinous, sanguinous, or purulent; (5) the presence or absence of odor in the wound (this should be determined after the wound is thoroughly cleaned); (6) describe the periwound tissues (eg, viable, macerated, inflamed, or hyperkeratotic); and (7) evidence of undermining (undermining is a separation of the tissues between the surface and the subcutaneous tissues).

PAIN MANAGEMENT

Pain is a major cause of immobility in older adults. Immobility, in turn, can exacerbate painful conditions and create a vicious cycle of pain, decreased mobility, and increased pain. The American Geriatrics Society has published recommendations of an expert panel for the management of persistent pain in older adults, and readers are referred to this publication for more details (AGS Panel on Persistent Pain in Older Persons, 2002). Pain is also discussed in Chap. 3 of this book.

Pain in older persons is commonly underdiagnosed and undertreated despite the availability of many assessment tools and effective therapeutic interventions. Pain is now viewed as a "fifth vital sign," and health professionals are encouraged to routinely inquire about pain. When pain is identified, it should be carefully characterized. In addition to the standard questions about location, timing, aggravating factors, and the like, a simple standardized pain scale can be helpful in rating the severity of pain. Several such scales are available in the American Medical Directors Association Clinical Practice Guideline on Pain Management (American Medical Directors Association Clinical Practice Guideline, 2006, available at www.amda.com/tools/guidelines.cfm). The degree to which pain interferes with ADL and sleep is especially important to explore. Recurrent or persistent pain can result in complications such as a predisposition to falling because of deconditioning, behavioral problems, depression, and impaired quality of life. Pain may present differently in older adults with cognitive impairment, and should be evaluated carefully using observational data rather than simply a subjective report. If appropriately evaluated older adults with cognitive impairment can reliably report pain and be evaluated for pain by observing for specific pain-related activities (agitation, moaning, or grimacing) (Feldt, 2000). Pain should be assessed on an ongoing basis to determine if it has been resolved following an intervention or if there is a need to alter the pain management regimen.

It is useful to differentiate between nociceptive pain, which includes somatic pain arising from the skin, bone, joint, muscle, or connective tissue and is often described as throbbing from visceral pain, which arises from internal organs such as the large intestine or pancreas, or neuropathic pain, which is pain sustained by abnormal processing of sensory input by the peripheral or central nervous system. Neuropathic pain is generally described as burning, tingling, shock-like, or shooting. Differentiating pain helps to guide management strategies and assures more efficient pain relief.

Pain management should consider nonpharmacological and pharmacological approaches. Nonpharmacological approaches include physical activity and exercise (Shih, 2006) to help manage chronic pain associated with arthritis, disuse, or positioning. Simple comfort measures such as listening to a book on tape, music, storytelling, or other types of distractions may be helpful. Additionally, heat, ice, stretching, massage, ultrasonography, and acupuncture can be considered and tried.

The mainstay of pain management is drug therapy. Table 10-9 lists drugs that can be helpful in managing pain in older adults. For persistent pain, most experts recommend initiating treatment with acetaminophen and the use of topical treatments such as capsaicin or ketamine gel, lidocaine patches, or local intra-articular corticosteroid injections. The use of NSAIDs can be very effective for short-term pain management. As noted above, the use of these agents in the long term may cause significant side effects. Alternatively, nonacetylated salicylates such as salsalate and trisalicylate may have less renal toxicity and antiplatelet activity than the nonsteroid anti-inflammatory agents and therefore may be a better option for older adults. Severe persistent pain often requires opioid therapy, which can be given alone or in combination with one of a number of adjuvant drugs (see Table 10-9). The side effects of opioids are well known and include such things as respiratory depression, sedation, constipation, nausea, vomiting, or delirium.

Nonopioid medications to treat persistent pain, used particularly for neuropathic pain, include tricyclic antidepressants, other classes of antidepressants such as the selective serotonin reuptake inhibitors, antiepileptic medications, and corticosteroids. The tricyclic drugs, while known to be effective for pain management

TABLE 10-9 TYPES OF PAIN, EXAMPLES, AND TREATMENT

TYPE OF PAIN AND EXAMPLES	SOURCE OF PAIN	TYPICAL DESCRIPTION	EFFECTIVE DRUG CLASSES AND TREATMENT
NOCICEPTIVE: SOMATIC			
Arthritis, acute postoperative, fracture, bone metastases	Tissue injury, eg, bones, soft tissue, joints, muscles	Well localized, constant; aching, stabbing, gnawing, throbbing	Nonopioids, NSAIDs, opioids Physical and cognitive-behavioral therapies
NOCICEPTIVE: VISCERAL			
Renal colic, bowel obstruction	Viscera	Diffuse, poorly localized, referred to other sites, intermittent, paroxysmal; dull, colicky, squeezing, deep, cramping; often accompanied by nausea, vomiting, diaphoresis	Nonopioids, NSAIDs, opioids Physical and cognitive-behavioral therapies
NEUROPATHIC			
Cervical or lumbar radiculopathy, post-herpetic neuralgia,	Peripheral or central nervous system	Prolonged, usually constant, but can be paroxysmal; sharp, burning, pricking, tingling,	Tricyclic antidepressants, anticonvulsants,

| trigeminal neuralgia, diabetic neuropathy, post-stroke syndrome, herniated intervertebral disc | squeezing; associated with other sensory disturbances, eg, paresthesias and dysesthesias; allodynia, hyperalgesia, impaired motor function, atrophy, or abnormal deep tendon reflexes | opioids, topical anesthetics Physical and cognitive-behavioral therapies |

UNDETERMINED

| Myofascial pain syndrome, somatoform pain disorders | Poorly understood No identifiable pathologic processes or symptoms out of proportion to identifiable organic pathology; widespread musculoskeletal pain, stiffness, and weakness | Antidepressants, antianxiety agents Physical, cognitive-behavioral, and psychological therapies |

Reprinted with permission from Reuben DB, Herr KA, Pacala JT, *et al. Geriatrics At Your Fingertips: 2008-2009, 10th ed.* New York, NY: The American Geriatrics Society; 2008:170.

(Ahmad and Goucke, 2002), commonly cause significant anticholinergic side effects including dry mouth, urinary retention, constipation, delirium, tachycardia, and blurred vision. Alternatively, other classes of antidepressants have been shown to be effective in the management of pain (Saarto and Wiffen, 2005; Schneider, 2005). Antiepileptic drugs, such as a carbamazepine, approved for some types of neuropathic pain, have fewer side effects although they may result in sedation, dizziness, weight gain, hyponatremia, or peripheral edema. Corticosteroids are long known to be effective in the management of pain, particularly when there is associated inflammation. Adverse effects with the short-term use of steroids include delirium, fluid retention, hyperglycemia, and immunosuppression.

A few drugs should be avoided when managing pain in older adults, unless no other alternative is effective. Propoxyphene can cause ataxia, dizziness, tremulousness, and seizures and has not been shown to be more effective than acetaminophen for pain management. Meperidine is metabolized to normeperidine, a substance that has no analgesic properties but may impair kidney function, cause tremulousness, myoclonus, and seizures. Tramadol, a drug that combines opioid-receptor binding and norepinephrine and serotonin reuptake inhibition, lowers the seizure threshold and should not be given when the individual is taking other medications with serotonergic properties.

EXERCISE

Exercise is a critical intervention for preventing immobility and its complications, and is also discussed in Chap. 5. Meta-analytic reviews have provided strong evidence that participation in either nonspecific physical activity or specific aerobic or resistive exercise is associated with decreased progression of DJD (Roddy et al., 2005), which is critical for maintaining mobility.

The specific amount of exercise needed to achieve the desired benefit varies based on individual goals and capabilities. Combining recommendations from the American College of Sports Medicine, the Centers for Disease Control and Prevention (CDC), and the National Institutes of Health (NIH), health-care providers should recommend that older adults engage in 30 minutes of physical activity DAILY, and this activity should incorporate aerobic activity (walking, dancing, swimming, biking), resistance training, and flexibility. Exercises can be done individually or in group settings depending on the individual's preference, cognitive ability, and motivational level.

In light of the many benefits of physical activity and the relatively low risk of serious adverse events associated with low- and moderate-intensity physical activity, current guidelines from a consensus group from the American Heart Association and the American College of Cardiology (United States Preventive

Services Task Force, 2004) no longer recommend routine stress testing for those initiating a physical activity. For sedentary older people who are asymptomatic, low-intensity physical activity can be safely initiated regardless of whether an older adult has had a recent medical evaluation. Screening of some type, however, is still frequently recommended for older adults to help assure them of the safety of exercise and to provide direction as to the appropriate exercise program in which to engage (Resnick et al., 2005). A new screening tool, referred to as the Exercising and Screening for You (EASY) (Resnick, et al., 2008) is one such tool that helps older individuals and their providers identify what physical activity program is appropriate for the individual, given their health status. EASY addresses six simple questions which, depending on responses, refer older individuals or their providers to appropriate exercise programs (ie, those for individuals with DJD, dizziness, or cardiovascular disorders).

REHABILITATION

The goal of rehabilitation is to restore function and prevent further disability. The goal of restorative care is to continue to focus on the restoration and/or maintenance of physical function by compensating for functional impairments so that the individual maintains their highest level of function and increases time spent in physical activity. Maintaining a restorative philosophy of care is therefore a core element of geriatric practice, especially for immobile elderly patients. Implementing this philosophy of care necessitates a team effort. Physiatrists, physical and/or occupational therapists can be very helpful in developing appropriate and optimal rehabilitative and restorative plans for older adults across the care continuum. It is beyond the scope of this text to provide a detailed discussion of rehabilitation in the older adult. Table 10-10 outlines some of the key principles. Careful assessment of a patient's function and underlying capability, the setting of realistic goals, prevention of secondary disabilities and complications of immobility, evaluation of the environment, and adapting the environment to the patients' abilities (and vice versa) are all essential elements of the rehabilitation process. Moreover, ongoing motivation of the older individual as well as the caregivers is critical to successful rehabilitation and restoration of function (Resnick, 2004).

The expertise of an interdisciplinary team, specifically physical and occupational therapists, can be extremely valuable in assessing, treating, motivating, and monitoring patients whose mobility is impaired. Physical therapists generally attend to the relief of pain, muscle strength and endurance, joint range of motion, and gait. They use a variety of treatment modalities (Table 10-11). Occupational therapists focus on functional abilities, especially as they relate to ADL. They

TABLE 10-10   BASIC PRINCIPLES OF REHABILITATION IN OLDER
                PATIENTS

Optimize the treatment of underlying diseases, nutrition and hydration, and
  psychosocial situation

Optimize the physical environment with regard to encouraging function and
  physical activity (eg, handrails, open access)

Optimize the care environment so that patient participation in functional
  activities and physical activities is optimized (eg, so that care is not task
  focused)

Prevent secondary disabilities and complications of immobility

Treat primary disabilities

Set realistic, individualized goals

Emphasize functional independence
    Set measurable goals related to functional performance
    Enhance residual functional capacities
    Provide adaptive tools to maximize function
    Adapt the environment to the patient's functional disabilities when
      feasible

Attend to motivation and other psychological factors of both patients and
  caregivers

Use a team approach

make detailed assessments of mobility and help patients improve or adapt to their
abilities to perform basic and instrumental activities of daily living. Even when
mobility and function remain impaired, occupational therapists can make life easier for these patients by performing environmental assessments and recommending modifications and assistive devices that will improve the patient's ability to
function independently (Table 10-12). Speech therapists are helpful in assessing
and implementing rehabilitation for disorders of communication and swallowing.
Nursing and informal caregivers have the responsibility of ongoing encouragement of older adults to engage in the activities recommended by these therapists
(ie, walking to the bathroom, participating in exercise classes, or completing specific strength training activities).

Rehabilitation services can occur in an acute hospital, skilled nursing facility,
in an outpatient clinical setting or at home. Rehabilitation provided at an acute
level of care, such as in stroke rehabilitation, is generally limited in terms of length

TABLE 10-11 PHYSICAL THERAPY IN THE MANAGEMENT
OF IMMOBILE OLDER PATIENTS

Objectives
  Relieve pain
  Evaluate, maintain, and improve joint range of motion
  Evaluate and improve strength, endurance, motor skills, and coordination
  Evaluate and improve gait and stability
  Assess the need for and teach the use of assistive devices for ambulation
    (wheelchairs, walkers, canes)
Treatment modalities
Exercise
  Active (isometric and isotonic)
  Passive
  Encourage sitting exercise programs
Heat
  Hot packs
  Paraffin
  Diathermy
  Ultrasound
Hydrotherapy
Ultrasound
Transcutaneous electrical nerve stimulation

of stay and depends on the older individual's goals and demonstration of progress toward goal achievement. At the acute level, rehabilitation includes 3 hours a day of therapy by at least two out of the three therapists (physical, occupational, or speech therapy). At this level of care, the patient is seen by a physician or designated provider daily, and receives 24-hour nursing rehabilitation care. Reimbursement is based on case-mix groups using the Functional Independence Measure. At the skilled level of care (Medicare Part A), rehabilitation is somewhat less rigorous although most Medicare intermediaries will require that a patient show significant rehabilitation potential and steady improvement toward some predetermined goal. At this level, a physician must supervise the care, but daily visits are not required. Reimbursement is based on prospective payment according to resource utilization groups (obtained from the Minimum Data Set). Once the older individuals' goals are achieved, continued rehabilitation services can occur under Medicare Part B 3 days a week at home or in institutional setting.

TABLE 10-12   OCCUPATIONAL THERAPY IN THE MANAGEMENT
OF IMMOBILE OLDER PATIENTS

Objectives
  Restore, maintain, and improve ability to function independently
  Evaluate and improve sensory and perceptual motor function
  Evaluate and improve ability to perform ADLs
  Fabricate and fit splints for upper extremities
  Improve coping and problem-solving skills
  Improve use of leisure time

Modalities
  Assessment of mobility
    Bed mobility
    Transfers
    Wheelchair propulsion

Assessment of other ADLs using actual or simulated environments
    Dressing
    Toileting
    Bathing and personal hygiene
    Cooking and cleaning

Visit home for environmental assessment and recommendations for adaptation

Provide task-oriented activities (eg, crafts, projects)

Recommend and teach use of assistive devices (eg, long-handled reachers,
  special eating and cooking utensils, sock aids)

Recommend and teach use of safety devices (eg, grab bars and railing,
  raised toilet seats, shower chairs)

ADLs, activities of daily living.

The benefit of rehabilitation services in one site, or at one level, versus the other has not been well established (Deutsch et al., 2006; Horn et al., 2005). Some of this may depend on the specific facility in which the care is provided and the philosophy of care that is implemented by the direct caregivers. For example, in inpatient rehabilitation settings, it is critical that the time spent outside of therapy should continue to implement a rehabilitation focus of care in which the older adults are encouraged to practice activities such as bathing, dressing, and ambulation in their real-world settings. If formal or informal caregivers provide the care (ie, bathe and dress) for the individual who has independent goals, it is unlikely that goal will be achieved. Similarly, exemplary rehabilitation services are of little value if following completion of rehabilitation the individual is no longer encouraged to do such things as walk to the dining room. While the caregivers may be well intended and believe that "helping" and demonstrating "caring" is best shown by providing hands-on care services, this type of care only creates deconditioning and dependency, along with contractures and the other sequelae of immobility. Regardless of site of service, therefore, a rehabilitative or restorative philosophy of care should be implemented so as to maintain and optimize the function of each older individual.

References

American Geriatrics Society Panel on Persistent Pain in Older Persons. The management of persistent pain in older persons. *Journal of the American Geriatrics Society.* 2000;50(6 Supple):S205-S224.

Ahmad M, Goucke CR. Management strategies for the treatment of neuropathic pain in the elderly. *Drugs Aging.* 2002;19:929-945.

American Heart Association and American College of Sports Medicine. (2007). Physical Activity and Public Health Guidelines, Available at: http://www.acsm.org. Last accessed July, 2008.

Andrianakos AA, Kontelis LK, Karamitsos DG, et al. Prevalence of symptomatic knee, hand, and hip osteoarthritis in Greece. The ESORDIG study. *J Rheumatol.* 2006;33(12):2507-2513.

Asikainen TM, Suni JH, Pasanen ME, et al. Effect of brisk walking in 1 or 2 daily bouts and moderate resistance training on lower-extremity muscle strength, balance, and walking performance in women who recently went through menopause: a randomized, controlled trial. *Phys Ther.* 2006;86(7):912-923.

Bauss F, Dempster DW. Effects of ibandronate on bone quality: preclinical studies. *Bone.* 2007;40(2):265-273.

Beloosesky Y, Hendel D, Weiss A, et al. Cytokines and C-reactive protein production in hip-fracture-operated elderly patients. *J Gerontol A Biol Sci Med Sci.* 2007;62(4):420-426.

Blomfeldt R, Tornkvist H, Eriksson K, et al. A randomised controlled trial comparing bipolar hemiarthroplasty with total hip replacement for displaced intracapsular fractures of the femoral neck in elderly patients. *J Bone Joint Surg Br.* 2007;89(2):160-165.

Bronte-Stewart H. Parkinson's disease: surgical options. *Curr Treat Options Neurol.* 2003;5(2):131-147.

Brouwer RW, van Raaij TM, Verhaar JA, et al. Brace treatment for osteoarthritis of the knee: a prospective randomized multi-centre trial. *Osteoarthr Cartil.* 2006;14(8):777-783.

Campbell PME, & Allain TJ. Muscle strength and vitamin D in older people. *Gerontology.* 2006;52:335-338.

Chang M, Cohen-Mansfield J, Ferrucci L, et al. Incidence of loss of ability to walk 400 meters in a functionally limited older population. *J Am Geriatr Society.* 2004;52(12): 2094-2098.

Chen G, Patten C. Treadmill training with harness support: selection of parameters for individuals with poststroke hemiparesis. *J Rehabil Res Dev.* 2006;43(4):485-498.

Chen JS, Cameron ID, Cumming RG, et al. Effect of age-related chronic immobility on markers of bone turnover. *J Bone Miner Res.* 2005;21(2):324-331.

Clegg DO. Treatment of ankylosing spondylitis. *J Rheumatol Suppl.* 2006;78:24-31.

Clinical Practice Guideline: Pain Management in the Long Term Care Settinghttp://www.amda.com/tools/cpg/chronicpain.cfm. Last accessed July, 2008.

Colombo R, Pisano F, Micera S, et al. Assessing mechanisms of recovery during robot-aided neurorehabilitation of the upper limb. *Neurorehabil Neural Repair.* 2007;3(1):111-115.

Colwell CW. Evidence-based guidelines for venous thromboembolism prophylaxis in orthopedic surgery. *Orthopedics.* 2007;30(2):129-135.

Cummings SR and Melton LJ. Epidemiology and outcomes of osteoporotic fractures. *Lancet.* 2002;359:1761-1767.

Deutsch A, Granger CV, Heinemann AW, et al. Poststroke rehabilitation: outcomes and reimbursement of inpatient rehabilitation facilities and subacute rehabilitation programs. *Stroke.* 2006 Jun;37(6):1477-1482.

Dhesi JK, Bearne LM, Moniz C, et al. Neuromuscular and psychomotor function in elderly subjects who fall and the relationship with vitamin D status. *Journal of Bone and Mineral Research.* 2002;17:891-897.

Di Monaco M, Vallero F, Di Monaco R, et al. Muscle mass and functional recovery in women with hip fracture. *Am J Phys Med Rehabil.* 2006;85(3):209-215.

Dillingham TR. Musculoskeletal rehabilitation: current understandings and future directions. *Am J Phys Med Rehabil.* 2007;86(1):S19-S28.

Dorsey ER, Constantinescu R, Thompson JP, et al. Projected number of people with Parkinson disease in the most populous nations, 2005 through 2030. *Neurology.* 2007;68(5):384-386.

Ensrud KE, Barrett-Connor EL, Schwartz A, et al. Randomized trial of effect of alendronate continuation versus discontinuation in women with low BMD: results from the Fracture Intervention Trial long-term extension. *J Bone Miner Res.* 2004;19(8):1259-1269.

Feldt KS. The checklist of nonverbal pain indicators (CNPI). *Pain Manag Nurs.* 2000;1(1): 13-21.

Gehlbach SH, Avrunin JS, Puleo E. Trends in hospital care for hip fractures. *Osteoporos Int.* 2007;18(5):585-591.

Gusi N, Raimundo A, Leal A. Low-frequency vibratory exercise reduces the risk of bone fracture more than walking: a randomized controlled trial. *BMC Musculoskelet Disord.* 2006;7:92.

Hedstrom M, Sjoberg K, Brosjo E, et al. Positive effects of anabolic steroids, vitamin D and calcium on muscle mass, bone mineral density and clinical function after a hip fracture. A randomised study of 63 women. *J Bone Joint Surg Br.* 2002;84(4): 497-503.

Herrero-Beaumont G, Ivorra JA, Blanco FJ, et al. Glucosamine sulfate in the treatment of knee osteoarthritis symptoms: a randomized, double-blind, placebo-controlled study using acetaminophen as a side comparator. *Arthritis Rheum.* 2007;56(2):555-567.

Horn SD, DeJong G, Smout RJ, et al. Stroke rehabilitation patients, practice, and outcomes: is earlier and more aggressive therapy better? *Arch Phys Med Rehabil.* 2005;18(12 suppl 2):S101-S114.

Host HH, Sinacore DR, Bohnert KL, et al. Training-induced strength and functional adaptations after hip fracture. *Phys Ther.* 2007;87(3):292-303.

Houston DK, Cesar M, Ferrucci L, et al. Association between vitamin D status and physical performance: the InCHIANTI study. *J Gerontol: Med Sci.* 2007;62A(4):440-446.

Jordan JM, Helmick CG, Renner JB, et al. Prevalence of knee symptoms and radiographic and symptomatic knee osteoarthritis in African Americans and Caucasians: the Johnston County Osteoarthritis Project. *J Rheumatol.* 2007;34(1):172-180.

Joseph C, Kenny AM, Taxel P, et al. Role of endocrine-immune dysregulation in osteoporosis, sarcopenia, frailty and fracture risk. *Mol Aspects Medicine.* 2005;26(3): 181-201.

Keating JF, Grant A, Masson M, et al. Randomized comparison of reduction and fixation, bipolar hemiarthroplasty, and total hip arthroplasty. Treatment of displaced intracapsular hip fractures in healthy older patients. *J Bone Joint Surg Am.* 2006;88(2):249-260.

Keysor JJ, Dunn JE, Link CL, et al. Are foot disorders associated with functional limitation and disability among community dwelling older adults? *J Aging Health.* 2005;17(6):734-752.

Mangione KK, Craik RL, Tomlinson SS, et al. Can elderly patients who have had a hip fracture perform moderate- to high-intensity exercise at home? *Phys Ther.* 2005;85(8):727-739.

Morely JE, Baumgartner RN, Roubenoff R, et al. Sarcopenia *Journal of laboratory Clinical Medicine.* 2001;137:231-241.

Mosekilde L. Vitamin D and the elderly. *Clinical Endocrinology.* 2005;62:265-281.

National Center for Health Statistics, & Centers for Disease Control and Prevention. (2006). National Nursing Home Survey (NNHS) Public-Use Data Files. Available at http://www.cdc.gov/nchs/products/elec_prods/subject/nnhs.htm. Last accessed July, 2008.

National Institute of Aging. Exercise: A Guide from the National Institute of Aging. http://www.nia.nih.gov/HealthInformation/Publications/ExerciseGuide/. Accessed September 2008.

Nixon J, Cranny G, Iglesias C, et al. Randomised, controlled trial of alternating pressure mattresses compared with alternating pressure overlays for the prevention of pressure ulcers: PRESSURE (pressure relieving support surfaces) trial. *BMJ.* 2006; 332(7555):1413-1415.

Petrella RJ, Jones TJ. Do patients receive recommended treatment of osteoporosis following hip fracture in primary care? *BMC Fam Pract.* 2007;7:31-37.

Prohaska T, Belansky E, Belza B, et al. Physical activity, public health, and aging: critical issues and research priorities. *J Gerontol B Psychol Sci Soc Sci.* 2006 Sep;61(5):S267-S73.

Rascol O, Brooks DJ, Korczyn AD, et al. Development of dyskinesias in a 5-year trial of ropinirole and L-dopa. *Mov Disord.* 2006;21(11):1844-1850.

Reich ML. Arthritis: avoiding diagnostic pitfalls. *Geriatrics.* 1982;37:46–54.

Resnick B. *Restorative Care Nursing for Older Adults*. New York, NY: Springer; 2004.

Resnick B, Orwig D, Yu-Yahiro J, et al. Testing the effectiveness of the exercise plus program in older women post-hip fracture. *Ann Behav Med*. 2007;34(1):67-76.

Resnick B, Ory M, Coday M, et al. Older adults' perspectives on screening prior to initiating an exercise program. *Prev Sci*. 2005;6(3):203-211.

Resnick B, Ory M, Hora K, et al. A new screening paradigm and tool: the Exercise/Physical Activity Assessment and Screening for You (EASY). *J Aging Phys Act*. In press.

Roddy E, Zhang W, Doherty M. Aerobic walking or strengthening exercise for osteoarthritis of the knee? A systematic review. *Ann Rheum Dis*. 2005;64(4):544-548.

Roddy E, Zhang W, Doherty M, et al. Evidence-based recommendations for the role of exercise in the management of osteoarthritis of the hip or knee—the MOVE consensus. *Rheumatology*. 2005;44(1):67-73.

Ryan T, Enderby P, Rigby AS. A randomized controlled trial to evaluate intensity of community-based rehabilitation provision following stroke or hip fracture in old age. *Clin Rehabil*. 2006;20(2):123-131.

Saarto T, Wiffen PJ. Antidepressants for neuropathic pain. *Cochrane Database Syst Rev*. 2005;CD005454.

Salvarani C, Macchioni P, Manzini C, et al. Infliximab plus prednisone or placebo plus prednisone for the initial treatment of polymyalgia rheumatica: a randomized trial. *Ann Intern Med*. 2007;146(9):461-469.

Schapira AH. Present and future drug treatment for Parkinson's disease. *J Neurol Neurosurg Psychiatr*. 2005;76(11):1472-1478.

Schneider JP. Chronic pain management in older adults: with coxibs under fire, what now? *Geriatrics Aging*. 2005;60(5):26-28, 30-31.

Sharp CA, McLaws ML. Estimating the risk of pressure ulcer development: is it truly evidence based? *Int Wound J*. 2006;3(4):344-352.

Shih M. Do patients with rheumatoid arthritis benefit from exercise? *Geriatrics Aging*. 2006;9(9):64-630.

Steier KJ, Singh G, Ullah A, et al. Venous thromboembolism: application and effectiveness of the American College of Chest Physicians 2001 guidelines for prophylaxis. *J Am Osteopath Assoc*. 2006;106(7):388-395.

Stenvall M, Olofsson B, Nyberg L, et al. Improved performance in activities of daily living and mobility after a multidisciplinary postoperative rehabilitation in older people with femoral neck fracture: a randomized controlled trial with 1-year follow-up. *J Rehabil Med*. 2007;39(3):232-238.

Suchowersky O. Treatment of Parkinson's disease—where do we go from here? *Nat Clin Pract Neurol*. 2006;2(9):461.

Sun BH, Wu CW, Kalunian KC. New developments in osteoarthritis. *Rheum Dis Clin North Am*. 2007;33(1):135-148.

The EASY Screening Group. The Exercise and Screening for You Tool. www://easyforyou.info. Accessed September 2008.

Toole T, Maitland CG, Warren E, et al. The effects of loading and unloading treadmill walking on balance, gait, fall risk, and daily function in Parkinsonism. *NeuroRehabilitation*. 2005;20(4):307-322.

Trivedi DP, Doll R, Khaw KT. Effect of four monthly oral vitamin D3 (cholecalciferol) supplementation on fractures and mortality in men and women living in the community; randomised double blind controlled trial. *BMJ.* 2003;326(7387);469.

United States Preventive Health Task Force. Screening for Osteoporosis in Postmenopausal Women: Recommendations and Rationale. http://www.guideline.gov/summary/summary. aspx?doc_id=3417. 2002. Accessed September 2008.

United States Preventive Services Task Force. Screening for coronary heart disease: recommendation statement. *Ann Intern Med.* 2004;140:569-572.

Unson CG, Litt M, Reisine S, et al. Adherence to calcium/vitamin D and estrogen protocols among diverse older participants enrolled in a clinical trial. *Contemp Clin Trials.* 2006; 27(3):215-226.

Unwin B. Polymyalgia rheumatica and giant cell arteritis. *Am Fam Physician.* 2006; 74(9):1547-1554.

Wise CM. Crystal associated arthritis in the elderly. *Rheum Dis Clin North Am.* 2007;33(1):33-55.

Yildizdas D, Topaloglu AK, Mungan NO, et al. Bone mineral changes in acute metabolic acidosis due to acute gastroenteritis. *Calcif Tissue Int.* 2004;75(5):380-383.

Zorowitz RD, Gross E, Polinski DM. The stroke survivor. *Disabil Rehabil.* 2002;24(13):666-679.

Suggested Readings

Immobility, General

Baumgarten M, Margolis DJ, Localio AR, et al. Pressure ulcers among elderly patients early in the hospital stay. *J Gerontol A Biol Sci Med Sci.* 2006;61(7):749-754.

Graf C. Functional decline in hospitalized older adults. *Am J Nurs.* 2007;106(1):58-67.

Musculoskeletal Disorders

McCarberg BH. Rheumatic diseases in the elderly: dealing with rheumatic pain in extended care facilities. *Rheum Dis Clin North Am.* 2007;33:87-103.

Tutuncu Z. Rheumatic disease in the elderly: rheumatoid arthritis. *Rheum Dis Clin North Am.* 2007;33:57-70.

Sun BH. New developments in osteoarthritis. *Rheum Dis Clin North Am.* 2007;33:135-148.

Parkinson Disease

Weiner WJ, Shulman LM, Lang AE. *Parkinson's Disease: A Complete Guide for Patients and Families. A Johns Hopkins Press Health Book.* Baltimore, MD: John Hopkins University Press; 2006.

Dennison AC, Noorigian JV, Robinson KM, et al. Falling in Parkinson disease: identifying and prioritizing risk factors in recurrent fallers. *Am J Phys Med Rehabil.* 2007;86(8):621-32.

Grosset KA, Grosset DG. Effect of educational intervention on medication timing in Parkinson's disease: a randomized controlled trial. *Br Med Clin Neurol.* 2007;16;7:20.

Pressure Ulcers

Jones KR, Fennie K. Factors influencing pressure ulcer healing in adults over 50: an exploratory study. *J Am Med Dir Assoc.* 2007;8(6):378-387.

Hengstermann S, Fischer A, Steinhagen-Thiessen E, et al. Nutrition status and pressure ulcer: what we need for nutrition screening. *J Parenter Enteral Nutr.* 2007;31(4):288-294.

Capon A, Pavoni N, Mastromattei A, et al. Pressure ulcer risk in long-term units: prevalence and associated factors. *J Adv Nurs.* 2007;58(3):263-272.

Ayello E, Rader C. Pressure Ulcers in Older Adults. Http://www.hartfordign.org/guides/Module7PressureUlcers.doc. Accessed September 2008.

Rehabilitation

Weiss CO, Hoenig HM, Fried LP. Compensatory strategies used by older adults facing mobility disability. *Arch Phys Med Rehabil.* 2007;88(9):1217-1220.

Hinkka K, Karppi SL, Pohjolainen T, et al. Network-based geriatric rehabilitation for frail elderly people: feasibility and effects on subjective health and pain at one year. *J Rehabil Med.* 2007;39(6):473-478.

Hershkovitz A, Kalandariov Z, Hermush V, et al. Factors affecting short-term rehabilitation outcomes of disabled elderly patients with proximal hip fracture. *Arch Phys Med Rehabil.* 2007;88(7):916-921.

Stroke

Centers for Disease Control and Prevention (CDC).Outpatient rehabilitation among stroke survivors—21 States and the District of Columbia, 2005. *MMWR Morb Mortal Wkly Rep.* 2007;56(20):504-507.

Siekierka EM, Eng K, Bassetti C, et al. New technologies and concepts for rehabilitation in the acute phase of stroke: a collaborative matrix. *Neurodegener Dis.* 2007;4(1):57-69.

Measures: Pain

Pain Assessment for Older Adults: Three Pain Scales: Faces pain scale, Numeric rating scale, and Verbal descriptor scale
www.hartfordign.org/publications/trythis/issue07.pdf

NIH Pain Consortium: Five Pain Scales: Numeric rating scale, Wong-Baker faces, COMFORT scale, CRIES pain scale, FLACC scale, Checklist of nonverbal indicators
http://painconsortium.nih.gov/pain_scales/

Function

Instrumental Activities of Daily Living Scale: www.abramsoncenter.org/PRI/documents/IADL.pdf

Activities of Daily Living scale (ADL): Katz ADL scale
www.fpnotebook.com/GER2.htm
www.hartfordign.org/publications/trythis/issue02.pdf
The Barthel Index: a measure of activities of daily living
www.fpnotebook.com/GER2.htm
www.hartfordign.org/publications/trythis/issue02.pdf

Pressure Ulcers

Braden Scale for Predicting Pressure Sore Risk: www.bradenscale.com/braden.PDF
Observation Protocol Pressure Ulcer Assessment and Documentation
www.aasa.dshs.wa.gov/Professional/ND/documents/SOP%20Pressure%20Sore%20Asses
sment.pdf

Exercise and Physical Activity Measures

Exercise Assessment and Screening for You: EASY Screening Tool and exercise recom-
mendations for older adults: http://www.easyforyou.info
Physical Activity Measures: www.drjamessallis.sdsu.edu/measures.html
Osteoporosis Screening Questionnaire: www.womensportsnutrition.com/questhp.html
The Osteoporosis Self-Assessment Screening Tool: www.ejbjs.org/cgi/content/full/89/4/765

Parkinson Disease

Hoehn and Yahr Staging of Parkinson Disease and the Unified Parkinson Disease Rating
Scale (UPDRS): www.neurosurgery.mgh.harvard.edu/Functional/pdstages.htm
Web pages for Additional Information:
Pressure Sore Prevention Tool: The Waterlow Pressure Sore Risk Assessment Tool and
Waterlow Scale Manual: www.judy-waterlow.co.uk/waterlow_downloads.htm
Veteran's Health Administration Handbook: Assessment and Prevention of Pressure
Ulcers: www1.va.gov/vhapublications/ViewPublication.asp?pub_ID=1447
Parkinson Disease: an overview appropriate for patients, families, and providers.
www.clevelandclinicmeded.com/medicalpubs/diseasemanagement/neurology/parkinsons/
parkinsons.htm
Clinical Assessment of Parkinson Disease from Brain Imaging Tests:
www.crump.ucla.edu/lpp/clinpetneuro/parkinsons.html

PART III

GENERAL MANAGEMENT STRATEGIES

CHAPTER 11

CARDIOVASCULAR DISORDERS

In older adults, heart disease is the leading cause of death worldwide and is the most common cause for hospitalization. Physiological changes of the cardiovascular system in aging may modify the presentation of cardiac disease.

PHYSIOLOGICAL CHANGES

In using data on physiological changes of the cardiovascular system, it is important to recognize the selection criteria of the population studied. Because the prevalence of coronary artery disease may be 50% in the eighth and ninth decades of life, screening to exclude occult cardiovascular disease may modify findings.

In a population screened for occult coronary artery disease, there is no change in cardiac output at rest over the third to eighth decades (Gerstenblith, Renlund, and Lakatta, 1987) (Table 11-1). There is a slight decrease in heart rate and a compensatory slight increase in stroke volume. This is in contrast to studies in unscreened individuals, where cardiac output falls from the second to the ninth decades. During maximal exercise, however, other changes are manifest even in the screened population (Table 11-2). Heart rate response to exercise is decreased in older adults compared to younger individuals, reflecting a diminished β-adrenergic responsiveness in aging. Cardiac output is decreased slightly. Cardiac output is maintained by increasing cardiac volumes—increasing end-diastolic and end-systolic volumes. With this increase in workload and the work of pumping blood against less-compliant arteries and a higher blood pressure, cardiac hypertrophy occurs even in the screened elderly population.

Because myocardial reserve mechanisms are used to maintain normal function in aging, older persons are more vulnerable to developing dysfunction when disease is superimposed.

Diastolic dysfunction—retarded left ventricular filling and higher left ventricular diastolic pressure—is present both at rest and during exercise in older persons. Older persons are more dependent on atrial contraction, as opposed to ventricular relaxation, for left ventricular filling, and thus are more likely to develop heart failure if atrial fibrillation ensues. Heart failure may occur in the absence of systolic dysfunction or valvular disease.

– 335 –

TABLE 11-1   RESTING CARDIAC FUNCTION IN PATIENTS AGED 30 TO
              80 YEARS COMPARED WITH THAT IN 30-YEAR-OLDS

	Unscreened for Occult CAD	Screened for Occult CAD
Heart rate	–	–
Stroke volume	– –	+
Stroke volume index	– –	0
Cardiac output	– –	0
Cardiac index	– –	0
Peripheral vascular resistance	+ +	0
Peak systolic blood pressure	+ +	+ +
Diastolic pressure	0	0

Key: CAD, coronary artery disease; +, slight increase; + +, increase; –, slight decrease; – –, decrease; 0, no difference.

TABLE 11-2   PERFORMANCE AT MAXIMUM EXERCISE IN SAMPLE
              SCREENED FOR CORONARY ARTERY DISEASE, AGE 30
              TO 80 YEARS

	Compared with 30-Year-Olds
Heart rate	– –
End-diastolic volume	+ +
Stroke volume	+ +
Cardiac output	–
End-systolic volume	+ +
Ejection fraction	– –
Total peripheral vascular resistance	0
Systolic blood pressure	0

Key: + +, increase; –, slight decrease; – –, decrease; 0, no difference.

HYPERTENSION

Hypertension is the major risk factor for stroke, heart failure, and coronary artery disease in older adults; all are important contributors to mortality and functional disability. Because hypertension is remediable and its control may reduce the incidence of coronary heart disease and stroke, increased efforts at detection and treatment of high blood pressure are indicated.

Hypertension is defined as a systolic blood pressure of 140 mm Hg or greater and/or a diastolic blood pressure of 90 mm Hg or greater. Isolated systolic hypertension is defined as a systolic pressure of 140 mm Hg or greater with a diastolic pressure of less than 90 mm Hg. With these definitions, as many as 67% of individuals older than age 60 may be hypertensive (Ostchega et al., 2007).

Despite the high prevalence of hypertension in older adults, it should not be considered a normal consequence of aging. Hypertension is the major risk factor for cardiovascular disease in older adults and that risk increases with each decade. Both elevation of systolic blood pressure and pulse pressure are better predicators of adverse events than diastolic pressure. This is particularly relevant to older individuals, where isolated systolic hypertension predominates and may be present in 90% of hypertensive patients over the age of 80 (reviewed in Chobanian, 2007).

Evaluation

The diagnosis should be made on serial blood pressures. In patients with labile hypertension, blood pressure should be averaged to make the diagnosis, because these patients are at no less risk than those patients with stable hypertension. The history and physical examination should be directed toward assessing the duration, severity, treatment, and complications of the hypertension (Table 11-3). Atherosclerosis may interfere with occlusion of the brachial artery by a blood pressure cuff, leading to erroneously elevated blood pressure determinations, or "pseudohypertension." Such an effect can be determined by the Osler maneuver. The cuff pressure is raised above systolic blood pressure. If the radial artery remains palpable at this pressure, significant atherosclerosis is probably present and may account for a 10- to 15-mm Hg pressure error. Standing blood pressure should also be determined. Initial laboratory evaluation should include urinalysis, complete blood cell count; measurements of blood electrolytes and calcium, estimated glomerular filtration rate, fasting glucose, and lipids; and 12-lead electrocardiogram (ECG).

Secondary forms of hypertension are uncommon in older adults, but should be considered in treatment-resistant patients and in those with diastolic pressures

TABLE 11-3   INITIAL EVALUATION OF HYPERTENSION IN OLDER ADULTS

History
Duration
Severity
Treatment
Complications
Other risk factors
Physical examination
Blood pressure, including Osler maneuver and standing determinations
Weight
Funduscopic, vascular, and cardiac examination for end-organ damage
Abdominal bruit
Neurological examination for focal deficits
Laboratory tests
   Urinalysis
   Electrolytes
   Estimated glomerular filtration rate
   Calcium
   Thyrotropin (TSH)
   Chest radiograph
   Electrocardiogram

greater than 115 mm Hg (Table 11-4). Pheochromocytoma is uncommon in older adults and is particularly unusual in those older than age 75. Atherosclerotic renovascular hypertension and primary hyperaldosteronism may occur more frequently in older persons. With the use of automated calcium determinations, the frequency of diagnosis of primary hyperparathyroidism is increasing, particularly in postmenopausal women. Because there is a causal link between this disorder and hypertension, the diagnosis and treatment of hyperparathyroidism may ameliorate the elevated blood pressure.

Estrogen therapy in the postmenopausal woman may be associated with hypertension. Such an association can be assessed by withdrawing estrogen therapy for several months and following the blood pressure response.

TABLE 11-4 SECONDARY HYPERTENSION IN OLDER PERSONS

Renovascular disease (atherosclerotic)

Primary hyperaldosteronism

Hyperparathyroidism (calcium)

Estrogen administration

Renal disease (decreased creatinine clearance)

Treatment

The issue of treatment of systolic/diastolic or isolated systolic hypertension in older individuals has been resolved. Multiple large trials have demonstrated that treating hypertension in older adults decreases morbidity and mortality from coronary artery disease and stroke (reviewed in Joint National Committee, 2003). Although there has been concern about the hazard of treating individuals with cerebrovascular disease, the evidence suggests that the presence of cerebrovascular disease is an indication for, rather than a contraindication to, hypertensive therapy.

Some of the treatment trials that have included individuals up to 84 years suggest that there should be no age cutoff above which high blood pressure is not treated. A study specifically directed to hypertensive patients (systolic blood pressure of 160 mm Hg or more) aged 80 years or older demonstrated a 30% reduction in the rate of fatal and nonfatal stroke, a 21% reduction in the rate of death from any cause, a 23% reduction in the rate of death from cardiovascular causes, and a 64% reduction in the rate of heart failure (Beckett et al., 2008). Relatively healthy older persons at any age should be treated unless they have severe comorbid disease that will clearly limit their life expectancy or unless the toxicity of treatment is so great that it outweighs potential benefits. The treatment goal for uncomplicated hypertension is a blood pressure less than 140/90 mm Hg.

Specific Therapy

Lifestyle changes are not easily accomplished but should be attempted, including maintaining ideal body weight, limiting dietary sodium intake, eating fruits and vegetables and low-fat dairy products, reducing saturated and total fats, and engaging in aerobic exercise. Foods rich in potassium, calcium, and magnesium should be consumed. Excess sodium intake and potassium deficit have adverse effects on arterial pressure and should be reversed as part of the management of all hypertensive patients (Adrorgue and Madias, 2007). Other

TABLE 11-5   THIAZIDE DIURETICS FOR ANTIHYPERTENSIVE THERAPY

ADVANTAGES	ADVERSE EFFECTS
Well tolerated	Hypokalemia
No central nervous system side effects	Volume depletion
Relatively inexpensive	Hyponatremia
Infrequent dosing	Hyperglycemia
Good response rate	Hyperuricemia
Orthostatic hypotension uncommon	Impotence
Can be used in conjunction with other agents	
Effective in advanced age	
Effective in systolic hypertension	

risk factors, such as smoking, dyslipidemia, and diabetes mellitus, should also be modified.

If dietary measures fail to control blood pressure, drug therapy should be considered. Physiological and pathological changes of aging should be considered in individualizing the therapy. Changes in volumes of distribution and hepatic and renal metabolism may alter pharmacokinetics (see Chap. 14). Changes in vessel elasticity and baroreceptor sensitivity may alter responses to posture and drug-induced falls in blood pressure.

Thiazide diuretics are usually the initial step in therapy, especially in older patients with isolated systolic hypertension. They are well tolerated, are relatively inexpensive, and can be given once a day (Table 11-5). Many older hypertensive patients can be treated with diuretics as the only medication. Low-dose thiazides, for example, 12.5 to 25 mg of chlorthalidone, are efficacious in lowering blood pressure, while minimizing metabolic side effects. Higher doses have a minimal additional effect on blood pressure with a more marked effect on hypokalemia. Thiazides are contraindicated in patients with gout. Postural hypotension is uncommon, but serum potassium should be monitored. Diabetics may have increased requirements for insulin or oral hypoglycemic agents.

Although β-blockers are also recommended as initial-step therapy, several meta-analyses have called this strategy into question (reviewed in Panjrath and Messerli, 2006). These meta-analyses indicate that traditional β-blockers do have efficacy in lowering blood pressure, but are not known to be effective in preventing coronary artery disease, cardiovascular mortality, or all-cause mortality in older adults. When compared to each other, thiazides are superior to β-blockers in older adults (MRC Working Party, 1992). In ALLHAT, thiazides were superior to angiotensin-converting enzyme (ACE) inhibitors in reducing cardiovascular disease, stroke, and heart failure (ALLHAT Collaborative Research Group, 2002). However, another trial suggests that ACE inhibitors are superior in older subjects, particularly men, in reducing cardiovascular events and mortality, but not stroke (Wing et al., 2003). β-Blocking agents may be used as the initial drug when another indication for their use exists, such as coronary heart disease, myocardial infarction (MI), heart failure, tachyarrhythmias, or essential tremor.

If thiazides alone do not control blood pressure, a second agent is added (Table 11-6) or a thiazide is added if one of the other agents has failed. The choice should be individualized and usually selected from among β-blockers, calcium-channel antagonists, ACE inhibitors, or angiotensin-receptor blockers (ARBs) (The Medical Letter, 2001). β-Blockers are indicated for treatment of angina, heart failure, previous MI, and tachyarrhythmias in association with hypertension. These agents are contraindicated in patients with cardiac conduction deficits, bradyarrhythmias, and reactive airways disease. The more water-soluble β-blockers may be well suited for the geriatric population because they enter the central nervous system less readily and thus have fewer of the central nervous system side effects such as somnolence and depression; this would be a particular advantage in the elderly. However, if cardiac output is decreased, renal perfusion and glomerular filtration rate may be affected. One concern with β-blockers is the production of bradycardia with reduced cardiac output. One simple test to monitor for this side effect is the patient's response to mild exercise after each dosage increase; a failure to increase pulse by at least 10 beats per minute is an indication to reduce the dosage. If a patient is to be taken off a β-blocking agent, withdrawal should be done slowly over a period of several days to avoid rebound of original symptoms.

Calcium-channel antagonists are peripheral vasodilators with the advantage of maintaining coronary blood flow. These agents appear to have increased potency with age, possibly as a result of the decreased reflex tachycardia and myocardial contractility in older adults as compared with younger individuals. Headache, sodium retention, negative inotropic effects—especially in combination with β-blockers—and conduction abnormalities may limit their use. Calcium-channel antagonists are effective in reducing stroke incidence in older patients with isolated systolic hypertension (Staessen et al., 1997). However, these drugs do not significantly reduce the risk of heart failure (Blood Pressure Lowering Treatment Trialists' Collaboration, 2000).

ACE inhibitors are effective and well tolerated for treatment of hypertension. They are both preload and afterload reducers and thus are particularly useful in the face of congestive heart failure. They prolong survival in patients with heart failure or left ventricular dysfunction after an MI. Long-acting agents may have an advantage in adherence. Renal function, which may deteriorate on administration of these agents, must be monitored carefully. These agents may

TABLE 11-6   ANTIHYPERTENSIVE MEDICATIONS

AGENT*	ADVANTAGES	DISADVANTAGES
β-Blockers	Useful in angina, previous myocardial infraction, heart failure Water-soluble agents have fewer central nervous system side effects Must be withdrawn slowly in presence of coronary artery disease	Contraindicated in cardiac conduction defects and reactive airways disease May cause bronchospasm, bradycardia, impaired peripheral circulation, fatigue, and decreased exercise tolerance
Calcium-channel blockers	Peripheral vasodilator Coronary blood flow maintained Potency increased with age or in systolic hypertension	Headaches Sodium retention Negative inotropic effect Conduction abnormality
Angiotensin-converting enzyme inhibitors	Preload and afterload reduction Use in congestive heart failure, diabetes mellitus, other nephropathy with proteinuria	Hyperkalemia Hypotension Decreased renal function Cough Angioedema
Angiotensin-receptor antagonists	Use in angiotensin-converting enzyme inhibitor–induced cough, congestive heart failure, diabetes mellitus, other nephropathy with proteinuria	Hyperkalemia Angioedema (rare)
Clonidine	Increased renal perfusion	Somnolence, depression Dry mouth, constipation Rarely, withdrawal hypertensive crisis
α-Blockers	Useful in benign prostatic hypertrophy	Orthostatic hypotension

TABLE 11-6   ANTIHYPERTENSIVE MEDICATIONS (*Continued*)

AGENT*	ADVANTAGES	DISADVANTAGES
Hydralazine	May be useful in systolic hypertension	Reflex tachycardia, aggravation of angina Lupus-like syndrome at high dosage
Eplerenone	Aldosterone-receptor antagonist Fewer side effects than spironolactone and avoidance of gynecomastia	Hyperkalemia Contraindicated in renal insufficiency (creatinine > 2.0) and in the presence of albuminuria

*With all these agents, initiation with low dosage and careful titration may minimize side effects

also induce hyperkalemia and should generally not be used with a potassium-sparing diuretic. Older adults are also more vulnerable to the hypotensive effects of these drugs.

ARBs are effective in lowering blood pressure without causing cough. They and ACE inhibitors are appropriate initial therapy in patients with diabetes mellitus, renal disease, or congestive heart failure (August, 2003). ARBs are superior to β-blockers in the treatment of patients with isolated systolic hypertension and left ventricular hypertrophy (Kjeldsen et al., 2002).

Clonidine may cause somnolence and depression, but it increases renal perfusion. The clonidine transdermal patch may lessen some of these adverse effects. However, local skin reactions may occur in about 15% of users. The once-per-week application of the patch may be an asset in improving adherence.

The major side effect of α-blockers is orthostatic hypotension; this is especially problematic with initial doses of prazosin. Newer agents with lesser hypotensive effects are now being used to treat symptomatic benign prostatic hypertrophy. In ALLHAT, the α-blocker arm was stopped early because of a higher incidence of congestive heart failure. Consequently, α-blockers are not recommended as monotherapy for hypertension.

Although hydralazine is usually a third-step drug, it may occasionally be used as a second-step drug in older adults because reflex tachycardia rarely occurs. If used with diuretics alone, it should be initiated in low doses, which should be increased slowly. It should not be used in the absence of a β-blocker if coronary artery disease is present.

A newer available agent is eplerenone, an aldosterone-receptor antagonist. It has a better side-effect profile than spironolactone, particularly the avoidance of gynecomastia in men, but needs to be used with caution with renal insufficiency and microalbuminuria, and potassium must be monitored for development of hyperkalemia.

With the newer, more effective agents, drug-resistant hypertension is unusual. In such cases, drug adherence should be monitored and sodium intake assessed. If such factors are not contributing to drug resistance, secondary causes of hypertension should be considered, especially renovascular disease and primary hyperaldosteronism.

STROKE AND TRANSIENT ISCHEMIC ATTACKS

Although the incidence of stroke is declining, it is still a major medical problem affecting approximately 50,000 individuals in the United States every year. It is the third leading cause of death and is also a major cause of morbidity, long-term disability, and hospital admissions. Stroke is clearly a disease of older adults; approximately 75% of strokes occur in those older than age 65. The incidence of stroke rises steeply with age, being 10 times greater in the 75- to 84-year-old age group than in the 55- to 64-year-old age group.

Table 11-7 lists the types and outcomes of stroke. In cerebral infarct, thrombosis, usually arteriosclerotic, is the commonest cause, with embolization from an ulcerated plaque or myocardial thrombosis less frequent. Table 11-8 lists outcomes for survivors.

Table 11-9 lists the modifiable risk factors for ischemic stroke. Hypertension is the major risk factor. Systolic hypertension is associated with a three- to five-fold increased risk for stroke. Hypertension accelerates the formation of atheromatous plaques and damages the integrity of vessel walls, predisposing to thrombotic occlusion and cerebral infarction. Hypertension also promotes growth

TABLE 11-7   STROKE

CAUSE	RELATIVE FREQUENCY %	MORTALITY RATE %
Subarachnoid hemorrhage	10	50
Intracerebral hemorrhage	15	80
Cerebral infarction (thrombosis and embolism)	75	40

TABLE 11-8 OUTCOME FOR SURVIVORS OF STROKE

OUTCOME	PERCENT
No dysfunction	10
Mild dysfunction	40
Significant dysfunction	40
Institutional care	10

of microaneurysms in segments of small intracranial arteries. Those lesions are sites of intracranial hemorrhage and lacunar infarcts.

Whether diabetes mellitus is a modifiable risk factor remains an unresolved issue. Tight glycemic control trials in type 2 diabetes have not shown improved outcomes for stroke.

Patients with a history of transient ischemic attacks (TIAs) are at substantial risk for subsequent stroke, particularly within the first few days. Completed stroke as a sequel of TIA is reported to occur in 12% to 60% or more of untreated TIA patients. In retrospective studies of patients with completed stroke, previous TIA is reported to have occurred in 50% to 75% of patients.

The keystone to the diagnosis of stroke is a clear history of sudden, acute neurological deficit. When the history is not clear, especially if the deficit could have had a gradual onset, consideration should be given to a mass lesion. Brain scanning with computed tomography (CT) or magnetic resonance imaging (MRI)

TABLE 11-9 MODIFIABLE RISK FACTORS FOR ISCHEMIC STROKE

Alcohol consumption (> 5 drinks/day)

Asymptomatic carotid stenosis (> 50%)

Atrial fibrillation

Elevated total cholesterol level

Hypertension

Obesity

Physical inactivity

Smoking

Modified from Straus et al., 2002.

is required to distinguish cerebral infarction from intracerebral hemorrhage. Laboratory testing should include glucose level, complete blood count, and prothrombin time and partial-thromboplastin time, especially if thrombolysis is considered. Electroencephalography (EEG) is only occasionally helpful in the differential diagnosis. An ECG should be performed routinely in cases of TIA or stroke because it may relate the episode to MI or cardiac arrhythmia. Invasive techniques are usually unnecessary in stroke patients.

In older adults, symptoms acceptable as evidence of cerebral ischemia are often misinterpreted. Table 11-10 lists the presenting symptoms for TIA in the carotid and vertebral–basilar systems.

Treatment

The FDA has approved and committees of the American Heart Association and the American Academy of Neurology have published guidelines endorsing the use of tissue plasminogen activator within 3 hours of onset of ischemic stroke. Thrombolytic therapy increases the risk for early death and intracranial hemorrhage but decreases the combined end point of death or dependency at 3 to 6 months. In two large randomized trials, the use of aspirin initiated within 48 hours after onset of stroke and continued for 2 weeks or until discharge reduced rates of death or dependency at discharge or at 6 months. A meta-analysis found no evidence that anticoagulants in the acute phase of stroke improve functional outcomes (therapies of acute stroke reviewed in van der Worp and van Gijn, 2007).

For primary prevention of stroke, adequate blood pressure reduction, smoking cessation, and treatment of hyperlipidemia; glucose control in patients with diabetes; use of antithrombotic therapy in patients with atrial fibrillation; and of antiplatelet therapy in patients with MI are effective and supported by evidence from several randomized trials (Straus, Majumdar, and McAlister, 2002). These same strategies are effective in secondary prevention of stroke, as is carotid endarterectomy in patients with severe carotid artery stenosis.

Lowering blood pressure in hypertensive individuals is effective in the prevention of hemorrhagic and ischemic stroke. The benefits of antihypertensive treatment extend to patients older than 80 years (Gueyffier et al., 1999). Thiazide diuretics, ACE inhibitors, and long-acting calcium-channel blockers reduce the incidence of stroke. β-Blockers are less efficacious. Selection of a specific class of drugs is discussed earlier in this chapter.

Patients with atrial fibrillation have a mortality rate double that of age- and sex-matched controls without atrial fibrillation. The risk of stroke with nonrheumatic atrial fibrillation is approximately 5% a year. Adjusted-dose warfarin and aspirin reduce stroke in patients with atrial fibrillation, and warfarin is substantially more efficacious than aspirin (Hart et al., 2007). Major extracranial hemorrhage is minimally increased in warfarin-treated patients. Excess bleeding risk with warfarin in elderly patients can be similar to the low rates achieved

TABLE 11-10   TIA: PRESENTING SYMPTOMS

SYMPTOM	CAROTID	VERTEBROBASILAR
Paresis	+ + +	+ +
Paresthesia	+ + +	+ + +
Binocular vision	0	+ + +
Vertigo	0	+ + +
Diplopia	0	+ +
Ataxia	0	+ +
Dizziness	0	+ +
Monocular vision	+ +	0
Headache	+	+
Dysphasia	+	0
Dysarthria	+	+
Nausea and vomiting	0	+
Loss of consciousness	0	0
Visual hallucinations	0	0
Tinnitus	0	0
Mental change	0	0
Drop attacks	0	0
Drowsiness	0	0
Light-headedness	0	0
Hyperacusia	0	0
Weakness (generalized)	0	0
Convulsion	0	0

Key: + + +, most frequent; 0, least frequent.

in the randomized trials (Caro et al., 1999; Fang et al., 2006). Therapy with clopidogrel plus aspirin is not an alternative to warfarin because it is less effective and significantly increases the risk of bleeding (ACTIVE, 2006). Strokes that occur in patients receiving warfarin or aspirin are not more severe than those occurring in placebo-treated patients. Stroke risks and benefits of antithrombotic therapy are similar for patients with paroxysmal or chronic atrial fibrillation (Hart et al., 2000).

The risk of ischemic stroke is increased after an MI, particularly in the first month. Aspirin reduces the risk of nonfatal stroke in patients who have experienced an MI (Antiplatelet Trialists' Collaboration, 2002). Aspirin decreases the risk of stroke in patients with previous TIA or stroke, and there appears to be no dose–response relationship in doses of 50 to 1500 mg/day. Clopidogrel is modestly more effective than aspirin in decreasing risk of the combined endpoint of stroke, MI, or vascular death (Straus, Majumdar, and McAlister, 2002).

Carotid endarterectomy decreases the risk of stroke or death in patients with symptomatic carotid disease and severe carotid artery stenosis (70% to 99%). In patients with symptomatic moderate carotid artery stenosis (50% to 69%) benefits were more marginal. Carotid stenting is less invasive than endarterectomy, but in a study of patients with symptomatic carotid stenosis of 60% or more, the rates of death and stroke at 1 and 6 months were lower with endarterectomy than with stenting (Mas et al., 2006). Patients with lesser degrees of stenosis (< 50%) may be harmed by surgery. For people with asymptomatic carotid disease, the optimal therapy is unclear. However, identifying carotid artery stenosis in asymptomatic individuals can involve expensive and invasive diagnostic procedures. The costs of screening large numbers of asymptomatic people outweigh the benefits to the number of individuals screening would identify.

Stroke Rehabilitation

Table 11-11 presents factors in the prognosis for rehabilitation of elderly stroke patients. Although the benefit of stroke rehabilitation is controversial, it should be initiated early in the course if it is to be of benefit. Stroke patients fare better in rehabilitative facilities than in skilled nursing facilities (Kane et al., 1996; Schlenker et al., 1997). Generally, most neurologic return occurs during the first month after the stroke. By the end of the third month, little, if any, further return can be expected. Not all dysfunctions result in the same level of disability. Motor loss is often the least disabling. Perceptual and/or sensory loss, aphasia, loss of

TABLE 11-11   FACTORS IN PROGNOSIS FOR REHABILITATION

Availability and implementation of sound program

Mentation

Motivation

Prognosis for neurological return

Vigor

TABLE 11-12   STROKE REHABILITATION

Acute phase
Change of patient's position at least every 2 h
Positioning of patient's joints to prevent contractures
Positioning of patient to prevent aspiration pneumonia
Range-of-motion exercises

Later phase
Activities of daily living training
Ambulation training
Functional activities for affected side
Muscle reeducation exercises
Perceptual training
Training in transfer technique

balance, hemicorporal neglect, hemianopsia, and/or cognitive damage may cause more severe and often untreatable disabilities.

In the immediate rehabilitation stage, treatment is directed toward avoiding complications such as pressure sores, contractures, phlebitis, pulmonary embolism, aspiration pneumonia, and fecal impaction.

In the next stage of rehabilitation, treatment is directed toward reeducating muscles (affected areas) and enhancing remaining capabilities (unaffected areas) (reviewed in Dobkin, 2005). Table 11-12 describes measures to be taken during this phase. In patients 3 to 9 months within a first stroke, constraint-induced movement therapy produced significant and clinically relevant improvements in arm motor function (Wolf, Winstein, and Miller, 2006).

When the patient stops making progress after intensive therapy, the goal of rehabilitation shifts to finding ways for the patient to cope with the dysfunction. At this stage, the patient is assessed for the need for braces and assistive devices for both ambulation and performance of activities of daily living. With a sound program of rehabilitation, the older patient who survives a stroke can return to the community.

CORONARY ARTERY DISEASE

The frequency of both coronary artery disease and MI increases with age. Elderly patients have more severe disease than younger patients, and mortality rate is higher after an acute MI.

Hypertension is the major risk factor for coronary artery disease in older adults. Hypercholesterolemia and cigarette smoking become less important risk factors in this age group, although they are still significant. Risk factor reduction should include treatment of hypertension and dyslipidemia, and smoking cessation.

Angina pectoris has a similar presentation in both older adults and in younger patients, with familiar pain characteristics and radiation. Pharmacologically, acute episodes of angina pectoris can be treated with sublingual nitroglycerin, which should be taken in the sitting position to avoid severe orthostatic hypotension. Primary therapy for chronic stable angina is aspirin and β-blockers. Both are underused in the elderly, especially after acute MI. Secondary therapy includes long-acting nitrates and calcium-channel blockers, but their use may be limited by orthostatic hypotension in older patients.

Younger patients with chronic symptomatic coronary artery disease benefit from revascularization. Procedure-related mortality increases with age both after coronary artery bypass graft (Alexander et al., 2000) and after percutaneous coronary intervention (Batchelor et al., 2000). In those without significant comorbidity, mortality approaches that seen in younger patients. One-year outcomes in elderly patients with chronic angina are similar with regard to symptoms, quality of life, and death or nonfatal infarction with invasive versus optimized medical strategies (Pfisterer et al., 2003). Elderly patients with angina refractory to standard drug therapy have a choice between an early invasive strategy that carries a certain early intervention risk and an optimized medical strategy that carries a chance of late hospitalization and revascularization. After 1 year, quality of life outcome and survival will be similar.

Elderly patients with an acute MI often present with symptoms other than chest pain (Table 11-13). Treatment of the older patient with acute MI is similar to that of the younger patient. Particular attention should be paid to avoiding drug toxicity and to beginning early mobilization when possible. Early mobilization may decrease deconditioning, orthostatic hypotension, and thrombophlebitis. No specific trials in the elderly have assessed percutaneous coronary intervention versus thrombolysis for treatment of acute MI. However, subgroup analyses indicate better outcomes with percutaneous coronary intervention (reviewed in Ting, Yang, and Rihal, 2006). Coronary artery surgery can be performed with excellent symptomatic results in older patients, but with increased morbidity and mortality. The strongest indication for surgery is angina pectoris refractory to medical management. In patients with left main coronary artery disease, surgery significantly improves survival over medical therapy. Patients with three-vessel disease may also have improved survival. In older adults, however, improved survival must be considered in the light of the patient's projected survival and the higher operative risk.

Long-term administration of β-blockers to patients after MI improves survival. Pooled analysis of intravascular ultrasound studies demonstrates that β-blockers can slow progression of coronary atherosclerosis (Sipahi et al., 2007).

TABLE 11-13   PRESENTING SYMPTOMS OF MYOCARDIAL INFARCTION

Chest pain

Confusion

Dyspnea

Rapid deterioration of health

Syncope

Worsening congestive heart failure

Despite these data, physicians are reluctant to administer β-blockers to many patients, such as older patients (Krumholz et al., 1998) and those with chronic pulmonary disease, left ventricular dysfunction, or non–Q-wave MI. However, all these subgroups benefit from β-blocker therapy after MI (Gottlieb, McCarter, and Vogel, 1998). Given the higher mortality rates in these subgroups, the absolute reduction in mortality was similar to or greater than that among patients with no specific risk factors. Other secondary prevention interventions should include aspirin, ACE inhibitors, lipid-lowering agents, and smoking cessation. Observational studies support that doses of aspirin greater than 75 to 81 mg do not enhance efficacy, whereas larger doses are associated with an increased incidence of bleeding events (reviewed in Campbell et al., 2007). Intensive low-density lipoprotein cholesterol-lowering therapy has been shown to be beneficial in high-risk older patients with established cardiovascular disease (Wenger et al., 2007). Current data do not support adding ezetimibe to statin therapy to lower cholesterol in prevention of vascular disease (Kastelein et al., 2008).

VALVULAR HEART DISEASE

Calcific Aortic Stenosis

Pathologically, degenerative calcification of the aortic and mitral valves is common among older adults; it is found at autopsy in approximately one-third of individuals older than age 75. For many years, degenerative aortic stenosis was thought to be caused by the passive accumulation of calcium on the surface of the aortic valve leaflet. Recent studies have demonstrated, however, that the etiology of aortic valve disease has a similar pathophysiology to that of vascular athero-sclerosis (Rajamannan, Bonow, and Rahimtoola, 2007). Aortic valve sclerosis is common in the elderly (29% in the Cardiovascular Health Study) and is associated with an increase in the risk of death from cardiovascular causes and the risk of MI, even in the absence of hemodynamically significant obstruction of left ventricular outflow (Otto et al., 1999). The frequency of aortic stenosis increases with age, appearing at autopsy in approximately 4% to 6% of those older than age 65. Isolated aortic stenosis is more common among men than women except in those older than age 80, where women predominate. Aortic insufficiency may coexist with calcific aortic stenosis, although regurgitation is usually mild and a regurgitant murmur is usually not heard.

The usual clinical presentation of aortic stenosis in older adults consists of fatigue, syncope, angina pectoris, and congestive heart failure. Because systolic murmurs are a frequent finding in older adults, differentiation of mitral regurgitation, aortic sclerosis, or aortic stenosis by auscultation is a challenge. The location of the murmur is usually along the lower left sternal border and apex and often does not radiate to the axilla or carotids. It is characteristically a crescendo–decrescendo late systolic murmur ending before the second heart sound. Table 11-14 describes aspects that may help differentiate mitral regurgitation from aortic murmurs.

Differentiating aortic stenosis from aortic sclerosis can be difficult in the elderly. The typical murmur and pulse of aortic stenosis may be modified in older adults. Systemic hypertension may shorten the systolic murmur of stenosis, giving it the characteristic of an aortic sclerosis murmur. Loss of vascular

TABLE 11-14 DIFFERENTIATION OF SYSTOLIC MURMURS

	POSTPER- CUTANEOUS CORONARY ANGIOPLASTY[*]	AMYL NITRATE	VALSALVA	SQUATTING
Aortic sclerosis	↑[†]	↑	↓	↑
Aortic stenosis	↑	↑↓	↓	↑
Idiopathic Hypertrophic Subaortic stenosis	↑	↑↑	↑↑	↓↓
Mitral regurgitation	—	↓	↓	—

[*]Best following a premature ventricular contraction.
[†]Effect of maneuver on intensity of murmur.

elasticity may modify the pulse pressure, so that the typical pulse contour of aortic stenosis is absent. Therefore, the physical examination alone is not reliable in diagnosing aortic stenosis in older adults. The addition of Doppler flow studies to echocardiography has improved the diagnostic accuracy of noninvasive procedures for aortic stenosis. Left ventricular catheterization remains the most reliable method of assessing aortic stenosis in older adults but should be reserved for patients who are symptomatic (angina, syncope, or dyspnea) and in whom surgery is contemplated.

Surgical mortality for valve replacement is higher in older individuals, but results have improved. Excellent early and late outcomes of aortic valve replacement in people aged 80 and older have been described (Filsoufi et al., 2008). Significant coexistent coronary artery disease should be treated with bypass surgery at the time of valve replacement. In general, a biological prosthetic valve is preferred.

Calcified Mitral Annulus

Mitral ring calcification is a disease of older adults and is most frequently found in patients older than age 70. It is reported in 9% of autopsies in individuals older than age 50 and has a striking increase with advancing age, particularly in women, in whom it rises from 3.2% in women younger than age 70 to 44% in women older than age 90.

This lesion often results in mitral insufficiency or conduction abnormalities and rarely in stenosis. It is an important contributing factor to congestive heart failure in older adults and is a site for endocarditis. As many as two-thirds of patients with mitral annulus calcification present with an apical systolic murmur of mitral regurgitation.

Echocardiography is the best technique for diagnosing mitral annulus calcification. Regurgitation is usually mild to moderate, and surgery is usually indicated only if endocarditis is superimposed. Recommendations for the prevention of bacterial endocarditis have been made by the American Heart Association (Dajani et al., 1997). There is a higher incidence of cerebral embolism in this disorder, and thus anticoagulation with Coumadin may be indicated.

Mitral Valve Prolapse

Mucoid degeneration affects mainly the mitral valve. This process allows stretching of the mitral valve leaflet under normal intracardiac pressure, with subsequent prolapse into the left atrium during systole.

Although the classic murmur is late systolic, the murmur can occur any time in systole. Mucoid degeneration of the mitral valve has been described in approximately 1% of autopsies on patients older than age 65. It is associated with mitral insufficiency; left atrial dilatation and regurgitant murmurs are common. Mitral insufficiency caused by this disorder is usually well tolerated and rarely requires surgery. Some patients with this syndrome have abnormal ECGs and chest pain suggestive of coronary artery disease; sudden death has been reported.

Death directly from the valve disease is usually related to rupture of the chordae tendineae. Mucoid degeneration also predisposes to infective endocarditis. Prophylaxis for subacute bacterial endocarditis is indicated, and recommendations of the American Heart Association should be followed (Dajani et al., 1997).

Idiopathic Hypertrophic Subaortic Stenosis

In older adults, idiopathic hypertrophic subaortic stenosis (IHSS) may be misdiagnosed as aortic valve stenosis or mitral regurgitation. Presenting symptoms are similar to those of aortic stenosis or coronary artery disease. The presence of a bisferious arterial pulse in the presence of a systolic ejection murmur and in the absence of an aortic regurgitation murmur should suggest IHSS. The IHSS murmur usually does not radiate to the carotids. Squatting, which increases left ventricular filling, usually decreases the murmur of IHSS. Factors that decrease left ventricular volume (Valsalva maneuver, standing) increase the intensity of the murmur.

Documentation of IHSS is accomplished by echocardiography.

Therapy usually relies on β-adrenergic antagonists. Symptoms may be worsened by cardiac glycosides, which increase myocardial contractility, and diuretics, which create volume depletion. Atrial fibrillation is poorly tolerated and may require cardioversion in the rapidly deteriorating patient. In the patients refractory to medical therapy, surgery should be considered after cardiac catheterization to assess severity of outflow obstruction and state of coronary artery flow.

ARRHYTHMIAS

Although the prevalence of arrhythmias increases with age, most of the older patients without clinical heart disease are in normal sinus rhythm.

Atrial fibrillation occurs in 5% to 10% of asymptomatic ambulatory older adults and more frequently in hospitalized patients. It is usually associated with underlying heart disease; the causes are the same as in younger individuals. Atrial fibrillation does, however, occur more frequently in older patients with thyrotoxicosis. Recently, pulse pressure has been demonstrated to be an important risk factor for incident atrial fibrillation (Mitchell et al., 2007). Further research is needed to determine whether interventions that reduce pulse pressure will limit the growing incidence of atrial fibrillation.

Patients with recent onset atrial fibrillation and hemodynamic instability or angina should undergo urgent cardioversion (Falk, 2001). If the patient's condition is stable, heart rate should be controlled with intravenous diltiazem, β-blocker, or digoxin. If atrial fibrillation persists and onset is ≤48 hours, cardioversion may be attempted after initiation of heparin therapy. If onset is more than 48 hours, treatment should include 3 weeks of anticoagulation prior to cardioversion, unless a transesophageal echocardiogram reveals no atrial thrombus at presentation. Anticoagulation for persistent and intermittent atrial fibrillation was discussed in the treatment of stroke and TIAs section of this chapter. For long-term rate control, verapamil, diltiazem, and β-blockers should be the initial drugs of choice. β-Adrenergic blockers are especially effective in the presence of thyrotoxicosis and increased sympathetic tone. Digoxin should be considered only in patients with congestive heart failure secondary to impaired systolic ventricular function or in those where β-blocker or calcium-channel blocker is limited by hypotension. In some patients, combinations of these drugs may be needed to control ventricular response. The maintenance dose of digoxin is usually lower in older adults because of decreased muscular mass and decreased renal clearance. In patients with recurrence of persistent atrial fibrillation after electrical cardioversion, rate control is not inferior to rhythm control (repeated cardioversion or antiarrhythmics) for prevention of death and morbidity from cardiovascular causes (Van Gelder et al., 2002; Marshall et al., 2004). Sinus rhythm can be maintained long-term by means of circumferential pulmonary-vein ablation with a significant decrease in both the severity of symptoms and the left atrial diameter (Oral et al., 2006; Wazni et al., 2005)

The incidence of premature ventricular contractions increases with age and occurs in approximately 10% of ECGs and in 30% to 40% of Holter monitorings. The decision to treat with antiarrhythmic therapy is difficult except in the immediate post-MI period, when it is recommended. Criteria for therapy in older patients are the same as for therapy in younger patients. The half-life of antiarrhythmic drugs is prolonged in the elderly. Therapy should be initiated at lower doses, and blood levels should be monitored (see Chap. 14).

The sick sinus syndrome is particularly common among older patients. Diagnosis is made by Holter monitor. Table 11-15 lists the symptoms of sick sinus syndrome, which are usually related to decreased organ perfusion. There is no satisfactory medical therapy. Symptomatic patients may require pacemakers, which do not seem to decrease mortality in this syndrome but can alleviate symptoms. A pacemaker may be indicated in patients with cardiac side effects from drugs used to control tachycardias in the bradycardia-tachycardia syndrome.

TABLE 11-15   MANIFESTATIONS OF SICK SINUS SYNDROME

Angina pectoris
Congestive heart failure
Dizziness
Insomnia
Memory loss
Palpitations
Syncope

CONGESTIVE HEART FAILURE

Although congestive heart failure is prevalent in older adults, it is often over-diagnosed. Pedal and pretibial edema is not sufficient to warrant the diagnosis. Venous stasis may produce a similar picture. Care is needed to establish the presence of other signs of congestive heart failure (eg, cardiac enlargement, S_3 heart sound, basilar crackles, jugular venous distention, enlarged liver). Determination of ejection fraction by echocardiography assists in the diagnosis.

More than 75% of cases of overt heart failure in older patients are associated with hypertension or coronary heart disease. Diastolic dysfunction, not systolic dysfunction, is the primary cause of heart failure in older patients, and is associated with marked increases in all-cause mortality (Redfield et al., 2003; Bursi et al., 2006). Diuretics should be used to treat pulmonary congestion or peripheral edema. In the absence of randomized controlled trials, ACE inhibitors, β-blockers, or calcium-channel blockers are recommended with reservation for the treatment of diastolic heart failure (Ahmed, 2003).

The mainstays of therapy for congestive heart failure as a result of systolic dysfunction in older patients, as in younger patients, are diuretics for fluid overload, ACE inhibitors or ARBs, β-blockers, and aldosterone blockers (reviewed in Yan, Yan, and Liu, 2005; Neubauer, 2007). To improve function and survival, all patients with chronic symptomatic congestive heart failure that is associated with reduced systolic ejection or left ventricular remodeling should be treated with ACE inhibitors. β-Blockers also improve symptoms and survival (Hjalmarson et al., 2000). Low doses, of spironolactone decrease mortality in severe heart failure (The Medical Letter, 1999). Statin use in adults with heart failure with or without coronary heart disease is associated with lower risk of death and hospitalization (Go et al., 2006).

Although low serum concentrations of digoxin (0.5-0.9 ng/mL) have been shown to reduce mortality and hospitalization in older heart failure patients, the use of digitalis preparations must be approached with caution (Ahmed, 2007). Patients once begun on digoxin tend to remain on it long after the indications have ceased. Subtle signs of toxicity may be missed, as the drug accumulates in the presence of decreased renal function. Because of decreases in lean body mass and glomerular filtration rate, lower doses of digoxin are generally required in the elderly. Initial maintenance doses should be lower; blood levels should be monitored to avoid toxic levels. Because the therapeutic window is narrowed in older adults, patients who have been on digoxin therapy for long periods of time after an acute episode of cardiac decompensation not related to arrhythmias should be considered for discontinuation of digoxin. Weight should be monitored closely so that digoxin can be reinstated before congestive symptoms occur. With such evaluation and monitoring, some older patients on chronic digoxin therapy for other than antiarrhythmic treatment may not require digoxin therapy.

PERIPHERAL VASCULAR DISEASE

The prevalence of peripheral vascular disease increases with age. Cigarette smoking and diabetes mellitus are the strongest risk factors. The risk of limb loss for patients without diabetes is low. Cardiovascular disease is the major cause of death (reviewed in White, 2007 from which this section was modified). Typical intermittent claudication is present in 20% of patients, and many patients present with atypical symptoms of leg fatigue, difficulty in walking, and atypical leg pain.

The examination should focus on pulses, hair loss, skin color, and trophic skin changes of the lower legs and feet. The initial screening test is calculation of the ankle-brachial index (Table 11-16). A result of 0.9 or less is adequate to make the

TABLE 11-16   CALCULATION OF THE ANKLE-BRACHIAL INDEX

Formula

   Ankle-brachial index = highest right (left)
   ankle pressure (mm Hg)/highest arm pressure (mm Hg)

Interpretation of Calculated Index

Above 0.90—normal

0.71-0.90—mild obstruction

0.41-0.70—moderate obstruction

0.00-0.40—severe obstruction

Modified with permission from White, 2007.

diagnosis of peripheral arterial disease. In uncertain diagnosis, further imaging with duplex ultrasound, computed tomographic angiography (CTA), or magnetic resonance angiography (MRA) may be useful. The gold standard is invasive digital-subtraction angiography if an endovascular intervention is planned.

Treatment is directed to risk-factor modification (smoking cessation, lowering lipids, controlling hypertension, and managing diabetes), an exercise program, and antiplatelet therapy. Antiplatelet therapy is initiated with low-dose aspirin. Clopidogrel may be considered as an alternative. Cilostazol (100 mg twice a day) has been shown to improve walking distance, where as pentoxifylline appears to be no better than placebo. If warranted for symptomatic relief, revascularization (endovascular or surgical) may be considered when the risk-benefit ratio is favorable.

EVIDENCE SUMMARY

DO'S

■ Treat hypertension in older adults including those over age 80.
■ Monitor standing blood pressure in patients on antihypertensive therapy.
■ Use adjusted dose warfarin in patients with atrial fibrillation.
■ Administer β-blockers to patients after an acute MI.

DON'TS

■ Use short-acting calcium-channel antagonists for long-term therapy of hypertension.
■ Use clopidogrel in combination with aspirin for stroke prevention for longer than 3 months.

CONSIDER

■ Limiting initial therapy with β-blockers in older patients with hypertension to those with compelling indications, such as coronary heart disease, MI, heart failure, or certain arrhythmias.
■ Thiazide diuretics or angiotensin-converting enzyme inhibitors as first line therapy of hypertension.
■ Percutaneous coronary intervention over thrombolysis for treatment of acute MI.
■ Aortic valve replacement for aortic stenosis, including those over age 80.

References

ACTIVE Writing Group on behalf of the ACTIVE Investigators. Clopidogrel plus aspirin versus oral anticoagulation for atrial fibrillation in the Atrial fibrillation Clopidogrel Trial with Irbesartan for prevention of Vascular Events (ACTIVE W): a randomised controlled trial. *Lancet.* 2006;367:1903-1912.

Adrogué HJ, Madias NE. Sodium and potassium in the pathogenesis of hypertension. *N Engl J Med.* 2007;356:1966-1978.

Ahmed A. American College of Cardiology/American Heart Association chronic heart failure evaluation and management guidelines: relevance to the geriatric practice. *J Am Geriatr Soc.* 2003;51:123-126.

Ahmed A. Digoxin and reduction in mortality and hospitalization in geriatric heart failure: importance of low doses and low serum concentrations. *J Gerontol A Biol Sci Med Sci.* 2007;62A(No. 3):323-329.

Alexander KP, Anstrom KJ, Muhlbaier LH, et al. Outcomes of cardiac surgery in patients > or = 80 years: results from the National Cardiovascular Network. *J Am Coll Cardiol.* 2000;1(35):731-738.

ALLHAT Collaborative Research Group. Major outcomes in high-risk hypertensive patients randomized to angiotensin-converting enzyme inhibitor or calcium channel blocker vs diuretic. The antihypertensive and lipid-lowering treatment to prevent heart attack trial (ALLHAT). *JAMA.* 2002;288:2981-2997.

Antiplatelet Trialists' Collaboration. Collaborative meta-analysis of randomized trials of antiplatelet therapy for prevention of death, myocardial infarction and stroke in high risk patients. *BMJ.* 2002;324:71-86.

August P. Initial treatment of hypertension. *N Engl J Med.* 2003;348:610-617.

Batchelor WB, Anstrom KJ, Muhlbaier LH, et al. Contemporary outcome trends in the elderly undergoing percutaneous coronary interventions: results in 7,472 octogenarians. National Cardiovascular Network Collaboration. *J Am Coll Cardiol.* 2000;36:723-730.

Beckett NS, Peters R, Fletcher AE, et al. Treatment of hypertension in patients 80 years of age or older. *N Engl J Med.* 2008;358:1-12.

Blood Pressure Lowering Treatment Trialists' Collaboration. Effects of ACE inhibitors, calcium antagonists, and other blood pressure-lowering drugs: results of prospectively designed overviews of randomized trials. *Lancet.* 2000;356:1955-1964.

Brown ML, Pellikka PA, Schaff HV, et al. The benefits of early valve replacement in asymptomatic patients with severe aortic stenosis. *J Thorac Cardiovasc Surg.* 2008;135:308-315.

Bursi F, Weston SA, Redfield MM, et al. Systolic and diastolic heart failure in the community. *JAMA.* 2006;296:2209-2216.

Campbell CL, Smyth S, Montalescot G, et al. Aspirin dose for the prevention of cardiovascular disease. *JAMA.* 2007;297:2018-2024.

Caro JJ, Flegel KM, Orejuela ME, et al. Anticoagulant prophylaxis against stroke in atrial fibrillation: effectiveness in actual practice. *CMAJ.* 1999;161:493-497.

Chobanian AV. Isolated systolic hypertension in the elderly. *N Engl J Med.* 2007;357:789-796.

Cohn JN. The management of chronic heart failure. *N Engl J Med.* 1996;335:490-498.

Dajani AS, Taubert KA, Wilson JW, et al. Prevention of bacterial endocarditis. Recommendations by the American Heart Association. *JAMA.* 1997;277:1794-1801.

Dobkin BH. Rehabilitation after stroke. *N Engl J Med.* 2005;352:1677-1684.

Falk RH. Atrial fibrillation. *N Engl J Med.* 2001;344:1067-1078.

Fang MC, Go AS, Hylek EM, et al. Age and the risk of warfarin-associated hemorrahage: the anticoagulation and risk factors in atrial fibrillation study. *J Am Geriatr Soc.* 2006;54:1231-1236.

Filsoufi F, Rahmanian PB, Castillo JG, et al. Excellent early and late outcomes of aortic valve replacement in people aged 80 and older. *J Am Geriatr Soc.* 2008;56:255-261.

Gerstenblith G, Renlund DG, Lakatta EG. Cardiovascular response to exercise in younger and older men. *Fed Proc.* 1987;46:1834-1839.

Go AS, Lee WY, Yang J, et al. Statin therapy and risks for death and hospitalization in chronic heart failure. *JAMA.* 2006;296:2105-2111.

Gottlieb SS, McCarter RJ, Vogel RA. Effects of beta-blockade on mortality among high-risk and low-risk patients after myocardial infarction. *N Engl J Med.* 1998;339:489-497.

Gueyffier F, Bulpitt C, Borssel JP, et al. Antihypertensive drugs in very old people: a subgroup meta-analysis of randomized controlled trials. *Lancet.* 1999;353:793-796.

Hart RG, Benavente O, McBride R, et al. Antithrombotic therapy to prevent stroke in patients with atrial fibrillation: a meta-analysis. *Ann Intern Med.* 1999;131:492-501.

Hart RG, Pearce LA, Rothbart RM, et al. Stroke with intermittent atrial fibrillation: incidence and predictors during ASA therapy. *J Am Coll Cardiol.* 2000;35:183-187.

Hart RG, Pearce LA, Aguilar MI, et al. Met-analysis: antithrombotic therapy to prevent stroke in patients who have nonvalvular atrial fibrillation. *Ann Intern Med.* 2007;146:857-867.

Hjalmarson A, Goldstein S, Fagerberg B, et al. Effects of controlled-release metoprolol on total mortality, hospitalizations, and well-being in patients with heart failure. The metoprolol CR/XL randomized intervention trial in congestive heart failure (MERIT-HF). *JAMA.* 2000;283:1295-1302.

Joint National Committee. *The Seventh Report of the Joint National Committee on Prevention, Detection, Evaluation, and Treatment of High Blood Pressure.* Bethesda, MD: National Institutes of Health; 2003.

Kane RL, Chen Q, Blewett LA, et al. Do rehabilitative nursing homes improve the outcomes of care? *J Am Geriatr Soc.* 1996;44:545-554.

Kastelein JJP, Akdim F, Stroes ESG, et al. for the ENHANCE INVESTIGATORS. Simvastatin with or without ezetimibe in familial hypercholesterolemia. *N Engl J Med.* 2008;358:1431-1443.

Kjeldsen SE, Dahlof B, Devereux RB, et al. Effects of losartan on cardiovascular morbidity and mortality in patients with isolated systolic hypertension and left ventricular hypertrophy. A losartan intervention for end point reduction (LIFE) substudy. *JAMA.* 2002;288:1491-1498.

Krumholz HM, Radford MJ, Wang Y, et al. National use and effectiveness of β-blockers for the treatment of elderly patients after acute myocardial infarction. *JAMA.* 1998;280:623-629.

MRC Working Party. Medical Research Council trial of treatment of hypertension in older adults: principal results. *BMJ* 1992;304:405-412.

Marshall DA, Levy AR, Vidaillet H, et al. and the AFFIRM and CORE Investigators. Cost-effectiveness of rhythm versus rate control in atrial fibrillation. *Ann Intern Med.* 2004;141:653-661.

Mas J-L, Chatellier G, Beyssen B, et al. for the EVA-3S Investigators. Endarterectomy versus stenting in patients with symptomatic severe carotid stenosis. *N Engl J Med.* 2006;355:1660-1671.

Mitchell GF, Vasan RS, Keyes MJ, et al. Pulse pressure and risk of new-onset atrial fibrillation. *JAMA.* 2007;297:709-715.

Neubauer S. The failing heart—an engine out of fuel. *N Engl J Med.* 2007;356:1140-1151.

Oral H, Pappone C, Chugh A, et al. Circumferential pulmonary-vein ablation for chronic atrial fibrillation. *N Engl J Med.* 2006;354:934-941.

Ostchega Y, Dillon CF, Hughes JP, et al. Trends in hypertension prevalence, awareness, treatment, and control in older U.S. adults: data from the National Health and Nutrition Examination Survey 1988 to 2004. *J Am Geriatr Soc.* 2007;55:1056-1065.

Otto CM, Lind BK, Kitzman DW, et al. Association of aortic-valve sclerosis with cardiovascular mortality and morbidity in the elderly. *N Engl J Med.* 1999;341:142-147.

Panjrath GS, Messerli FH. β-Blockers for primary prevention in hypertension: era bygone? *Science Direct.* 2006;2(Issue 2):76-87.

Pfisterer M, Buser P, Osswald S, et al. Outcome of elderly patients with chronic symptomatic coronary artery disease with an invasive vs optimized medical treatment strategy. One-year results of the randomized TIME trial. *JAMA.* 2003;289:1117-1123.

Rajamannan NM, Bonow RO, Rahimtoola SH. Calcific aortic stenosis: an update. *Nat Clin Pract Cardiovasc Med.* 2007;4(No. 5):254-262.

Redfield MM, Jacobsen SJ, Burnett JC, et al. Burden of systolic and diastolic ventricular dysfunction in the community. Appreciating the scope of the heart failure epidemic. *JAMA.* 2003;289:194-202.

Schlenker RE, Kramer AM, Hrincevich CA, et al. Rehabilitation costs: implications for prospective payment. *Health Serv Res.* 1997;32:651-668.

Sipahi I, Tuzcu M, Wolski KE, et al. β-Blockers and progression of coronary atherosclerosis: polled analysis of 4 intravascular ultrasonography trials. *Ann Intern Med.* 2007;147:10-18.

Staessen JA, Fagard R, Thijs L, et al. Morbidity and mortality in the placebo-controlled European trial on isolated systolic hypertension in the elderly. *Lancet.* 1997;350:757-764.

Straus SE, Majumdar SR, McAlister FA. New evidence for stroke prevention. Scientific review. *JAMA.* 2002;288:1388-1395.

The Medical Letter. Spironolactone for heart failure. *Med Lett Drugs Ther.* 1999;41:81-84.

The Medical Letter. Drugs for hypertension. *Med Lett Drugs Ther.* 2001;43:17-22.

Ting HH, Yang E, Rihal CS. Narrative review: reperfusion strategies for ST-segment elevation myocardial infarction. *Ann Intern Med.* 2006;145:610-617.

van der Worp HB, van Gijn J. Acute ischemic stroke. *N Engl J Med.* 2007;357:572-579.

Van Gelder IC, Hagens VE, Bosker HA, et al. A comparison of rate control and rhythm control in patients with recurrent persistent atrial fibrillation. *N Engl J Med.* 2002;347:1834-1840.

Wazni OM, Marrouche NF, Martin DO, et al. Radiofrequency ablation vs antiarrhythmic drugs as first-line treatment of symptomatic atrial fibrillation. *JAMA.* 2005;293:2634-2640.

Wenger NK, Lewis SJ, Herrington DM, et al. for the Treating to New Targets Study Steering Committee and Investigators. Outcomes of using high- or low-dose atorvastatin in patients 65 years of age or older with stable coronary disease. *Ann Intern Med.* 2007;147:1-9.

White C. Intermittent claudication. *N Engl J Med.* 2007;356:1241-1250.

Wing LMH, Reid CM, Ryan P, et al. A comparison of outcomes with angiotensin-converting-enzyme inhibitors and diuretics for hypertension in the elderly. *N Engl J Med.* 2003;348:583-592.

Wolf SL, Winstein CJ, Miller JP, et al. for the EXCITE Investigators: effect of constraint-induced movement therapy on upper extremity function 3 to 9 months after stroke. *JAMA.* 2006;296:2095-2104.

Yan AT, Yan RT, Liu PP. Narrative review: parmacotherapy for chronic heart failure: evidence from recent clinical trials. *Ann Intern Med.* 2005;142:132-145.

Suggested Readings

Carabello BA. Aortic stenosis. *N Engl J Med.* 2002;346:677-682.

Ezekowitz MD, Levine JA. Preventing stroke in patients with atrial fibrillation. *JAMA.* 1999;281:1830-1835.

Frohlich ED. Treating hypertension—what are we to believe? *N Engl J Med.* 2003;348:639-641.

Gage BF, Fihn SD, White RH. Warfarin therapy for an octogenarian who has atrial fibrillation. *Ann Intern Med.* 2001;134:465-474.

Haider AW, Larson MG, Franklin SS, et al. Systolic blood pressure, diastolic blood pressure, and pulse pressure as predictors of risk for congestive heart failure in the Framingham heart study. *Ann Intern Med.* 2003;138:10-16.

Hart RG, Halperin JL. Atrial fibrillation and thromboembolism: a decade of progress in stroke prevention. *Ann Intern Med.* 1999;131:688-695.

Kitzman DW, Little WC, Brubaker PH, et al. Pathophysiological characterization of isolated diastolic heart failure in comparison to systolic heart failure. *JAMA.* 2002;288:2144-2150.

Man-Son-Hing M, Nichol G, Lau A, et al. Choosing antithrombotic therapy for elderly patients with atrial fibrillation who are at risk for falls. *Arch Intern Med.* 1999;159:677-685.

Rich MW. Epidemiology, pathophysiology, and etiology of congestive heart failure in older adults. *J Am Geriatr Soc.* 1997;45:968-974.

Weber KT. Aldosterone in congestive heart failure. *N Engl J Med.* 2001;345:1689-1697.

CHAPTER 12

DECREASED VITALITY

Among older adults, decreased vitality is a common complaint; it has a host of underlying causes. This chapter deals with metabolic factors that may lead to decreased energy in the older adults: endocrine disease, anemia, poor nutrition, lack of exercise, and infection.

ENDOCRINE DISEASE

Carbohydrate Metabolism

Approximately 50% of older people have glucose intolerance with normal fasting blood sugar levels. Although poor diet, obesity, and lack of exercise may account for some of these findings, aging itself is associated with deteriorating glucose tolerance. Most data suggest a change in peripheral glucose utilization as the major factor in this phenomenon, although beta-cell dysfunction and decreased insulin secretion are also contributing factors. Glucose intolerance should not be diagnosed as diabetes mellitus. However, such individuals are at increased risk of developing diabetes mellitus. Prediabetes is identified as impaired fasting glucose (fasting plasma glucose level 100 to 125 mg/dL) or as impaired glucose tolerance (plasma glucose level 140 to 199 mg/dL 2 hours after 75 g of glucose). Lifestyle modification, including weight loss and exercise, prevents or forestalls the development of type 2 diabetes in individuals with glucose intolerance (Diabetes Prevention Program Research Group, 2002; reviewed in Gillies et al., 2007). Both the US Preventive Services Task Force (USPSTF) and the American Diabetes Association (ADA) recommend these interventions for patients at risk for diabetes (US Preventive Services Task Force, 2003).

By the age of 75 years, approximately 20% of the population has developed diabetes mellitus (Meneilly and Tessier, 2001). At least half of these patients are unaware that they have the disease. The USPSTF concludes that the evidence is insufficient to recommend for or against routinely screening asymptomatic adults for type 2 diabetes, except that those with hypertension or hyperlipidemia should be screened as an approach to reducing cardiovascular risk. The ADA recommends that screening should begin at age 45 at 3-year intervals, but at shorter intervals in high-risk patients. The diagnosis of diabetes should be made on the basis of fasting plasma glucose of 126 mg/dL or greater on at least two occasions. Initial evaluation in patients with type 2 diabetes should include glycosylated hemoglobin level, fasting lipid profile, basic metabolic panel, urine dipstick for overt proteinuria or screen for microalbuminuria, and electrocardiography.

The therapeutic goal for most of the older diabetic patients is the same as that for younger patients: normal fasting plasma glucose without hypoglycemia A HbA1c value of less than 7% is often defined as optimal control. However, in those with short life expectancies (including many nursing home residents), the therapeutic goal may be modified to eliminate symptoms associated with hyperglycemia and to enhance quality of life. This can be accomplished by lowering the blood sugar to levels that avoid glycosuria. The age at which tight control is no longer indicated has not been defined; however, studies that demonstrated benefit of tight control were 4 to 6 years in duration.

Because most patients with adult-onset diabetes are obese, weight reduction should be attempted, although only approximately 10% will maintain a prolonged weight loss. Dietary fats should be reduced. Aerobic exercise is of benefit in both delaying the onset of type 2 diabetes mellitus and in improving insulin resistance in individuals with established disease (Boule et al., 2001).

Several groups of oral hypoglycemic agents, each with a different mechanism of action, are now available. Sulfonylureas act primarily by increasing beta-cell insulin secretion. They increase circulating insulin levels and are frequently associated with weight gain and may cause hypoglycemia. HbA1c reduction is in the 1% to 2% range. Although package inserts carry a warning on the increased risk of cardiovascular disease, the UK Prospective Diabetes Study (UKPDS) Group reported no adverse cardiovascular outcomes in sulfonylurea-treated patients (UK Prospective Diabetes Study Group, 1998a).

Acarbose reduces postprandial plasma glucose by inhibiting small intestine brush-border α-glucosidases. It has a small effect on metabolic control (HbA1c reduction of 0.5%-1%) and causes frequent gastrointestinal distress with bloating and flatulence.

Metformin, a biguanide, exerts its major metabolic effect by inhibiting hepatic glucose production. Metformin leads to significant improvement in glucose control when used alone (HbA1c reduction of 1%-2%) or in combination with a sulfonylurea (Inzucchi et al., 1998). Unlike sulfonylureas, which often lead to weight gain, metformin therapy is associated with weight loss, a benefit to most type 2 diabetic patients. Weight should be monitored closely in thin diabetic patients. A serious side effect of metformin is lactic acidosis. It should not be used in patients with renal insufficiency or chronic heart failure. In patients 80 years or older, creatinine clearance should be measured before therapy is initiated. Metformin should be discontinued during illnesses associated with volume depletion and prior to surgery.

Thiazolidinediones lower blood sugar by improving target-cell insulin sensitivity. Besides the potential for hepatic toxicity, which requires frequent liver function testing, thiazolidinedione therapy may be associated with marked weight gain. Fluid retention occurs more frequently in combination with insulin and in heart failure, making these conditions contraindications for the use of these agents. Recent studies have suggested that the thiazolidinedione, rosiglitazone, is associated with an increased risk of heart failure, acute myocardial infarction, and death (Lipscombe et al., 2007; Singh, Loke, and Furberg, 2007). This appears to be limited to rosiglitazone, for, although pioglitazone is associated with an increased risk for serious heart failure, it is not associated with increased risk for death, myocardial infarction, or stroke (Lincoff et al., 2007).

Meglitinide analogues (nateglinide and repaglinide) are nonsulfonylurea insulin secretagogues. They have a shorter onset of action and half-life than sulfonylureas, have a greater decrease in postprandial glucose level, and a lower risk of hypoglycemia. They may be good choices for individuals with irregular mealtimes, but are more expensive than other oral diabetes drugs and morbidly and mortality effects are unknown (reviewed in Black et al., 2007).

Two new classes of agents have been recently approved: incretin mimetics and dipeptidyl peptidase IV (DPP-4) inhibitors (reviewed in Amori, Lau, and Pittas, 2007). The first incretin mimetic, exenitide, has the same glucoregulatory action as glucagon-like peptide-1 (GLP-1), a naturally occurring incretin hormone (reviewed in Drucker, 2007). It enhances glucose-dependent insulin secretion, suppresses inappropriately high glucagon secretion, slows gastric emptying, decreases food intake, promotes beta-cell proliferation and neogenesis, reduces adiposity, and increases insulin-sensitizing effects. It is administered by subcutaneous injection twice daily, with a major side-effect of nausea and vomiting. In 2006, the FDA approved sitagliptin, a DPP-4 inhibitor. By inhibiting the breakdown of GLP-1 and glucose-dependent insulinotropic polypeptide, it leads to a lower blood glucose, stimulates insulin secretion, and decreases levels of circulating glucagon. It does not inhibit gastric emptying or promote satiety, and does not lead to weight loss. It is well tolerated without nausea or vomiting. Sitagliptin is one of the less effective glycemia-lowering drugs (HbA1c reduction of 0.5%-0.9%) (Nathan, 2007). Because these are new agents with small, short-term studies, and no specific data in older adults, treatment should be directed to maximizing glycemic control with other currently available therapeutic interventions.

Table 12-1 presents a step-care approach to the treatment of type 2 diabetes.

Because of the results of the UKPDS study, close control of blood glucose in type 2 diabetes is now in vogue. Intensive blood-glucose control with sulfonylureas or insulin decreased the risk of microvascular complications, but not macrovascular disease. Intensive treatment did increase the risk of hypoglycemia. Intensive blood-glucose control with metformin in overweight patients decreased the risk of both microvascular and macrovascular complications, and was associated with less weight gain and fewer hypoglycemic attacks than insulin and sulfonylureas (UK Prospective Diabetes Study Group, 1998b). Metformin is recommended as the first-line pharmacological therapy in overweight patients. It is important to observe patients closely for hypoglycemic reactions and their ability

TABLE 12-1   STEP-CARE APPROACH TO THE TREATMENT OF TYPE 2 DIABETES

STEP	CRITERIA AND RECOMMENDATION	MONITORING
Step 1: Evaluation and nonpharmacologic approaches	Newly diagnosed or current therapy ineffective: initiate or reinforce diet, exercise, home blood glucose monitoring, formal diabetes education Current therapy effective: continue therapy	Success: continue step 1 Failure after 2-3 months: go to step 2*
Step 2: Oral monotherapy	Obese or dyslipidemic: first line—metformin; second line—thiazolidinedione or acarbose Nonobese: first line—sulfonylurea or metformin; second line— acarbose	Success: continue step 2 Failure: go to step 3
Step 3: Oral combination therapy	Previously on metformin: add sulfonylurea Previously on sulfonylurea: add metformin or thiazolidinedione Previously on thiazolidinedione: add sulfonylurea Previously on acarbose, obese: add metformin Previously on acarbose, nonobese: add sulfonylurea	Success: continue step 3 Failure: go to step 4
Step 4: Insulin initiation or insulin + oral therapy	FBG <200-240: eliminate one drug and always thiazolidinedione, start bedtime glargine FBG >200-240: eliminate one drug, start bedtime glargine and preprandial lispro†	Success: continue step 4 Failure: consult specialist

*Severe hyperglycemia (fasting blood glucose > 300) may require initiation of insulin therapy.
†Other long-acting soluble insulin may be substituted for glargine for basal control. Other rapid-acting insulin may be substituted for lispro for prandial control.

to respond to this stress as any of these regimens is prescribed. Although each agent is effective as monotherapy, the majority of patients need multiple therapies to attain glycemic target levels in the longer term (Turner et al., 1999).

Patients who do not achieve adequate glycemic control with a combination of oral medications are candidates for insulin treatment. Insulin therapy may be combined with oral therapy to better achieve target glucose control. Glucose monitoring is essential for titrating the insulin dose. Multiple insulin regimens are possible but most begin with a basal insulin of once-daily glargine or twice daily NPH or Lente. Fast-acting insulin may be added with meals (reviewed in Mooradian, Bernbaum, and Albert, 2006).

Pramlintide has been approved for use with mealtime insulin. It is a synthetic form of the hormone amylin which is produced and secreted along with insulin by pancreatic beta-cells. It enhances insulin action and is administered subcutaneously before each meal. Again as with other new agents, there are no long-term morbidity or mortality data.

Diabetics are at increased risk of macrovascular disease. Other atherosclerotic risk factors such as smoking, dyslipidemia, and hypertension should be eliminated or treated. Therapy of these risk factors may be of greater benefit than tight glucose control in older diabetics. Tight blood pressure control reduces both micro- and macrovascular complications in type 2 diabetes (UK Prospective Diabetes Study Group, 1998c). A meta-analysis of cholesterol-lowering and blood pressure–lowering trials demonstrated large, significant effects on reducing macrovascular disease in type 2 diabetes (Huang, Meigs, and Singer, 2001). The target blood pressure for patients with diabetes is 130/85 mm Hg or lower. Angiotensin-converting enzyme (ACE) inhibitors and angiotensin-receptor blockers (ARBs) attenuate progression of nephropathy in both type 1 and type 2 diabetic patients with hypertension and in normotensives with microalbuminuria. They also attenuate decline in renal function in normotensive, normoalbuminuric type 2 diabetic patients (reviewed in Strippoli et al., 2006). The antihypertensive regimen of diabetics should include an ACE inhibitor or ARB, and such therapy should be initiated in normotensive albuminuric patients. Intensified multifactorial intervention with tight glucose regulation and the use of renin-angiotensin system blockers, aspirin, and lipid-lowering agents has been shown to reduce the risk of nonfatal cardiovascular disease, and rates of death from cardiovascular causes and death from any causes (Gaede et al., 2008).

The diagnosis, screening, prevention, evaluation, and treatment of type 2 diabetes have been recently reviewed (Laine and Wilson, 2007).

The goals for glycemic control are less well established for hospitalized than for ambulatory patients. However, data suggest that maintaining blood glucose at 80 to 110 mg/dL in critically ill patients reduces mortality, and hyperglycemia adversely effects wound healing and increases the risk for infection (reviewed in Inzucchi, 2006). Although sliding scale insulin regimens are frequently used in hospitalized patients with diabetes, it is the opinion of the authors that they should not be used. The University of Washington has developed an algorithm to replace sliding scale insulin orders (Fig. 12-1).

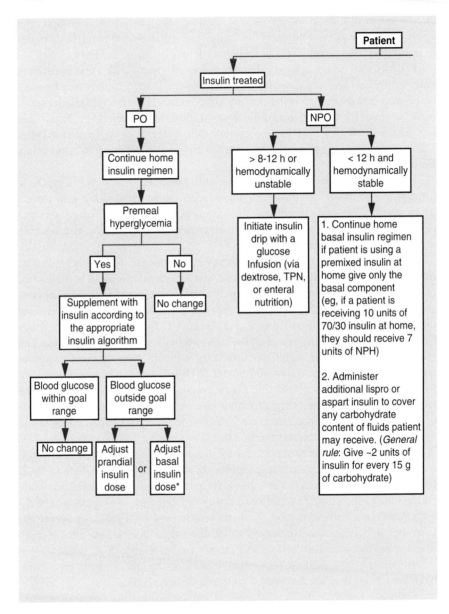

— FIGURE 12-1 — Flow diagram for treatment of hospitalized (non-intensive care
neutral protamine Hagedorn (insulin); NPO, nothing by mouth; PO, by mouth;

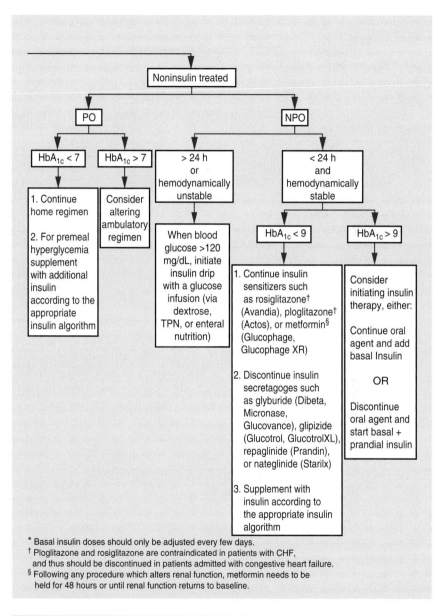

Under "> 24 h or hemodynamically unstable":

When blood glucose >120 mg/dL, initiate insulin drip with a glucose infusion (via dextrose, TPN, or enteral nutrition)

Under "HbA₁c < 9":

1. Continue insulin sensitizers such as rosiglitazone† (Avandia), ploglitazone† (Actos), or metformin§ (Glucophage, Glucophage XR)

2. Discontinue insulin secretagoges such as glyburide (Dibeta, Micronase, Glucovance), glipizide (Glucotrol, GlucotrolXL), repaglinide (Prandin), or nateglinide (Starilx)

3. Supplement with insulin according to the appropriate insulin algorithm

Under "HbA₁c > 9":

Consider initiating insulin therapy, either:

Continue oral agent and add basal Insulin

OR

Discontinue oral agent and start basal + prandial insulin

* Basal insulin doses should only be adjusted every few days.
† Ploglitazone and rosiglitazone are contraindicated in patients with CHF, and thus should be discontinued in patients admitted with congestive heart failure.
§ Following any procedure which alters renal function, metformin needs to be held for 48 hours or until renal function returns to baseline.

unit) patients with type 2 diabetes mellitus. CHF, congestive heart failure; NPH, TPN, total parenteral nutrition. (From Ku, 2002.)

Older adults have an increased incidence of hyperosmolar nonketotic (HNK) coma. Characteristic symptoms and signs help the physician distinguish this syndrome from diabetic ketoacidotic (DKA) coma. Table 12-2 compares HNK and DKA. Whereas DKA frequently develops over hours, HNK typically develops over days to weeks. Focal or generalized seizures are common in HNK and unusual in uncomplicated DKA. The fluid deficit is greater in HNK, thus leading to a higher serum sodium and more marked rise in blood urea nitrogen. Therapy in HNK must therefore address the volume and hyperosmolar state of the patient. Because these patients may be quite sensitive to insulin, lowering of glucose should be done cautiously. Volume replacement should be initiated with normal saline. This therapy alone may reduce blood glucose levels, as renal perfusion is enhanced and glucose is lost in the urine. If, after 1 hour of volume repletion, blood glucose levels are not reduced, a bolus of 20 U of regular insulin should be administered intravenously. If glucose levels do not respond, an insulin drip may be started. Such an approach should allow repletion of volume without lowering serum osmolarity too rapidly.

Thyroid

The changes with aging in the hypothalamic-pituitary-thyroid axis have been recently reviewed (Habra and Sarlis, 2005). Although thyroid function is generally normal in aging, the physician should be aware of the norms for thyroid function tests for this age group (Table 12-3). The majority of data indicate that T_4 levels are normal. T_3 levels may be lower in healthy older people when compared to younger individuals, but are still in the normal range. It has been suggested that

TABLE 12-2   HYPEROSMOLAR NONKETOTIC (HNK) COMA
AND DIABETIC KETOACIDOSIS (DKA)

	HNK*	DKA
Time of development	Days to weeks	Hours
Seizures	Common	Uncommon
Fluid deficit	Marked	Present
Serum sodium	↑↑	↑
Blood urea nitrogen	↑↑	↑

*Double arrow signifies a higher increase than for a single arrow. Correction factor for sodium: 100 mg/dL of glucose = 1.6 mEq/L of sodium.

TABLE 12-3   THYROID FUNCTION IN THE NORMAL ELDERLY

NORMAL	DECREASED
T_4	TSH response to TRH in males
Free T_4	Thyroid hormone production rate
T_3	Metabolic clearance rate of thyroid hormone
TSH	

TRH, thyroid-releasing hormone; TSH, thyroid-stimulating hormone.

the lower T_3 levels reported in several studies are caused by undiagnosed illness and the low-T_3 syndrome described below. Thyroid-stimulating hormone (TSH) levels are also normal, while the TSH response to thyroid-releasing hormone (TRH) is decreased in males and normal in females. Thus, the TRH test is less valuable in older males. Metabolic clearance of thyroid hormones is decreased in aging. With intact feedback loops, normal thyroid function is maintained despite this change. However, with exogenous replacement of thyroid hormone, such regulatory mechanisms are not maintained; thyroid replacement doses in older adults should be lower to take into account the lower metabolic clearance. Laboratory evaluation tests most useful in thyroid disease are summarized in Table 12-4.

Hypothyroidism   Hypothyroidism is primarily a disease of those aged 50 to 70 years. Goiter is rarely seen with hypothyroidism in the elderly except when it is iodide induced. Diagnosis is usually made by a low free T_4 and an elevated TSH. Because total T_4 levels may be depressed in seriously ill patients, diagnosis of hypothyroidism should not be made on the basis of low T_4 levels alone. Table 12-5 lists laboratory characteristics of the low-T_4 syndrome associated with nonthyroidal illness. Not all free-T_4 methods distinguish the low-T_4 syndrome from hypothyroidism; physicians should be aware of the type of determination and interpretation used in their laboratory. Because the T_3 level may be in the normal range in hypothyroidism, this is not a helpful test. The low T_3 level associated with a host of acute and chronic nonthyroidal illnesses also contributes to the poor specificity of this test in hypothyroidism. Approximately 75% of circulating T_3 is derived from peripheral conversion from T_4. The enzymes that convert T_4 to T_3 or reverse T_3 are under metabolic control. During illness, more T_4 is converted to reverse T_3, leading to the characteristic laboratory findings of the low-T_3 syndrome.

The radioactive iodine uptake is also not helpful because normal values are so low that they overlap with hypothyroidism. The TRH stimulation test can be used in females, but decreased responsiveness to TRH in older males does not allow

TABLE 12-4   LABORATORY EVALUATION OF THYROID DISEASE
IN THE ELDERLY

	HYPOTHYROIDISM	HYPERTHYROIDISM
T_4	E	E
TSH	E	E
Free T_4	E	E
T_3	O	D
Radioactive iodine uptake	O	D
TRH test	D (Females)	D (Females)
	O (Males)	O (Males)
Reverse T_3	D	D
TSH stimulation	D	O
T_3 suppression	O	O

E, test for initial evaluation; D, helpful in confirming diagnosis or in differentiation of difficult cases; O, not helpful in diagnosis or not indicated; TRH, thyroid-releasing hormone; TSH, thyroid-stimulating hormone.

TABLE 12-5   THYROID-FUNCTION TESTS IN NONTHYROIDAL
ILLNESS

	LOW-T_4 SYNDROME	LOW-T_3 SYNDROME
T_4	Decreased	Normal
Free T_4	Normal or increased	Normal
T_3	Decreased	Decreased
Reverse T_3	Normal or increased	Normal or increased
Thyroid-stimulating hormone	Normal	Normal

this test to distinguish normal from pathological states. In males, a TSH stimulation test may help to confirm the presence of hypothyroidism.

Hypothyroidism may be accompanied by other laboratory abnormalities. Creatine phosphokinase (CPK) levels may be elevated. A normocytic, normochromic anemia, which responds to thyroid hormone replacement, may be present. There is an increased incidence of pernicious anemia in hypothyroidism, but the microcytic anemia of iron deficiency remains the commonest anemia associated with hypothyroidism.

The symptoms and signs of hypothyroidism may be overlooked when such complaints as fatigue, memory loss, and decreased hearing are ascribed to aging without further investigation. The prevalence of undiagnosed hypothyroidism in healthy older people has varied from 0.5% to 2% in multiple studies; consequently, a general screening program is not cost-effective. The prevalence among older adults who are ill, however, is sufficient to support screening for hypothyroidism in this population, comprising individuals who have already presented themselves for care.

Therapy for hypothyroidism should be started at 0.025 to 0.05 mg of sodium levothyroxine (Synthroid) per day and increased by the same dose at 1- to 3-week intervals. The decreased metabolic clearance rate of thyroid hormone in aging may lead to a lower maintenance dose of T_4. The physician should monitor heart rate response and symptoms of angina and, in the laboratory, the TSH level. When indicated for symptomatic cardiovascular disease, a β-blocker may be added to the T_4 regimen. In patients with coronary artery disease, therapy can be initiated with tri-iodothyronine 5 μg/day and increased by 5 μg at weekly intervals to a level of 25 μg/day, at which time the patient can be converted to T_4 therapy. Because T_3 has a shorter half-life than T_4, symptoms will remit more rapidly after discontinuance of therapy if the patient develops cardiovascular complications. A β-blocker can also be added to the T_3 regimen. T_4 monotherapy, rather than T_4-T_3 combination, should remain the treatment of choice for clinical hypothyroidism (Grozinsky-Glasberg et al., 2006).

Subclinical Hypothyroidism   Subclinical hypothyroidism is characterized by increased serum TSH concentrations with normal free T_4 and free T_3 levels. It occurs in 10% to 15% of the general population. The presentation is nonspecific and symptoms are usually subtle. In a prospective follow-up study, based on the initial TSH level (4 to 6/ > 6 to 12/ > 12), the incidence of overt hypothyroidism after 10 years was 0%, 42.8%, and 76.9%, respectively (Huber et al., 2002). The incidence of overt disease was increased in those with positive microsomal antibodies. Subclinical hypothyroidism has been described as an independent risk factor for atherosclerosis and myocardial infarction (Hak et al., 2000), and associated with left ventricular diastolic dysfunction that is improved with T_4 therapy (Biondi et al., 1999). Others have not found an association of subclinical hypothyroidism with cardiovascular disorders or mortality (Cappola et al., 2006). The decision to treat patients remains controversial (Fatourechi, 2007). Contributing to this controversy is the question of the age-specific distribution of TSH (Surks and Hollowell, 2007). This is further complicated by recent data showing reduced mortality risk in untreated mild hypothyroid subjects aged > 85 years (Mariotti and Cambuli, 2007). However, if therapy is contemplated, an algorithm for the management of subclinical hypothyroidism has been proposed (Fig. 12-2).

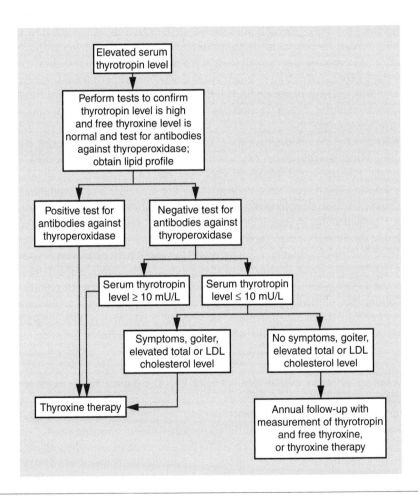

— FIGURE 12-2 — An algorithm for the management of subclinical hypothyroidism. LDL = low-density lipoprotein. (Reproduced with permission from Cooper DS: Clinical Practice. Subclinical hypothyroidism. *N Engl J Med.* 2001;345: 260-265.)

Myxedema Coma   Most patients with myxedema coma are older than age 60 (Table 12-6). In approximately 50% of the cases, the coma is induced in the hospital by treating hypothyroid patients with hypnotics. A neck scar, from previous thyroid surgery, is a clue to the cause of coma. Because patients with this disorder die of respiratory failure, hypercapnia requires prompt attention. These patients should be treated in an intensive care setting, with intubation and respiratory assistance instituted at the first sign of respiratory failure. The cerebrospinal fluid protein level is often more than 100 mg/dL and should not in itself be used as an indicator of other central nervous system pathology. Therapy includes a large initial dose (200 to 300 μg) of T_4 intravenously. Although studies have not been done to demonstrate the efficacy of glucocorticoids in this syndrome, it is generally recommended that these patients receive 50 mg of hydrocortisone every 6 hours for the first 1 or 2 days. Patients with concomitant adrenal insufficiency will require continued steroid therapy.

Hyperthyroidism   Approximately 20% of hyperthyroid patients are older adults; 75% have classic signs and symptoms. Ophthalmopathy is infrequent. Approximately one-third have no goiter. Toxic multinodular goiter is more frequent than in the young. Severe nonthyroidal disease may disguise thyrotoxicosis (apathetic hyperthyroidism). Congestive heart failure (CHF), stroke, and infection are common disorders associated with masked hyperthyroidism. There should be a high threshold of suspicion for hyperthyroidism in older adults. Unexplained heart failure or tachyarrhythmia, recent onset of a psychiatric disorder, or profound myopathy should raise questions about masked hyperthyroidism. The triad of weight loss, anorexia, and constipation, which may raise the possibility of neoplastic disease, occurs in 15% of older thyrotoxic patients. Diagnosis is made by T_4, T_3, and/or radioactive iodine uptake (see Table 12-4). The ultrasensitive TSH assays can differentiate hyperthyroidism from normal. In the absence of acute nonthyroidal disease, this test alone may confirm the clinical diagnosis of

TABLE 12-6   MYXEDEMA COMA

Usually older than age 60 years

50% induced by hypnotics

Neck scar

Hypothermia

Delayed relaxation of tendon reflex

Respiratory failure and apnea

hyperthyroidism. In the presence of acute illness, concomitant determination of TSH and free T_4 may be more appropriate. A T_3 suppression test should not be done in older adults because of the risk of angina or myocardial infarction.

Therapy is usually by radioactive iodine ablation. Often patients are first treated with antithyroid medications to control hyperthyroidism and deplete the thyroid gland of hormone prior to the radioactive iodine treatment (reviewed in Cooper, 2005). Surgery is reserved for patients with thyroid glands that are causing local obstructive symptoms.

Severe thyrotoxicosis is treated with antithyroid drugs (preferably propylthiouracil because it blocks peripheral conversion of T_4 to T_3) to inhibit new hormone synthesis, iodides to block thyroid hormone secretion, and β-blockers to decrease the peripheral manifestations of thyroid hormone action. In older adults with underlying cardiac disease, β-blocker therapy may be a problem; thus the cardiovascular response must be closely monitored. In patients allergic to antithyroid medications or where β-blockers are contraindicated, calcium ipodate (Oragrafin), 3 g every 3 days, can be used because it inhibits peripheral conversion of T_4 to T_3. Dexamethasone 2 mg every 6 hours inhibits peripheral conversion of T_4 to T_3 and may be added to any of the above regimens.

Subclinical Hyperthyroidism   Subclinical hyperthyroidism is defined as a combination of undetectable serum TSH and normal serum T_3 and T_4. Subclinical hyperthyroidism is associated with the development of atrial fibrillation (Cappola et al., 2006). Subclinical hyperthyroidism caused by multinodular goiter often progresses to overt hyperthyroidism, and ablative therapy with iodine-131 is usually recommended (Toft, 2001). In older patients with atrial fibrillation or osteoporosis that may be related to the mild excess of thyroid hormone, ablative therapy is also the best initial option. In patients with subtle, nonspecific symptoms in the absence of a multinodular goiter, an antithyroidal medication should be tried for a 6-month period. If symptoms improve, ablative therapy should be considered.

Hyperparathyroidism

One-third of patients with hyperparathyroidism are older than age 60. Symptoms are the same in older adults as in those who are younger, but may be overlooked. Bone demineralization, weakness, and joint complaints may be ascribed to aging when they may actually indicate parathyroid disease. Primary hyperthyroidism is common in postmenopausal women with forearm fracture and low bone mineral density (Bergstrom, Landgreen, and Freyschuss, 2007). Basic laboratory screening is indicated in these individuals. An NIH Workshop has developed guidelines for surgery in patients with asymptomatic primary hyperthyroidism (Summary Statement from a Workshop on Asymptomatic Primary Hyperparathyroidism, 2002). Surgery is recommended if one of the following is

TABLE 12-7   LABORATORY FINDINGS IN METABOLIC BONE DISEASE

DISEASE	CA	P	ALK	PTH
Hyperparathyroidism	High	Low/normal	High/normal	High
Osteomalacia	Low/normal	Low	High/normal	High
Hyperthyroidism	High	High	High/normal	Low
Osteoporosis	Normal	Normal	Normal	Normal/high
Paget disease	Normal/high	Normal/high	High	Normal

Alk, alkaline phosphatase; Ca, calcium; P, phosphorus; PTH, parathyroid hormone.

present: serum calcium concentration greater than 1.0 mg/dL above upper limit of normal; 24-hour urinary calcium greater than 400 mg; creatinine clearance reduced by 30%: Bone mineral density T-score lower than −2.5 at any site: age less than 50 years. In those older than 50, surgery can be delayed with monitoring for the above criteria.

Table 12-7 contrasts some of the basic patterns of the common laboratory tests in hyperparathyroidism with those of other metabolic bone diseases that are common in older adults.

Vasopressin Secretion

Basal vasopressin levels are unaltered in normal older individuals. Infusion of hypertonic saline, however, leads to a greater increase in plasma vasopressin in older as compared with younger persons. In contrast to the response to the hyperosmolar challenge, volume changes related to the assumption of upright posture are associated with less of a vasopressin response in older subjects as compared with the young. Both these findings might be explained by impaired baroreceptor input to the supraoptic nucleus. Volume expansion decreases osmoreceptor sensitivity. Hypertonic saline infusion results in volume expansion and thus decreases osmoreceptor sensitivity. If baroreceptor input is impaired in older adults, volume expansion would lead to a lesser dampening effect, and thus the vasopressin response to hyperosmolar stimuli would be increased.

Hyponatremia is a serious and often overlooked problem of the older patient (reviewed in Miller, 2006). This syndrome is often associated with one of three general causes: (1) decreased renal blood flow with a decreased ability to excrete a water load; (2) diuretic administration leading to water intoxication (this condition is rapidly corrected by discontinuing diuretics); and (3) excess vasopressin secretion. Although a host of pulmonary disorders (eg, pneumonia, tuberculosis, tumor) and central nervous system disorders (eg, stroke, meningitis, subdural hematoma) are associated with the syndrome of inappropriate secretion of antidiuretic hormone (SIADH) in any age group, older adults seem more prone to develop this complication. Certain drugs, such as chlorpropamide and barbiturates, may cause this syndrome more frequently in older individuals.

In addition to treatment directed at correcting the underlying cause, water restriction and hypertonic saline are indicated when the patient is symptomatic or the sodium level is below 120 mEq/L. Demethylchlortetracycline therapy may be needed in resistant patients with SIADH. This agent induces a partial nephrogenic diabetes insipidus and thus corrects the hyponatremia. Serum creatinine and blood urea nitrogen should be closely monitored.

Anabolic Hormones

Aging is associated with a decline in anabolic hormones (Lamberts, van den Beld, and van der Lely, 1997). The declining activity of the growth hormone insulin-like growth factor-1 (IGF-1) axis with advancing age may contribute to the decrease in lean body mass and the increase in mass of adipose tissue that occur with aging. Increased lean body mass and decreased fat mass have been demonstrated to occur in men and women with growth hormone treatment. Men had marginal improvement of muscle strength and maximum oxygen consumption (Vo_{2max}), but women had no significant change. Adverse effects were frequent, including glucose tolerance and diabetes (Blackman et al., 2002).

Normal male aging is accompanied by a decline in testicular function, including a fall in serum levels of total testosterone and bioavailable testosterone. Only some men become hypogonadal. Androgens have many important physiological actions, including effects on muscle, bone, and bone marrow. However, little is known about the effects of the age-related decline in testicular function on androgen target organs. Studies of testosterone supplementation in older males demonstrate significant increases in lean body mass and significant decreases in biochemical parameters of bone resorption with testosterone treatment. Testosterone supplementation in older men with low normal testosterone concentration did not affect functional status or cognition (Emmelot-Vonk et al., 2008). However, there was a significant increase in hematocrit and a sustained stimulation of prostate-specific antigen (Gruenewald and Matsumoto, 2003). Based on these results, growth hormone administration and testosterone supplementation cannot be recommended at this time for older men with normal or low normal levels of these anabolic hormones. Although clinical trials data are limited, current practice guidelines recommend testosterone replacement therapy in symptomatic men with low testosterone levels to improve bone mineral density, muscle mass and strength, sexual function, and quality of life (Kazi, Geraci, and Koch, 2007).

ANEMIA

Anemia is common in older adults, but should not be attributed simply to old age. Increased weakness, fatigue, and a mild anemia should not be dismissed as a manifestation of aging. In healthy older individuals, there is generally no change in normal levels of hemoglobin from younger adult values. A low hemoglobin concentration at old age signifies disease and is associated with increased mortality, disability, and hospitalization (Izaks, Westerndrop, and Koch, 1999; Longo, 2005; Maraldi et al., 2006; Penninx et al., 2006), although the actual mechanism has not been elucidated.

Signs and symptoms of anemia may be subtle. Table 12-8 lists some of these manifestations. Anemia should be considered in these circumstances. If anemia is present, a diagnostic evaluation is indicated to define the cause. The appearance of the peripheral blood smear along with the history and physical examination should direct the diagnostic evaluation as described below.

Iron Deficiency

Iron deficiency is the most common cause of anemia in older adults. Laboratory findings include hypochromia, microcytosis, low reticulocyte count, decreased serum iron, increased total iron-binding capacity (TIBC), low transferrin saturation, and absent bone marrow iron stores. A low serum iron and elevated TIBC indicate iron deficiency even in the absence of changes in red cell morphology. Because transferrin is reduced in many diseases, the TIBC may be normal or low in older patients with iron deficiency. However, a transferrin saturation

TABLE 12-8   SIGNS AND SYMPTOMS OF ANEMIA

Weakness	Ischemic chest pain
Postural hypotension	Congestive heart failure
Syncope	Exertional dyspnea
Falls	Pallor
Confusion	Tachycardia
Worsened dementia	

of less than 10% would suggest iron deficiency even in the presence of a low TIBC. A low serum ferritin level is valuable in confirming the diagnosis because serum ferritin levels are below 12 mg/L in iron-deficiency anemia. Because inflammatory disease can elevate ferritin levels and liver disease can influence ferritin levels in either direction, the diagnosis of iron deficiency on the basis of a ferritin level must be made with a knowledge of the clinical situation.

Once iron deficiency is identified, it should be treated, and the cause of the anemia must be identified and corrected. Poor dietary intake of iron may contribute to iron deficiency in older adults. A dietary evaluation is important, both for foods that contain iron and for substances such as tea, which inhibit iron absorption. However, even in the presence of poor nutrition, evaluation for a bleeding lesion must be completed.

The stool should be examined for occult blood. Evaluation for a gastrointestinal lesion should be carried out in a patient with unexplained iron deficiency, even if the stool is negative for occult blood. Although gastrointestinal bleeding may be caused by drugs (especially certain analgesics, steroids, and alcohol), a gastrointestinal lesion must be excluded. Diverticulosis is a common cause of bleeding. Vascular ectasia of the cecum and ascending colon is increasingly a recognized cause of bleeding in older adults.

Replacement of iron should usually be by daily oral administration. The hemoglobin should improve in 10 days and be normal in approximately 6 weeks. Normal bone marrow iron stores should occur in an additional 4 months. If the anemia does not improve, one should consider nonadherence, continued bleeding, or an incorrect diagnosis. In unreliable patients, or when oral iron is not tolerated, parenteral iron replacement with iron dextran is indicated. Tolerance should be monitored with a test dose, and the patient should be closely observed for an acute reaction. Severe reactions occur less frequently with ferric gluconate, but a test dose should be used as well. Parenteral iron should not be used routinely but it is an important therapeutic modality in the appropriate patient.

Chronic Disease

The anemia of chronic disease (ACD) may display many similarities with iron deficiency (reviewed in Weiss and Goodnough, 2005). In older adults, this anemia is frequently associated with chronic inflammatory diseases or neoplasia. There is a defect in bone marrow red cell production and a shortening of erythrocyte life span. The finding of hypochromia, low reticulocyte count, and low serum iron may lead to confusion with iron deficiency. When a high TIBC does not confirm the presence of iron deficiency, a ferritin level can differentiate the two anemias. It is low in iron deficiency and high-normal or elevated in the ACD. Treatment is addressed to the underlying chronic illness, because there is no specific therapy for this type of anemia.

Sideroblastic Anemia

Sideroblastic anemia should be considered in an older patient with hypochromic anemia who does not have iron deficiency or a chronic disease. Serum iron and transferrin saturation are increased. Hence, synthesis is defective, leading to increased iron stores and the diagnostic finding of ringed sideroblasts in the marrow.

In older adults, sideroblastic anemia is commonly of the acquired type. The idiopathic group is usually refractory; only a few patients have a partial response to pyridoxine, but all should have a trial of pyridoxine. Although the prognosis is fairly good, approximately 10% of patients develop acute myeloblastic leukemia. Secondary sideroblastic anemia may be associated with underlying diseases such as malignancies and chronic inflammatory diseases. Certain drugs and toxins can induce sideroblastic anemia (eg, ethanol, lead, isoniazid, chloramphenicol). The drug-induced syndromes are corrected by administering pyridoxine. Table 12-9 lists the tests that will assist in the differential diagnosis of hypochromic anemias.

Vitamin B_{12} and Folate Deficiency

Both vitamin B_{12} and folate deficiency may occur on a nutritional basis, although folate deficiency is more common. Older people who live alone or who are alcoholics are most likely to have poor nutrition. Poor dietary intake of fresh fruits and vegetables may lead to folate deficiency; lack of meat, poultry, fish, eggs, and dairy products may lead to vitamin B_{12} deficiency. Vitamin B_{12} deficiency also

TABLE 12-9   DIFFERENTIAL TESTS IN HYPOCHROMIC ANEMIA

ITEM	IRON DEFICIENCY	CHRONIC DISEASE	SIDEROBLASTIC ANEMIA
Serum iron	Low	Low	High
Total iron-binding capacity	Usually increased*	Low	Normal
Transferrin saturation	Low	Low	High
Ferritin	Low	High	Normal
Bone marrow iron	Absent	Adequate	Increased ringed sideroblasts

*May be normal or even low in older adults.

occurs with the loss of intrinsic factor (pernicious anemia) and in gastrointestinal disorders associated with malabsorption of vitamin B_{12}.

The laboratory findings are similar in the two deficiencies and include macrocytosis, hyperchromasia, hypersegmented neutrophils, and megaloblasts in the marrow. Leukopenia and thrombocytopenia may be present, and serum lactic dehydrogenase and bilirubin may be increased. The two are differentiated by measuring serum vitamin B_{12} and folate levels.

Treatment is with vitamin B_{12} or folic acid, as appropriate. However, because folate will correct the hematological disorder but not the neurological abnormalities of vitamin B_{12} deficiency, a correct diagnosis is essential before treatment.

Erythropoietin

A longitudinal analysis of erythropoietin (Epo) levels in the Baltimore Longitudinal Study on Aging revealed a significant rise in Epo levels with age (Ershler et al., 2005). Subjects who developed anemia but did not have hypertension or diabetes had the greatest slope in Epo rise over time, whereas those with hypertension or diabetes had the lowest slope. In very advanced age or in those with compromised renal function, an inadequate compensatory mechanism leads to anemia.

Epo effectively corrects the anemia in patients with chronic kidney disease (CKD) who do not yet require dialysis, and may improve anemia-induced symptoms, cardiovascular function, and perhaps decrease mortality (Jones et al., 2004). An adequate response to Epo requires the maintenance of sufficient iron stores. Iron status should be evaluated and iron supplements given when there is evidence of iron deficiency. The FDA recommendation indicates that patients with CKD, who are not on dialysis, should have a hemoglobin count of 10 g/dL prior to starting treatment. However, better outcomes have been demonstrated with Hgb values above 11 g/dL (Hct of 33%). There is also evidence for little benefit and potential risk for maintaining Hgb levels of 13 g/dL or higher (Hct 39%). The recommended target is Hgb levels between 11 and 12 g/dL. Future recommendations may be lower because of the boxed warning to adjust Epo dose to maintain the Hgb level necessary to avoid the need for blood transfusion.

The FDA has issued a black box safety alert, indicating that treating the anemia of cancer with Epo in patients who are not receiving chemotherapy offers no benefit and may cause serious harm (Steensma, 2008). As in CKD, the FDA recommendation is to gradually increase the Hgb concentration to the lowest level sufficient to avoid blood transfusions in patients who are receiving chemotherapy.

The preferred therapy for the ACD is correction of the underlying disorder, rather than transfusion or Epo therapy. Studies in humans of therapy with Epo in ACD have been limited. Although one of the hallmarks of ACD is reduced bone marrow response to endogenous or exogenous Epo, some patients may respond.

Epo has been helpful in ACD in patients with rheumatoid arthritis or AIDS who have low Epo levels (< 500 mU/mL).

With the present FDA recommendations and cautions, Epo therapy in older adults should be reserved for those who meet the criteria for therapy described above.

NUTRITION

A discussion of nutrition and aging is limited by the lack of adequate studies, defined methods, and standards. Although it is generally accepted that intake moderately above recommended allowances is optimal, animal studies demonstrate increased longevity with lower caloric levels than recommended. In establishing nutritional requirements in humans, we must contend with the multiple factors that confine interpretation of available data, for example, genetic factors, social environment, economic status, selection of food, and weak methods of assessing nutritional status.

Several national surveys have been performed to assess nutrition in older adults. Taken as a whole, these surveys do not indicate poor nutritional status or marked deficiency among older individuals in the United States, and suggest that intake relates more to health and poverty than to age. However, because folate and B$_{12}$ deficiencies are associated with an increased incidence of coronary artery disease, vitamin D deficiency is associated with osteoporosis, and vitamins A, C, and E have antioxidant effects that may be beneficial in prevention of certain chronic diseases, and because most people do not consume an optimal amount of all vitamins alone, some authors recommend that all adults take vitamin supplements (Fletcher and Fairfield, 2002).

Vitamins, Protein, and Calcium

Table 12-10 summarizes nutritional requirements in older adults and demonstrates that there is no general increase in vitamin requirements with age. Studies on vitamin metabolism and requirements reveal no correlation between age and the requirement for vitamins A, B$_1$, B$_2$, or C. Vitamin B$_6$ and vitamin B$_{12}$ requirements also do not increase with age.

Studies on protein requirements are not in agreement. Based on nitrogen balance studies, estimates of protein requirement varied from 0.5 to more than 1.0 g/kg daily. Data on amino acid requirements are also conflicting: some data show increased requirements with age, and other data show no change.

For calcium, estimated requirements vary from 850 to 1020 mg/day, and some recommendations are as high as 1500 mg/day for postmenopausal women. Data on the correlation of dietary calcium intake and osteoporosis are conflicting.

TABLE 12-10   NUTRITIONAL REQUIREMENTS IN OLDER PERSONS

Vitamins	Unchanged in older persons
Protein	0.5 to > 1.0 g/kg/day
Amino acids	Unchanged to increased
Calcium	850-1020 mg/day
Calories	Declines by 12.4 cal/day/year (maturity to senescence)

However, calcium and vitamin D supplementation do improve postmenopausal osteoporosis. It may be necessary to use calcium and vitamin D supplements to ensure adequate intake.

Nutritional Deficiency and Physiological Impairments

There is little evidence to correlate age-associated nutritional deficiency with clinical findings. In a study on the consequences of vitamin A levels, there was no significant correlation with dark adaptation, epithelial cells excreted, or percent of keratinization. In other studies, there was no correlation between vitamin C levels and gingivitis or vitamin B_{12} and lactic acid, lactic dehydrogenase, or hematocrit. Older people with limited sun exposure may be at risk of vitamin D deficiency. Studies of older individuals in nursing homes suggest that these patients require 800 IU of vitamin D per day, double the usual recommended daily requirement. Total 25-hydroxy vitamin D levels should be measured and maintained in the 30 to 40 ng/mL range. Until recently, vitamin D was only considered as one of the calciotropic hormones. Recent data have demonstrated that vitamin D has an important role in cell differentiation, function, and survival (Montero-Odasso and Duque, 2005). Muscle and bone are significantly affected by the presence or absence of vitamin D. In bone, vitamin D stimulates bone turnover while protecting osteoblasts from apoptosis, whereas in muscle it maintains the function of type II fibers, preserving strength and preventing falls. Both osteoporosis and sarcopenia have been linked to the development of frailty in older adults. Although data on the effect of vitamin D supplementation have been conflicting, a recent meta-analysis demonstrated a benefit of vitamin D in preventing falls (Jackson et al., 2007). Data are conflicting on correlation of dietary calcium intake and osteoporosis. Problems in assessing this correlation include reduced calcium intake in older adults, altered calcium and phosphorus ratio, decreased protein intake, and acid–base balance.

Reversal of Deficiency by Supplementation

There is no impairment of vitamin or protein absorption in older adults. Data demonstrate conclusively that low vitamin levels in older adults can be reversed by administration of oral supplementation. Because these deficiencies can be corrected by dietary supplementation, they are most likely related to decreased intake.

Caloric Needs

A study of 250 individuals aged 23 to 99 demonstrated an age-associated decline in total caloric intake at the rate of 12.4 cal/day for a year. A yearly decline in basal metabolic rate accounted for 5.23 cal/day, while 7.6 cal/day related to reduction in other requirements, including physical exercise (McGandy et al., 1966).

Dietary Restriction and Food Additives

Rats, mice, *Drosophila*, and other lower organisms have demonstrated that caloric restriction delays maturation and increases life span. The mechanism, however, is not understood, but studies suggest that it may be related to decreased levels of IGF-1. Animals fed isocaloric diets but decreased protein have an increased life span. Based on the free radical theory of aging, it has been proposed that reducing agents would prolong life. Although the data are conflicting, some studies support this hypothesis. In certain animal models, caloric restriction decreases the incidence and delay onset of disease, including chronic glomerulonephritis, muscular dystrophy, and carcinogenesis. In humans, however, body weight below ideal is not associated with increased life span. In animal experiments, nutrition is maintained during caloric variation. This may not be true in humans, and thus may lead to the differing results.

Although the influence of dietary fiber on colonic carcinoma and diverticular disease is controversial, the use of dietary fiber to maintain bowel regularity has significant support, especially in older adults, where constipation may present a difficult clinical problem. When dietary intake of fiber is low, bran can be used as a supplement, particularly in cereals, breads, or as bran powder. Intake of bran can be adjusted to maintain normal bowel movements. Adequate fluid intake should also be assured.

Although the food industry is slowly responding, most canned foods still contain large amounts of added sodium and sugar. Because some of these are less expensive than fresh or frozen foods, older adults with limited incomes may use such prepared foods exclusively. When refined carbohydrates or sodium need to be restricted, these patients should be educated about the use of canned products.

Obesity

The prevalence of obesity among older persons is growing (reviewed in Jensen and Rogers, 1998). Although increased mortality rate from all causes extends into the seventh decade, controversy exists about the potential harms of obesity in older adults and the relation between obesity in old age and total or disease specific mortality (Zamboni et al., 2005). A recent meta-analysis indicated that a body mass index (BMI) in the overweight range (BMI 25-29.9 kg/m^2) is not associated with a significantly increased risk of mortality in older adults, while a BMI in the moderately obese range (BMI > 30 kg/m^2) is only associated with a modest (10%) increase in mortality risk (Janssen and Mark, 2007). Central fat and relative loss of fat-free mass may become relatively more important than BMI in determining the health risk associated with obesity in older ages. However, obesity causes serious medical complications, impairs quality of life, can exacerbate the age-related decline in physical function, and lead to frailty (Villareal et al., 2005). The prevalence of many of the medical complications associated with obesity, for example, hypertension, diabetes, cardiovascular disease, and osteoarthritis, increases with age. All components of the metabolic syndrome are prevalent in older populations. High BMI is associated with an increased risk of knee osteoarthritis in older persons. Obesity is associated with pulmonary function abnormalities, obesity-hypoventilation syndrome, and obstructive sleep apnea. An increase in urinary incontinence is associated with increased BMI. Obesity is associated with an increased risk of several types of cancer including breast, colon, pancreas, renal, bladder, and prostate. Self-reported functional capacity, particularly mobility, is markedly diminished in overweight and obese compared with lean older adults. Older persons who are obese (BMI > 30) have a greater rate of nursing home admissions than those who are not obese. Obesity impairs quality of life in older persons. Beneficial effects of obesity include an increased bone mineral density and decreased osteoporosis and hip fracture in older men and women.

Weight-loss therapy improves physical function, quality of life, and the medical complications associated with obesity in older persons (Villareal et al., 2005). Weight-loss therapy that minimizes muscle and bone losses is recommended for older persons who are obese and who have functional impairments or metabolic complications that can benefit from weight loss. The primary approach is to achieve lifestyle change. Modest goals are key components of a weight management program for older adults. A modest reduction in energy intake (500-700 kcal/day) is recommended. Regular physical activity is particularly important in obese older persons to improve physical function and help preserve muscle and bone mass. The available data are insufficient to determine the efficacy and safety of pharmacotherapy for obesity in older persons. Bariatric surgery is the most effective weight-loss therapy for obesity. Perioperative morbidity and mortality is greater, whereas relative weight loss and improvement in obesity-related medical complications are lower in older than in younger patients. Bariatric surgery should be reserved for a select group of older subjects who have disabling obesity that can be ameliorated with weight loss and who meet the criteria for surgery.

INFECTIONS

Although it is proposed that alterations in host defense mechanisms predispose older adults to certain infections, there is little evidence to support this hypothesis. It may well be that environmental factors, physiological changes in other than the immune system, and specific diseases are the major elements in the increased frequency of certain infections in older adults (Table 12-11).

TABLE 12-11   FACTORS PREDISPOSING TO INFECTION IN OLDER ADULTS

More frequent and longer hospital stays
    Nosocomial infections
        Gram-negative bacilli
        Staphylococcus aureus

Physiological changes
    Lung
    Bladder
    Skin
    Glucose homeostasis

Chronic disease
    Malignancy
        Multiple myeloma and leukemia
        Immunosuppression from therapy

Diabetes mellitus
    Urinary tract infection
    Soft-tissue infections
    Osteomyelitis

Prostatic hypertrophy
    Urinary tract infection

Host defenses
    Phagocytosis unaltered
    Complement unaltered
    Cellular and humoral immunity diminished

Because the elderly more often have acute and chronic illnesses necessitating hospitalization and have longer hospital stays, they are at greater risk for nosocomial infections. Such hospitalizations put older patients at greater risk for gram-negative and *Staphylococcus aureus* infections. Physiological alterations (Chap. 1)—in the lungs, bladder function, and the skin—and glucose homeostasis may also predispose older adults to infections.

The incidence of malignancies is increased in older adults. Many of these neoplastic disorders, especially those of the hematological system, are associated with a higher frequency of infection. Immunosuppression during therapy is also a predisposing factor. The prevalence of diabetes mellitus is higher in older adults, thus predisposing them to more frequent urinary tract, soft-tissue, and bone infections. Prostatic hypertrophy with obstruction predisposes the older male to urinary tract infections.

Phagocytic function appears to be unaltered in aging, as is the complement system. Cell-mediated immunity and, to a lesser extent, humoral immunity, is diminished in aging. The role that these changes play in predisposing older individuals to infection has not been well defined.

Many infections occur more frequently in older adults and are often associated with a higher morbidity and mortality. Atypical presentation of infection in some older patients may delay diagnosis and treatment. Underreporting of symptoms, impaired communication, coexisting diseases, and altered physiological responses to infection may contribute to altered presentations.

As an example, failure of patients to seek medical evaluation is one factor in the higher morbidity and mortality of appendicitis in the elderly. Difficulties in communication may also alter presentation. Infections not directly involving the central nervous system may cause confusion in the elderly, particularly in individuals with preexisting dementia. The mechanism by which this occurs has not been defined. Acute unexplained functional deterioration should also alert the physician to a potential acute infectious process.

Existing chronic disease may mask an acute infection. Septic arthritis usually occurs in a previously abnormal joint. It may be difficult to distinguish clinically between exacerbation of the underlying arthritis and acute infection. Therefore, the physician should not be hesitant to examine synovial fluid in elderly patients with acute exacerbation of joint disease.

Febrile response may be blunted or absent in some older individuals with bacterial infections. This may obscure diagnosis and delay therapy. A poor febrile response may also be a negative prognostic factor. Conversely, a febrile response is more likely to indicate a bacterial rather than viral illness in older patients, particularly in the very old. The absence of leukocytosis in older patients should also not exclude consideration of a bacterial infection.

Antibiotic therapy in older adults, as in the young, is directed to the specific organism isolated. However, when empiric antimicrobial therapy is initiated, consideration should be given to including a third generation cephalosporin and/or aminoglycoside because gram-negative infections are more common regardless of the site. With all antibiotics, but particularly with the aminoglycosides, renal function must be considered and monitored for toxicity. Monitoring of drug blood level and renal function is mandatory with the aminoglycosides.

The spectrum of pathogens, causing common infections in the elderly, is often different than that in younger adults (Table 12-12). The frequency of gram-negative bacilli increases in each category. Pneumonia is the most frequent cause of death caused by infection in geriatric patients. *Streptococcus pneumoniae* is the most common cause of pneumonia in the elderly, but gram-negative bacilli increase in prevalence, particularly in the nursing home setting (Yoshikawa, 1999). Annual immunization against influenza, and at least one pneumococcal vaccine, are recommended for all persons 65 years of age and older. Nearly 50% of infective endocarditis cases occur in older adults. The underlying cardiac lesion is often caused by atherosclerotic and degenerative valve diseases, as well as by prosthetic valves. Bacterial meningitis is an infection primarily of early childhood and late adulthood. Mortality in the elderly ranges from 50% to 70%. *S pneumoniae* is the most frequent pathogen, but older patients may be infected with *Listeria monocytogenes* or gram-negative bacilli.

TABLE 12-12   PATHOGENS OF COMMON INFECTIONS IN OLDER ADULTS

INFECTION	COMMON PATHOGENS IN ADULTS	COMMON PATHOGENS IN OLDER ADULTS
Pneumonia	*Streptococcus pneumoniae* Anaerobic bacteria	*Streptococcus pneumoniae* Anaerobic bacteria *Haemophilus influenzae* gram-negative bacilli
Urinary tract	*Escherichia coli*	*Escherichia coli* *Proteus* sp. *Klebsiella* sp. *Enterobacter* sp. Enterococcus
Meningitis	*Streptococcus pneumoniae* *Neisseria meningitidis*	*Streptococcus pneumoniae* *Listeria monocytogenes* gram-negative bacilli
Septic arthritis	*Neisseria gonorrhoeae* *Staphylococcus aureus*	*Staphylococcus aureus* gram-negative bacilli

The incidence of tuberculosis is on the rise again. Older persons of both sexes among all racial and ethnic groups are especially at risk for tuberculosis. This cohort has lived through a period of higher incidence of tuberculosis, has probably not been treated with isonicotinic acid hydrazide (INH) prophylaxis, and may have predisposing factors such as physiological changes, malnutrition, and underlying disease that may lead to reactivation. Older patients are also at increased risk for primary infection. This is particularly the case for older patients in long-term care institutions.

Tuberculosis screening programs should be implemented in long-term care facilities because of this increased risk and because of the potential to prevent active disease among patients whose skin test converts to a strongly positive reaction (see Chap. 16). The American Thoracic Society now recommends preventive therapy for certain types of patients regardless of age, including insulin-dependent diabetic patients, those on steroids and other immunosuppressive treatment, patients with end-stage renal disease, and patients who have lost a large amount of weight rapidly. A useful rule in geriatric care is to suspect tuberculosis when a patient is inexplicably failing.

Several studies suggest that bacteriuria is associated with increased mortality in the elderly. However, other studies do not confirm this finding. Most of these nonconfirming studies did not differentiate between the effect of bacteriuria and age and/or concomitant disease on mortality. When adjusted for age, fatal diseases associated with bacteriuria account for the increase in mortality among older patients with bacteriuria.

Several previous studies in elderly hospitalized or institutionalized patients have not revealed antimicrobial therapy for bacteriuria to be effective because of the high rate of recurring infection. One study in older ambulatory nonhospitalized women with asymptomatic bacteriuria demonstrated that short-course antimicrobial therapy is effective in eliminating bacteriuria in most of the women for at least a 6-month period. Survival was not an outcome measure.

Bacteriuria in older persons is common and usually asymptomatic. At present, in the absence of obstructive uropathy, no evidence exists to support the routine use of antimicrobial therapy for asymptomatic bacteriuria in older persons. Among bacteriuric patients with urinary incontinence and no other symptoms of urinary tract infection, the bacteriuria should be eradicated as part of the initial assessment of the incontinence (see Chap. 8).

The incidence of herpes zoster (HZ) increases with aging. In a prospective vaccine trial, the incidence of herpes was 11.8 cases per 1000 persons per year in those more than 60 years of age, whereas the incidence rate in all ages is 1.2 to 3.4 per 1000 persons per year (reviewed in Schmader, 2007). Increasing age is also the strongest risk factor for developing postherpetic neuralgia (PNH). Acyclovir, famciclovir, and valacyclovir reduce acute pain and the duration of chronic pain if started within 72 hours of rash onset. Analgesics for relief of acute pain are important. Those with moderate to severe pain may require opioids. The addition of corticosteroids of gabapentin may be considered if pain persists. Corticosteroids have not been shown to reduce the incidence of PNH in the elderly. Topical lidocaine patch, gabapentin, and pregabalin are FDA approved for treatment of PNH, but nortriptyline and opioids have also been shown to be of benefit. In some cases, combination therapy may be necessary. Alive, attenuated varicella-zoster vaccine has been developed and shown to reduce the incidence of HZ, PNH, and duration of pain (Oxman et al., 2005).

DISORDERS OF TEMPERATURE REGULATION

Temperature dysregulation in the elderly demonstrates the narrowing of homeostatic mechanisms that occurs with advancing age. Older adults may have a mean oral body temperature lower than 37°C, and older nursing home residents may have lower body temperature and fail to demonstrate a diurnal rise (Gomolin et al., 2005). Older persons are less able to adjust to extremes of environmental temperatures. Hypo- and hyperthermic states are predominantly disorders of older adults. Despite underreporting of these disorders, there is evidence that morbidity and mortality increase during particularly hot or cold periods, especially among ill elderly. Much of this illness is caused by an increased incidence of cardiovascular disorders (myocardial infarction and stroke) or infectious diseases (pneumonia) during these periods.

Hypothermia is a common finding among older adults during the winter, when homes are heated at less than 21°C (70°F).

Pathophysiology

Impaired temperature perception, diminished sweating in hyperthermia, and abnormal vasoconstrictor response in hypothermia are major pathophysiological mechanisms in these disorders.

Hypothermia

Hypothermia is defined as a core temperature (rectal, esophageal, tympanic) below 35°C (95°F). Essential to the diagnosis is early recognition with a low-recording thermometer.

Table 12-13 illustrates the clinical spectrum of hypothermia. Because early signs are nonspecific and subtle, a high index of suspicion must exist to allow an early diagnosis. A history of known or potential exposure is helpful, but older patients can become hypothermic at modest temperatures. Frequently the most difficult differential diagnosis in more severe hypothermia is hypothyroidism. A previous history of thyroid disease, a neck scar from previous thyroid surgery, and a

TABLE 12-13 CLINICAL PRESENTATION OF HYPOTHERMIA

EARLY SIGNS (89.6°-95°F [32°-35°C])	LATER SIGNS (82.4°-86°F [28°-30°C])	LATE SIGNS (< 82.4°F [28°C])
Fatigue	Cold skin	Very cold skin
Weakness	Hypopnea	Rigidity
Slowness of gait	Cyanosis	Apnea
Apathy	Bradycardia	No pulse—ventricular fibrillation
Slurred speech	Atrial and ventricular arrhythmias	Areflexia
Confusion		
Shivering (±)	Hypotension	Unresponsiveness
Cool skin	Semicoma and coma	Fixed pupils
Sensation of cold (±)	Muscular rigidity Generalized edema Slowed reflexes Poorly reactive pupils Polyuria or oliguria	

delay in the relaxation phase of the deep tendon reflexes may assist in diagnosing hypothyroidism. Patients may sometimes be mistaken for dead. Case reports reveal patients who have survived after being discovered without respiration and pulse.

The most significant early complications are arrhythmias and cardiorespiratory arrests. Later complications involve the pulmonary, gastrointestinal, and renal systems. Electrocardiogram (ECG) abnormalities are frequent. The most specific ECG finding is the J wave (Osborn wave) following the QRS complex. This abnormality disappears as temperature returns to normal.

General supportive therapy for severe hypothermia consists of intensive care management of complicated multisystem dysfunctions. Every attempt should be made to assess and treat any contributing medical disorder (eg, infection, hypothyroidism, hypoglycemia). Hypothermia in older patients should promptly be treated as sepsis unless proven otherwise. While patients should have continuous ECG monitoring, central lines should be avoided if possible because of myocardial irritability. Because there is delayed metabolism, most drugs have little effect on a severely hypothermic patient, but they may cause problems once the patient is rewarmed. It is preferable to stabilize the patient and immediately undertake specific rewarming techniques. Serious arrhythmias, acidosis, and fluid and electrolyte disorders will usually respond to therapy only after rewarming has been accomplished.

Passive rewarming is generally adequate for those with mild hypothermia (>32°C [>89.6°F]). Active external rewarming has been associated with increased morbidity and mortality because cold blood may suddenly be shunted to the core, further decreasing core temperature; peripheral vasodilatation can precipitate hypovolemic shock by decreasing circulatory blood volume. For more severe hypothermia (<32°C [<89.6°F]), core rewarming is necessary. Several techniques for core rewarming have been used, but positive results have been reported only from small, uncontrolled studies. Peritoneal dialysis and inhalation rewarming may be the most practical techniques in the majority of institutions.

Mortality is usually greater than 50% for severe hypothermia. It increases with age and is particularly related to underlying disease.

Hyperthermia

Heat stroke is defined as a failure to maintain body temperature and is characterized by a core temperature of >40.6°C (>105°F), severe central nervous system dysfunction (psychosis, delirium, coma), and anhidrosis (hot, dry skin). The two groups primarily affected are older adults who are chronically ill and the young undergoing strenuous exercise. Mortality is as high as 80% once this syndrome is manifest.

There are multiple predisposing factors for heat stroke in older adults, but most often there is a prolonged heat wave (reviewed in O'Malley, 2007). The diagnosis requires a high level of suspicion. In view of the poor survival, efforts must be directed toward prevention. Older patients should be cautioned about the dangers of hot weather. For those at particularly high risk, temporary relocation to more protected environments should be considered.

Early manifestations of heat exhaustion are nonspecific (Table 12-14). Later, severe central nervous system dysfunction and anhidrosis develop.

Table 12-15 lists some of the more serious complications resulting from heat damage to organ systems. Once the full syndrome has developed for any length of time, the prognosis is very poor. While management at this stage requires intense multisystem care, the key is rapid specific therapy consisting of cooling to 38.9°C (102°F) within the first hour. Ice packs and ice-water immersion are superior to convection cooling with alcohol sponge baths or electric fans.

Prevention appears to be the most appropriate approach to management of temperature dysregulation in older adults. Education of older adults to their susceptibility to hypo- and hyperthermia in extremes of environmental temperature, education as to appropriate behavior in such conditions, and close monitoring of the most vulnerable older adults should help reduce the morbidity and mortality from these disorders.

TABLE 12-14   CLINICAL PRESENTATION OF HYPERTHERMIA

EARLY SIGNS	LATER SIGNS
Dizziness	Central nervous system dysfunction
Weakness	Psychosis
Sensation of warmth	Delirium
Anorexia	Coma
Nausea	Anhidrosis
Vomiting	Hot, dry skin
Headache	
Dyspnea	

TABLE 12-15   COMPLICATIONS OF HEAT STROKE

Myocardial damage
    Congestive heart failure
    Arrhythmias
Renal failure (20%-25%)
Cerebral edema
    Seizures
    Diffuse and focal findings
Hepatocellular necrosis
    Jaundice
    Liver failure
Rhabdomyolysis
    Myoglobinuria
Bleeding diathesis
    Disseminated intravascular coagulation
Electrolyte disturbances
Acid–base disturbances
    Metabolic acidosis
    Respiratory alkalosis
Infection
    Aspiration pneumonia
    Sepsis
Dehydration and shock

EVIDENCE SUMMARY

Do's

- Screen patients with hypertension or hyperlipidemia for diabetes.
- Use metformin as first-line therapy in overweight diabetic patients.
- Treat other atherosclerotic risk factors (smoking, dyslipidemia, hypertension) in diabetic patients.
- Screen ill older patients for hypothyroidism.
- Screen older adults for vitamin D deficiency.
- Primary hyperparathyroidism in patients with fracture and low bone mineral density.

Don'ts

- Use metformin in patients with renal insufficiency or heart failure.
- Use thiazolidinediones in patients with heart failure.
- Recommend testosterone supplementation in older men with low normal testosterone concentrations.

Consider

- Life expectancy and quality of life in setting goals for glucose control.

References

Amori RE, Lau J, Pittas AG. Efficacy and safety of incretin therapy in type 2 diabetes. *JAMA*. 2007;298(2):194-206.

Bergström I, Landgren BM, Freyschuss B. Primary hyperparathyroidism is common in postmenopausal women with forearm fracture and low bone mineral density. *Acta Obstet Gynecol Scand*. 2007;861:61-64.

Bilezikian JP, Potts JT, Fuleihan GE-H, et al. Summary Statement from a Workshop on Asymptomatic Primary Hyperparathyroidism. *J Clin Endocrinol Metab*. 2002;87: 5353.

Biondi B, Fazio S, Palmieri EA, et al. Left ventricular diastolic dysfunction in patients with subclinical hypothyroidism. *J Clin Endocrinol Metab*. 1999;84:2064-2067.

Black C, Donnelly P, McIntyre L, et al. Meglitinide analogues for type 2 diabetes mellitus. *Cochrane Database Syst Rev*. 2007;18:CD004654.

Blackman MR, Sorkin JD, Munzer T, et al. Growth hormone and sex steroid administration in healthy aged women and men: a randomized controlled trial. *JAMA*. 2002;288:2282-2292.

Boulé NG, Haddad E, Kenny GP, et al. Effects of exercise on glycemic control and body mass in type 2 diabetes mellitus: a meta-analysis of controlled clinical trials. *JAMA.* 2001;286:1218-1227.

Cappola AR, Fried LP, Arnold AM, et al. Thyroid status, cardiovascular risk, and mortality in older adults. *JAMA.* 2006;295:1033-1041.

Cooper DS. Antithyroid drugs. *N Engl J Med.* 2005;352:905-917.

Cooper DS. Subclinical hypothyroidism. *N Engl J Med.* 2001;345:260-265.

Diabetes Prevention Program Research Group. Reduction in the incidence of type 2 diabetes with lifestyle intervention or metformin. *N Eng J Med.* 2002;346:393-403.

Drucker DJ. The role of gut hormones in glucose homeostasis. *J Clin Invest.* 2007;117:24-32.

Emmelot-Vonk MH, Verhaar HJ, Nakhai Pour HR, et al. Effect of testosterone supplementation on functional mobility, cognition, and other parameters in older men: a randomized controlled trail. *JAMA.* 2008;2(299):39-52.

Fatourechi V. Upper limit of normal serum thyroid-stimulating hormone: a moving and now and aging target? *Endo Journal.* 2007;92:4560-4562.

Ershler WB, Sheng S, McKelvey J, et al. Serum Erythropoietin and aging: a longitudinal analysis. *J Am Geriatr Soc.* 2005;53:1360-1365.

Fletcher RH, Fairfeild KM. Vitamins for chronic disease prevention: clinical applications. *JAMA.* 2002;287:3127-3129.

Gaede P, Lund-Anderson H, Parving H-H, et al. Effect of a multifactorial intervention on mortality in type 2 diabetes. *N Engl J Med.* 2008;358:580-591.

Gillies CL, Abrams KR, Lambert PC, et al. Review: lifestyle or pharmacologic interventions prevent or delay type 2 diabetes in impaired glucose tolerance. *BMJ.* 2007;334:299-307.

Gomolin IH, Aung MM, Wolf-Klein G, et al. Older is colder: temperature range and variation in older people. *J Am Geriatr Soc.* 2005;53:2170-2172.

Grozinsky-Glasberg S, Fraser A, Nahshoni E, et al. Thyroxine-triiodothyronine combination therapy versus thyroxine monotherapy for clinical hypothyroidism: meta-analysis of randomized controlled trials. *J Clin Endocrinol Metab.* 2006;91:2592-2599.

Gruenewald DA, Matsumoto AM. Testosterone supplementation therapy for older men: potential benefits and risks. *J Am Geriatr Soc.* 2003;51:101–115.

Habra M, Sarlis NJ. Thyroid and aging. *Endo & Metabolic Disorders.* 2005;6:145-154.

Hak AE, Pols HAP, Visser TJ, et al. Subclinical hypothyroidism is an independent risk factor for atherosclerosis and myocardial infarction in elderly women: the Rotterdam study. *Ann Intern Med.* 2000;132:270-278.

Huang ES, Meigs JB, Singer DE. The effect of interventions to prevent cardiovascular disease in patients with type 2 diabetes mellitus. *Am J Med.* 2001;111:633-642.

Huber G, Staub J-J, Meier C, et al. Prospective study of the spontaneous course of subclinical hypothyroidism: prognostic value of thyrotropin, thyroid reserve, and thyroid antibodies. *J Clin Endocrinol Metab.* 2002;87:3221-3226.

Inzucchi SE. Management of hyperglycemia in the hospital setting. *N Engl J Med.* 2006;355:1903-1911.

Inzucchi SE, Maggs DG, Spollett GR, et al. Efficacy and metabolic effects of metformin and troglitazone in type II diabetes mellitus. *N Engl J Med.* 1998;338:867-872.

Izaks GJ, Westendorp RG, Knook DL. The definition of anemia in older persons. *JAMA*. 1999;281:1714-1717.

Jackson C, Gaugris S, Sen SS, et al. The effect of cholecalciferol (vitamin D3) on the risk of fall and fracture: a meta-analysis. *QJM*. 2007;100:185-192.

Janssen I, Mark AE. Elevated body mass index and mortality risk in the elderly. *Obesity Rev*. 2007;8:41-59.

Jensen GL, Rogers J. Obesity in older persons. *J Am Diet Assoc*. 1998;98:1308-1311.

Jones M, Ibels L, Schenkel B, et al. Impact of epoetin alfa on clinical end points in patients with chronic renal failure: a meta-analysis. *Kidney Int*. 2004;65:757-767.

Kazi M, Geraci SA, Koch CA. Considerations for the diagnosis and treatment of testosterone deficiency in elderly men. *Am J Med*. 2007;120:835-840.

Ku S. Algorithms replace sliding scale insulin orders. *Drug Ther Topics*. 2002;31:49-53.

Laine C, Wilson JF. Type 2 diabetes. *Ann Intern Med*. 2007;146:ITC1-ITC15.

Lamberts SWJ, van den Beld AW, van der Lely A-J. The endocrinology of aging. *Science*. 1997;278:419-424.

Lincoff AM, Wolski K, Nicholls SJ, et al. Pioglitazone and risk of cardiovascular events in patients with type 2 diabetes mellitus. *JAMA*. 2007;298:1180-1188.

Lipscombe LL, Gomes T, Lévesque LE, et al. Thiazolidinediones and cardiovascular outcomes in older patients with diabetes. *JAMA*. 2007;298:2634-2643.

Longo DL. Closing in on a killer: anemia in elderly people. *J Gerontol Biol Sci Med Sci*. 2005;60A:727-728.

Maraldi C, Ble A, Zuliani G, et al. Association between anemia and physical disability in older patients: role of comorbidity. *Aging Clin Exp Res*. 2006;8:485-492.

Mariotti S, Cambuli VM. Cardiovascular risk in elderly hypothyroid patients. *Thyroid*. 2007;17:1067-1073.

McGandy RB, Barrows CH Jr, Spanias A, et al. Nutrient intakes and energy expenditures in men of different ages. *J Gerontol*. 1966;21:581-587.

Miller M. Hyponatremia and arginine vasopressin dysregulation: mechanisms, clinical consequences, and management. *J Am Geriatr Soc*. 2006;54(2):345-53.

Meneilly GS, Tessier D. Diabetes in elderly adults. *J Gerontol A Biol Sci Med Sci*. 2001;56A:M5-M13.

Montero-Odasso M, Duque G. Viamin D in the aging musculoskeletal system: an authentic strength preserving hormone. *Mol Aspects Med*. 2005;26:203-219.

Mooradian AD, Bernbaum M, Albert SG. Narrative review: a rational approach to starting insulin therapy. *Ann Intern Med*. 2006145:125-134.

Nathan DM. Finding new treatments for diabetes—how many, how fast . . . how good? *N Engl J Med*. 2007;356:437-536.

O'Malley PG. Commentary on heat waves and heat-related illness. *JAMA*. 2007;298:917-919.

Oxman MN, Levin MJ, Johnson GR, et al. A vaccine to prevent herpes zoster postherpetic neuralgia in older adults. *N Engl J Med*. 2005;352:2271-2284.

Penninx BWJH, Pahor M, Woodman RC, et al. Anemia in old age is associated with increased mortality and hospitalization. *J Gerontol Biol Sci Med Sci*. 2006;61A: 474-479.

Schmader K. Herpes zoster and postherpetic neuralgia in older adults. *Clin Geriatr Med.* 2007;23:615-632.

Singh S, Loke YK, Furberg CD. Long-term risk of cardiovascular events with rosiglitazone. *JAMA.* 2007;298:1189-1195.

Steensma DP. Is anemia of cancer different from chemotherapy induced anemia? *J Clin Oncol.* 2008;26:1022-1024.

Strippoli GF, Craig MC, Schena FP, et al. Review: ACE inhibitors delay onset of microalbuminuria in diabetes without nephropathy and reduce mortality in diabetic nephropathy. *J Am Soc Nephrol.* 2006;17:S153-S155.

Surks MI, Hollowell JG. Age-specific distribution of serum thyrotropin and antithyroid antibodies in the US population: implications for the prevalence of subclinical hypothyroidism. *J Clin Endocrinol Metab.* 2007;92;4575-4582.

Toft AD. Subclinical hyperthyroidism. *N Engl J Med.* 2001;345:512-516.

Turner RC, Cull CA, Frighi V, et al. Glycemic control with diet, sulfonylurea, metformin, or insulin in patients with type 2 diabetes mellitus. *JAMA.* 1999;281:2005-2012.

UK Prospective Diabetes Study (UKPDS) Group. Intensive blood-glucose control with sulphonylureas or insulin compared with conventional treatment and risk of complications in patients with type 2 diabetes (UKPDS 33). *Lancet.* 1998a;352:837-852.

UK Prospective Diabetes Study (UKPDS) Group. Effect of intensive blood-glucose control with metformin on complications in overweight patients with type 2 diabetes (UKPDS 34). *Lancet.* 1998b;352:854-865.

UK Prospective Diabetes Study (UKPDS) Group. Tight blood pressure control and risk of macrovascular and microvascular complications in type 2 diabetes: UKPDS 38. *BMJ.* 1998c;317:703-712.

US Preventive Services Task Force. Screening for type 2 diabetes mellitus in adults: recommendations and rationale. *Ann Intern Med.* 2003;138:212-214.

Villareal DT, Apovian CM, Kushner RF, et al. Obesity in older adults: technical review and position statement of the American Society for Nutrition and NAASO, The Obesity Society. *Am J Clin Nutr.* 2005;82:923-934.

Weiss G, Goodnough LT. Anemia of chronic disease. *N Engl J Med.* 2005;352:1011-1023.

Yoshikawa TT. State of infectious diseases health care in older persons. *Clin Geriatr Med.* 1999;7:55-58.

Zamboni M, Mazzali G, Zoico E, et al. Health consequences of obesity in the elderly: a review of four unresolved questions. *Int J Obesity.* 2005;29:1011-1029.

Suggested Readings

Anonymous. Antimicrobial prophylaxis in surgery. *Med Lett Drugs Ther.* 1999;41:75-80.

Anonymous. The choice of antibacterial drugs. *Med Lett Drugs Ther.* 1999;41:95-104.

Treatment of hypothermia. *Med Lett Drugs Ther.* 1986;28:123-124.

Bartlett JG. Antibiotic-associated diarrhea. *N Engl J Med.* 2002;346:334-339.

Belshe RB. Influenza prevention and treatment: current practices and new horizons. *Ann Intern Med.* 1999;131:621-623.

Bentley DW, Bradley S, High K, et al. Practice guideline for evaluation of fever and infection in long-term care facilities. *J Am Geriatr Soc.* 2001;49:210-222.

Bouchama A, Knochel JP. Heat stroke. *N Engl J Med.* 2002;346:1978-1988.

Brady MA, Perron WJ. Electrocardiographic manifestations of hypothermia. *Am J Emerg Med.* 2002;20:314-326.

Chandalia M, Garg A, Lutjohann D, et al. Beneficial effects of high dietary fiber intake in patients with type 2 diabetes mellitus. *N Engl J Med.* 2000;342:1392-1398.

Davis PJ, Davis FB. Hyperthyroidism in patients over the age of 60 years. *Medicine (Baltimore).* 1974;53:161-181.

Elia M, Ritz P, Stubbs RJ. Total energy expenditure in the elderly. *Eur J Clin Nutr.* 2000;54:S92-S103.

Federman DD. Hyperthyroidism in the geriatric population. *Hosp Pract.* 1991;26:61-76.

Gambert SR. Effect of age on thyroid hormone physiology and function. *J Am Geriatr Soc.* 1985;33:360-365.

Gress TW, Nieto J, Shahar E, et al. Hypertension and antihypertensive therapy as risk factors for type 2 diabetes mellitus. *N Engl J Med.* 2000;342:905-912.

Lipschitz DA. An overview of anemia in older patients. *Older Patient.* 1988;2:5-11.

Mahler RJ, Adler ML. Type 2 diabetes mellitus: update on diagnosis, pathophysiology, and treatment. *J Clin Endocrinol Metab.* 1999;84:1165-1171.

Morley JE, Mooradian AD, Silver AJ, et al. Nutrition in the elderly. *Ann Intern Med.* 1988;109:890-904.

Mylonakis E, Calderwood SB. Infective endocarditis in adults. *N Engl J Med.* 2001;345: 1318-1330.

Sawin CT, Castelli WP, Hershman JM, et al. The aging thyroid: thyroid deficiency in the Framingham Study. *Arch Intern Med.* 1985;145:1386-1388.

Stead WW, To T, Harrison RW, et al. Benefit-risk considerations in preventive treatment for tuberculosis in elderly persons. *Ann Intern Med.* 1987;107:843-845.

Thomas FB, Mazzaferi EL, Skillman TB. Apathetic thyrotoxicosis: a distinctive clinical and laboratory entity. *Ann Intern Med.* 1970;72:679-685.

Trevino A, Bazi B, Beller BM, et al. The characteristic electrocardiogram of accidental hypothermia. *Arch Intern Med.* 1971;127:470-473.

Trivalle C, Doucet J, Chassagne P, et al. Differences in the signs and symptoms of hyperthyroidism in older and younger patients. *J Am Geriatr Soc.* 1996;44:50-53.

Tuomilehto J, Lindstrom J, Eriksson JG, et al. Prevention of type 2 diabetes mellitus by changes in lifestyle among subjects with impaired glucose tolerance. *N Engl J Med.* 2001;344:1343-1350.

UK Prospective Diabetes Study Group. Efficacy of atenolol and captopril in reducing risk of macrovascular and microvascular complications in type 2 diabetes: UKPDS 39. *BMJ.* 1998;371:713-719.

Walsh JR. Hematologic disorders in the elderly. *West J Med.* 1981;135:445-446.

Yoshikawa TT. Infectious diseases. *Clin Geriatr Med.* 1992;8:701-945.

Yoshikawa TT. Tuberculosis in aging adults. *J Am Geriatr Soc.* 1992;40:178-187.

CHAPTER 13

SENSORY IMPAIRMENT

Because as many as 75% of older adults have significant visual and auditory dysfunction not reported to their physicians, adequate screening for these problems is important. These disorders may limit functional activity and lead to social isolation and depression. Correction of remediable conditions may improve ability to perform daily activities.

VISION

Physiologic and Functional Changes

The visual system undergoes many changes with age (Table 13-1). Decreases in visual acuity in old age may be caused by morphological changes in the choroid, pigment epithelium, and retina, or by decreased function of the rods, cones, and other neural elements. Older patients frequently have difficulties turning their eyes upward or sustaining convergence. Intraocular pressure slowly increases with age.

The refractive error may become either more hyperopic or more myopic. In the young, hyperopia may be overcome by the accommodative power of the ciliary muscle on the young lens. However, with age, this latent hyperopia becomes manifest because of loss of accommodative reserve.

Other older patients may show an increase in myopia with age, caused by changes within the lens. The crystalline lens increases in size with age as old lens fibers accumulate in the lens nucleus. The nucleus becomes more compact and harder (nuclear sclerosis), increasing the refractive power of the lens and worsening the myopia.

Another definitive refractive change of aging is the development of presbyopia from nuclear sclerosis of the lens and atrophy of the ciliary muscle. As a result, the closest distance at which one can see clearly slowly recedes with age. At approximately age 45, the near point of accommodation is so far that comfortable reading and near work become cumbersome and difficult. Corrective lenses are then needed to enable the patient to move that point closer to the eyes.

TABLE 13-1   PHYSIOLOGICAL AND FUNCTIONAL CHANGES OF THE EYE

FUNCTIONAL CHANGE	PHYSIOLOGICAL CHANGE
Visual acuity	Morphological change in choroid, pigment epithelium, or retina Decreased function of rods, cones, or other neural elements
Extraocular motion	Difficulty in gazing upward and maintaining convergence
Intraocular pressure	Increased pressure
Refractive power	Increased hyperopia and myopia Presbyopia Increased lens size Nuclear sclerosis (lens) Ciliary muscle atrophy
Tear secretion	Decreased tearing Decreased lacrimal gland function Decreased goblet cell secretion
Corneal function	Loss of endothelial integrity Posterior surface pigmentation

Diminished tear secretion in many older patients, especially postmenopausal women, may lead to dryness of the eyes, which can cause irritation and discomfort. This condition may endanger the intactness of the corneal surface. The treatment consists mainly in substitution therapy, with artificial tears instilled at frequent intervals.

The corneal endothelium often undergoes degenerative changes with aging. Because these cells seldom proliferate during adult life, the cell population is decreased. This may leave an irregular surface on the anterior chamber side, where pigments may accumulate. This type of endothelial dystrophy is frequently seen in older patients, and dense pigment accumulation may slightly decrease visual acuity. In some patients, the endothelial dystrophy will spontaneously progress and lead to corneal edema. Such cases require corneal transplants.

Blindness

The prevalence of visual problems and blindness increases with age (Fig. 13-1). The most common causes of blindness are cataracts, glaucoma,

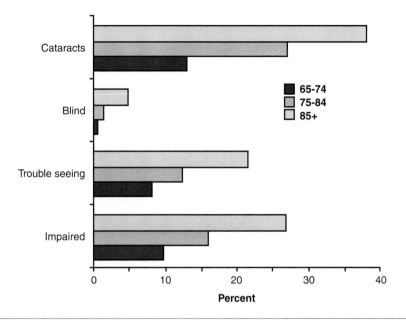

— FIGURE 13-1—   Prevalence of vision problems in older persons, 1984. (From Havlik, 1986.)

macular degeneration, and diabetic retinopathy. Screening for these disorders should include testing visual acuity, performing an ophthalmoscopic evaluation, and checking intraocular pressure (Table 13-2).

Senile Cataract   Opacification of the crystalline lens is a frequent complication of aging. In the Framingham Eye Study, the prevalence of cataracts was associated with age and reached 46% at ages 75 to 85 (Kini et al., 1978).

The cause of age-related cataracts is unknown, but the opacifications in the lens are associated with the breakdown of the g-crystalline proteins.

TABLE 13-2   OPHTHALMOLOGICAL SCREENING

Visual acuity	Ability to read newspaper-sized print
Lens, fundus	Ophthalmoscopic examination
Intraocular pressure	Tonometry
	Visual fields

Epidemiological data and basic research suggest that ultraviolet light may be a contributing factor in cataract development. The pathological process may occur in either the cortex or the nucleus of the lens. Cortical cataracts have various stages of development. Early in the process, opacities are in the periphery and do not decrease visual acuity. At the mature stage, opacifications are more widespread and involve the pupillary area, leading to a slow decrease in visual acuity. In the mature stage, the entire lens becomes opaque. The nuclear cataract does not have these stages of development, but is a slowly progressing central opacity, which frequently shows a yellowish discoloration, therefore preventing certain colors from reaching the retina.

Cataracts of mild degree may be managed by periodic examination and optimum eyeglasses for an extended period. Ultraviolet lenses may be of benefit. When a cataract progresses to the point where it interferes with activities, cataract surgery is generally indicated. The surgeon may use several methods to remove it, and the decision regarding the best method for each patient should be made by the ophthalmologist.

In intracapsular cataract extractions, the entire cataract and surrounding capsule are removed in a single piece. This removes the entire opacity. In extracapsular cataract extractions, the cataractous lens material and a portion of the capsule are removed. The posterior capsule is left in place to hold an intraocular lens implant.

After cataract removal, the eye has decreased refractive power. Three methods of restoring useful vision are available: eyeglasses, contact lenses, and intraocular lenses (Table 13-3). Approximately 95% of those who undergo cataract surgery now receive intraocular lens implants.

Eyeglasses required after surgery are usually thick and heavy. These correct the focus of the eye and permit excellent vision through the central portion. However, they increase the apparent size of an object by approximately 25%, introduce optical distortion, and interfere with peripheral vision. Patients must learn to turn their head instead of their eyes to see clearly to the side. Eyeglasses can be used for patients who have had surgery on both eyes or surgery on one eye and decreased vision in the other. However, eyeglasses cannot usually be used for patients who have had surgery in one eye and have normal vision in the other eye because of the difference in image size.

Contact lenses correct the focus of the eye, permit both central and peripheral vision, and increase apparent object size by 6%. However, handling contact lenses is difficult for some individuals, and most lenses must be removed and inserted daily. Extended-wear contact lenses are available, and approximately 50% to 70% of elderly patients are able to wear them after surgery. Contacts are useful in patients who have had cataract surgery in one or both eyes. The lenses correct for distant vision, but eyeglasses are required for reading.

The intraocular lens is surgically placed inside the iris and is expected to remain permanently in place. This lens corrects the focus of the eyes and permits

TABLE 13-3   METHODS OF RESTORING VISION AFTER CATARACT
              SURGERY

EYEGLASSES
Are thick and heavy
Provide good central vision
Interfere with peripheral vision
Introduce optical distortion
Increase image size by 25%
Cannot be used after surgery on one eye if other eye is normal

CONTACT LENSES
Correct central and peripheral vision
Increase image size by 6%
Are difficult for some patients to handle
Most require daily insertion and removal
Approximately 50%-70% can use extended-wear lenses
Can be used after surgery on one or both eyes
Require reading glasses

INTRAOCULAR LENSES
Correct central and peripheral vision
Increase image size by 1%
Can be used after surgery on one or both eyes
Are useful for older adults unable to wear contact lenses
Require bifocal eyeglasses
Introduce added surgical and postsurgical complications

central and peripheral vision; object size is increased by only 1%. It is appropriate for patients with cataracts in one or both eyes and is particularly useful for patients unable to wear a contact lens. Because the lens cannot change shape to accomodate, bifocal eyeglasses are usually required to aid distant or near vision.

Glaucoma   The glaucomas are a group of eye disorders characterized by increased intraocular pressure, progressive excavation of the optic nerve head with damage to the nerve fibers, and a specific loss in the visual field. Most cases of primary glaucoma occur in older patients. In the Framingham Eye Study, prevalence of open-angle glaucoma increased with age to 7.2% at ages 75 to 85, with men having much higher rates than women (Kini et al., 1978).

Angle-closure glaucoma is an acute and relatively infrequent type of glaucoma, characterized by a sudden painful attack of increased intraocular pressure accompanied by a marked loss in vision. The treatment consists of normalizing the intraocular pressure by the application of miotic eye drops or other medication (such as carbonic anhydrase inhibitors or osmotic agents). The definitive treatment, however, is surgical excision of a peripheral piece of iris or, more frequently now, by laser iridectomy, ensuring free flow of aqueous humor. Because the disease is usually bilateral, some physicians propose prophylactic iridectomy on the second eye.

Chronic open-angle glaucoma is the more frequent variety of primary glaucoma. It is characterized by an insidious onset, slow progression, and the appearance of typical defects of the visual fields. Early in the disease, intraocular pressure is only moderately elevated, and optic nerve head excavation progresses slowly and sometimes asymmetrically. While central visual acuity may remain normal for a long time, the defects in the peripheral visual field are characteristic and gradually progressive. Initially, there is a paracentral scotoma, which may coalesce. A nasal step of the visual field is another important sign. Finally, the entire field will constrict and eventually involve the visual centers.

The treatment is usually medical, with miotics of various kinds used first. β-Blocking agents may also be used and have the advantage of not changing the diameter of the pupil. However, care should be taken because these agents may be systemically absorbed. In severe cases, combination drops may be used with systemic medications such as carbonic anhydrase inhibitors. Surgery or laser therapy is indicated only if disease progresses on maximal medical therapy.

Age-Related Macular Degeneration   The macular area of the retina lying at the posterior pole of the globe is the site of highest visual acuity. This area depends entirely on choriocapillaries for nutrition.

Any disturbance in the vessel wall of the choroidal capillaries, in the permeability or thickness of the Bruch membrane, or in the retinal pigment epithelium may interfere with the exchange of nutrients and oxygen from the choroidal blood to the central retina. Such disturbances occur frequently in older patients. Senile degeneration of the macula is one of the most frequent causes of visual loss in older adults and is the commonest cause of legal blindness (20/200 or worse). In the Framingham Eye Study, the prevalence was 28% at ages 75 to 85 years, with a higher rate in women than in men (Kini et al., 1978). In addition to older age, risk factors include family history of the disorder, cigarette smoking, low dietary intake or plasma concentrations of antioxidant vitamins and zinc, and white race for "wet" lesions (Fine et al., 2000). Age-related macular degeneration (AMD) is a common disease caused by the interplay of genetic predisposition and exposure to modifiable risk factors. Two susceptibility genes have been identified (*CFH* and *LOC387715*). Carrying the susceptibility alleles of either increases the risk between 3- and 8-fold, whereas having two copies of the susceptibility alleles in both genes increases the risk 50-fold (Schaumerg et al., 2007). The combined effect of these polymorphisms carries an attributable risk of 60% (Haines and Pericak-Vance, 2007). Cigarette smoking and obesity multiplied the risks associated with these variants.

Ophthalmoscopic findings vary and do not always parallel loss of vision. In the "dry" (atrophic) form of degeneration, there are areas of depigmentation alternating with zones of hyperpigmentation caused mainly by changes in the retinal pigment epithelium. In another form, the degeneration involves the Bruch membrane, leading to the pigmentation of well-circumscribed, roundish yellow areas.

The second type of degeneration is an exudative or "wet" (neovascular, exudative) type. Here there is an elevated focus in the macular area, which at first contains serous fluid but later contains blood derived from blood vessels sprouting from the choroid to the subretinal space. The blood may become organized and form a plaque. Wet AMD is more common in those with advanced disease. Dry AMD may produce a slow deterioration of central vision. Wet AMD can cause a rapid distortion and loss of central vision. Most patients who progress to legal blindness have the neovascular form.

In all these cases, central visual acuity will be markedly affected. These patients will gradually lose the ability to read or see any other details. The atrophic type has no proven treatment or prevention. Verteporfin photodynamic (PTD) has been shown to be beneficial in the treatment of advanced wet type AMD (reviewed in Bourla and Young, 2006). PTD therapy combines the intravenous infusion of the light-sensitive dye verteporfin with low-intensity laser targeted to the neovascular tissue, causing occlusion of the abnormal choroidal vessels. However, recent therapy has been directed to vascular endothelial growth factor (VEGF) antagonism (reviewed in The Medical Letter, 2006). VEGF may play a critical role in the pathogenesis of neovascularization. Several VEGF antagonists, both systemic and intraocular injections, are available, but ranibizumab given monthly by intravitreal injection is the first drug demonstrated to not only slow progression but to improve vision in patients with wet AMD. Total blindness does not occur, as patients retain peripheral vision and therefore are able to perform activities that do not necessitate acute central vision. Visual rehabilitation is an important part of therapy for AMD. Patients may benefit from reading glasses or magnification devices. Clinical depression may occur as a consequence of reductions in quality of life and should be treated.

Diabetic Retinopathy   In the geriatric population, a significant amount of visual loss is attributed to diabetic retinopathy. The Framingham Eye Study showed an age-associated increase in prevalence up to 7% at ages 75 to 85 years (Kini et al.,1978). In the adult-onset diabetes with background changes, the visual loss is usually related to vascular changes in and around the macula. Leakage of serous fluid from vessels surrounding the macula leads to macular edema and deterioration of visual acuity. This may respond to laser photocoagulation.

Hemorrhages within the macula may lead to more permanent visual loss. A loss of retinal capillaries may lead to macular ischemia and poor prognosis of visual recovery.

Intensive blood-glucose control and tight blood pressure control reduce the risk of microvascular disease, including retinopathy in type 2 diabetes (see Chap. 12). Pan-retinal and focal retinal laser photocoagulation reduces the risk of visual loss in patients with severe diabetic retinopathy and macular edema, respectively (reviewed in Mohamed, Gillies, and Wong, 2007). There is currently insufficient evidence for routine use of other treatments, such as VEGF antagonists.

General Factors

Table 13-4 summarizes the general patterns of signs and symptoms associated with common visual problems of older adults. In addition to the specific treatment discussed above, some simple techniques, such as use of a magnifying device, large-print reading material, lighting intensifiers, and reduction of glare, can help maximize visual function (see Table 13-5).

Health-care providers should also be aware of the significant systemic absorption of ophthalmic medications (Anand and Eschmann, 1988). These agents may lead to other organ systems' dysfunction and interact with other medications (Table 13-6). The patient's other medical problems and medications should be assessed and the minimum dose to achieve the desired effect should be used. Patients should also be monitored for systemic toxicity.

HEARING

This section covers four areas related to hearing problems in older adults: a review of the major parts of the auditory system, tests used to evaluate the hearing system, effects of aging on hearing performance, and specific pathologic disorders affecting the auditory system.

Hearing problems are common in the elderly, especially in a highly industrialized society where noise and age interact to cause hearing loss (Fig. 13-2). In the National Health and Nutrition Examination Survey, hearing loss was present in 35.1% of those surveyed aged 55 to 74 years (Reuben et al., 1998). Screening is endorsed by most professional organizations, including the US Preventive

TABLE 13-4   SIGNS AND SYMPTOMS ASSOCIATED WITH COMMON VISUAL PROBLEMS IN OLDER ADULTS

Signs and Symptoms	Cataract	Open-Angle Glaucoma	Angle-Closure Glaucoma	Macular Degeneration	Temporal Arteritis	Diabetic Retinopathy
Pain			x		x	
Red eye			x			
Fixed pupil			x			
Retinal vessel changes					x	x
Retinal exudates				x	x	x
Optic disk changes		x			x	
Sudden visual loss			x		x	
Loss of peripheral vision		x				
Glare intolerance	x					
Elevated intraocular pressure		x	x			
Loss of visual acuity	x			x		x

TABLE 13-5 AIDS TO MAXIMIZE VISUAL FUNCTION

Magnifying device

Lighting intensifiers without glare

Tinted glasses to reduce glare

Night light to assist in adaptation

Large-print newspapers, books, and magazines

TABLE 13-6 POTENTIAL ADVERSE EFFECTS OF OPHTHALMIC SOLUTIONS

DRUG	ORGAN SYSTEM	RESPONSES
β-Blockers (eg, timolol)	Cardiovascular	Bradycardia, hypotension, syncope, palpitation, congestive heart failure
	Respiratory	Bronchospasm
	Neurologic	Mental confusion, depression, fatigue, light-headedness, hallucinations, memory impairment, sexual dysfunction
	Miscellaneous	Hyperkalemia
Adrenergics (eg, epinephrine, phenylephrine)	Cardiovascular	Extrasystoles, palpitation, hypertension, myocardial infarction
	Miscellaneous	Trembling, paleness, sweating
Cholinergic/ anticholinesterases (eg, pilocarpine, echothiophate)	Respiratory	Bronchospasm
	Gastrointestinal	Salivation, nausea, vomiting, diarrhea, abdominal pain, tenesmus
	Miscellaneous	Lacrimation, sweating
Anticholinergics (eg, atropine)	Neurologic	Ataxia, nystagmus, restlessness, mental confusion, hallucination, violent and aggressive behavior
	Miscellaneous	Insomnia, photophobia, urinary retention

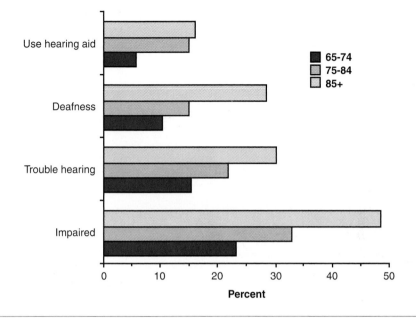

— FIGURE 13-2—   Prevalence of hearing problems in older persons, 1984. (From Havlik, 1986.)

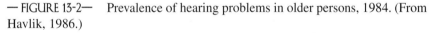

Services Task Force. Screening tests that reliably detect hearing loss are use of an audioscope, a hand-held combination otoscope and audiometer, and a self-administered questionnaire, the Hearing Handicap Inventory for the Elderly-Screening (reviewed in Yueh et al., 2003 and Bogardus, Yueh, and Shekelle, 2003). Hearing loss in the elderly is usually of the sensorineural type, caused by damage of the hearing organ, the peripheral nervous system, and/or the central nervous system. These hearing problems are not usually amenable to medical or surgical intervention, and thus require hearing aids, aural rehabilitation, and understanding as the major avenues of remediation.

The Auditory System

On a functional basis, the auditory system can be divided into three major parts: peripheral, brainstem, and cortical areas (Table 13-7). Each part of the hearing system has unique functions, which combine to allow hearing and understanding of speech. Table 13-8 lists these functions.

The main functions of the peripheral auditory system are to change sound into a series of electrical impulses and to transmit those to the brainstem. The major brainstem function is binaural interaction. Binaural interaction allows localization

TABLE 13-7   PERIPHERAL AND CENTRAL AUDITORY NERVOUS SYSTEM

A. External ear and peripheral hearing mechanism
  1. Auricle
  2. Tympanic membrane
  3. Ossicular chain
  4. Eustachian tube
  5. Cochlea
    a. Bony labyrinth
    b. Membranous labyrinth
  6. Cochlear nerve
B. Auditory areas in the brainstem
  1. Entrance of the eighth cranial nerve
  2. Cochlear nucleus
  3. Superior olivary complex
  4. Lateral lemniscus
  5. Inferior colliculus
  6. Medial geniculate
  7. Auditory radiations (brainstem-to-cortex tract)
C. Auditory areas in the cortex
  1. Temporal lobe
  2. Parietal lobe
  3. Corpus callosum

of sound and extraction of a signal from a noisy environment. The cortex brings sound to consciousness and allows interpretation of speech and initiation of appropriate reactions to sound signals.

Assessment

Assessment of hearing function can be divided into three kinds of hearing tests: standard, binaural, and difficult speech. The standard tests are useful for evaluating the peripheral system, binaural tests for evaluating the brainstem, and difficult speech tests for evaluating cortical problems (Table 13-9). Standard tests are performed by presenting pure tones or single words at varying intensity. An audiometer (AudioScope, Welch-Allyn, Inc.) that will deliver pure tones is available for the office screening of hearing deficits.

TABLE 13-8   FUNCTIONAL COMPONENTS OF THE AUDITORY SYSTEM

A. Transmission of signals in the periphery
   1. Molecular motion (ear canal)
   2. Mechanical vibration (eardrum and ossicles)
   3. Hydromechanical motion (inner ear)
   4. Electrical impulse (eighth nerve)
B. Binaural interaction in the brainstem
   1. Localization and lateralization of sound
   2. Extraction of signals from environmental noise
C. Speech processing in the cortex
   1. Conscious sensation of hearing
   2. Interpretation of speech
   3. Initiation of response to sound

Tympanic membrane movement is assessed with a probe. Loudness comparison assesses the individual's ability to balance intensity of sound coming from both ears; lateralization tests the individual's ability to fuse sounds from both ears; and masking level differences assesses the ability to pick out specific sounds from a background of noise. Monotic degraded tasks present difficult sounds such as noise background, filtered sound, and time-compressed speech; dichotic tasks

TABLE 13-9   ASSESSMENT OF HEARING FUNCTION

A. Standard test measures
   1. Sensitivity for tones and speech
   2. Speech discrimination/understanding
   3. Movement of tympanic membrane
B. Binaural tests
   1. Loudness comparison
   2. Lateralization
   3. Masking level differences
C. Difficult speech tests
   1. Monotic degraded tasks
   2. Dichotic tasks

TABLE 13-10   EFFECTS OF AGING ON THE HEARING MECHANISM

Atrophy and disappearance of cells in the inner ear

Angiosclerosis in the inner ear

Calcification of membranes in the inner ear

Bioelectric and biomechanical imbalances in the inner ear

Degeneration and loss of ganglion cells and their fibers in
the eighth cranial nerve

Eighth nerve canal closure, with destruction of nerve fibers

Atrophy and cell loss at all auditory centers in the brainstem

Reduction of cells in auditory areas of the cortex

simultaneously present sense and nonsense speech, which the individual is asked
to repeat.

Aging Changes

Many changes in the peripheral and central auditory system during aging have
effects on the hearing mechanism (Table 13-10). These changes lead to diminished performance by older subjects (Table 13-11), including the loss of sensitivity and distortion of signals that succeed in passing to higher levels, difficulty in

TABLE 13-11   HEARING PERFORMANCE IN OLDER ADULTS

A. Peripheral pathology
  1. Hearing loss for pure tones
  2. Hearing loss for speech
  3. Problems understanding speech

B. Brainstem pathology
  1. Problems localizing sounds
  2. Problems in binaural listening

C. Cortical pathology
  1. Problems with difficult speech
  2. Language problems

localizing signals and in taking advantage of two-ear listening, difficulty under-standing speech under unfavorable listening conditions, and problems with lan-guage, especially when aging is compounded by stroke.

Three major factors enhance the progression of hearing loss with advancing age: previous middle-ear disease, vascular disease, and exposure to noise. These factors alone, however, do not account for the hearing loss of old age, called *pres-bycusis*. Although clinically and pathologically complex, this is a distinct pro-gressive sensorineural hearing loss associated with aging. The deterioration is not limited to the peripheral sensory receptor. Presbycusis affects 60% of individuals older than age 65 in the United States. However, only a fraction of these have a functional deficit necessitating aural rehabilitation.

Sensitivity

Beginning with the third decade of life, there is a deterioration in the hearing threshold. At first, sensitivity at the high frequencies declines gradually. This age-associated loss has been confirmed in populations not exposed to high levels of noise. This gradual impairment is sensorineural and can be tested by pure-tone audiometry, which reveals useful information about the physiological condition of hearing, but does not disclose some important aspects of deterioration.

Speech

Although there is a close relationship between pure tone loss and the ability to hear speech, the audiogram does not precisely measure hearing for speech. To assess this auditory function, speech audiometry can be performed by presenting the undistorted test words above threshold intensities in the absence of background noise.

Older people with hearing impairment may have difficulty understanding speech under less-favorable conditions, as with background noise, under poor acoustic conditions, or when speech is rapid. This difficulty may be caused in part by the longer time required by higher auditory centers to identify the message. Such hearing loss may necessitate testing of desired signals with the presentation of a competing signal. This will more accurately reflect hearing of speech in social cir-cumstances.

Speech occurring in rooms that cause long reverberations is also much less intelligible to the elderly. Auditory temporal discrimination and auditory reaction time and frequency discrimination also decline with age. Because consonant sounds are of higher frequency and shorter duration, the loss of high-frequency hearing in the elderly may affect these sounds, which encode much of speech information. Lipreading may compensate to some extent for this effect on under-standing speech, but other factors of processing information still remain.

Loudness

A common auditory problem of the elderly is abnormal loudness perception. This can occur as hypersensitivity to sounds of high intensity and appears as increased "loudness recruitment," in which gradually increasing loudness, such as amplified sound, is unpleasantly harsh and difficult to tolerate. In older adults with hearing impairment, this abnormality is manifest when a speaker is asked to speak louder or the output of a hearing aid is increased. It may result from a sensorineural loss attributable to changes in the hair cells of the inner ear.

Localization

Sound localization contributes to effectiveness of signal detection and helps with discrimination. Loss of directional hearing results in greater hearing difficulty in a noisy environment. Localization is disturbed in older adults with hearing loss and may be partly caused by the aging brain's deranged processing of interaural intensity differences and time delays. A strongly asymmetrical hearing loss also disturbs localization.

Tinnitus

Tinnitus, an internal noise generated within the hearing system, occurs in many types of hearing disorders at all ages, but is much more frequent in older adults. Tinnitus, however, is not necessarily associated with hearing loss and may occur in older adults without hearing impairment. Estimates of prevalence of tinnitus in the United States are about 10%, with the majority of persons with tinnitus being 40 to 80 years of age (Peifer, Rosen, and Rubin, 1999). Treatment is generally unsatisfactory.

Other Hearing Disorders

One of the most easily treatable but too easily overlooked causes of hearing loss is cerumen that occludes the external auditory canal (Table 13-12). Cerumen usually affects low-frequency sounds and complicates existing hearing impairments.

Hearing loss in the geriatric patient may be caused by scarring of the tympanic membrane. In tympanosclerosis, there is calcification of the tympanic membrane that results in stiffening of the drumhead.

Otosclerosis may cause fixation of the ossicular chain and lead to a conduction hearing loss. The bony capsule may also be affected, leading to sensorineural loss. Paget disease may also lead to both kinds of hearing loss and should be evaluated radiologically and by an alkaline phosphatase determination.

Ototoxic medication is an acquired cause of hearing loss producing cochlear damage. The aminoglycoside antibiotics require special caution. At high doses, ethacrynic acid and furosemide may be ototoxic.

TABLE 13-12 DISORDERS OF HEARING IN OLDER ADULTS

Cerumen plug

Tympanosclerosis

Otosclerosis

Paget disease

Ototoxic medications

Sound trauma

CNS lesions

Pseudo-deafness (depression)

High doses of aspirin may cause a reversible hearing impairment. Unfortunately, except for aspirin, removal of the offending drug usually does not reverse the sensorineural loss.

Sound trauma is an environmental factor with neurosensory consequences. Superimposed on the changes of aging, sound trauma can have a severe impact on a patient's communicative ability.

Vascular or mass lesions may affect hearing at one of several levels, including the middle and inner ear, auditory nerve, brainstem, and cortex.

Aural Rehabilitation

Every individual who has communication difficulties caused by a permanent hearing loss should have an ear, nose, and throat evaluation to rule out remediable disease and then an audiological evaluation to assess the roles of amplification and aural rehabilitation. Table 13-13 lists the factors that should be considered during the evaluation for a hearing aid. In the severely impaired, in addition to a hearing aid, aural rehabilitation with speech reading may be necessary.

Patient and family counseling may improve use of and satisfaction with a hearing aid. Realistic expectations should be explained to the patient. Hearing aids are most useful in one-on-one conversations and are less effective in noisy, group settings. They are also less useful in improving understanding of less-familiar accents and languages, for example, a British accent in a movie or television production. Such understanding can be improved by use of the closed caption feature on television. Facing the speaker and lipreading also improves understanding. Improvements and modifications in design and construction of hearing aids have enabled a greater proportion of the hearing-impaired population to profit from

TABLE 13-13   FACTORS IN EVALUATION FOR A HEARING AID

Exclude contraindicating medical or other correctable problem

Greatest satisfaction is achieved with aid if loss is 55-80 dB; there is only partial help if loss is > 80 dB

Less satisfaction is achieved when poor discrimination is present

Aid is specifically designed for face-to-face conversation; patient's expectations should be realistic

Aid may need to be combined with lipreading

Loudness perception abnormalities may make aid unacceptable

More severe hearing loss requires aid worn on the body rather than behind-the-ear device

Assess for monaural or binaural aids

Assess for patient's ability to handle aid independently

Assess patient's motivation for using an aid

---

amplification. The old adage that hearing aids will not help people with sensorineural loss is simply not true. The aid can be adjusted to a specific frequency rather than all frequencies, thus decreasing loudness problems, improving discrimination, and making the aid more acceptable. Binaural aids improve sound localization and discrimination.

The hearing aid that is worn on the body provides the greatest amplification but is necessary only for patients with the most severe hearing loss. The controls are large and therefore more easily managed by some elderly persons. However, many elderly people prefer behind-the-ear or in-the-ear devices. The in-the-ear devices are small, cosmetically more acceptable, but more difficult to manipulate.

Although expensive, cochlear implants can restore hearing in individuals with severe hearing loss not corrected by hearing aids.

TASTE

During aging there is a significant loss of lingual papillae and an associated diminution of ability to taste. Salivary secretion also diminishes, thus decreasing solubilization of flavoring agents. Upper dentures may cover secondary taste sites and decrease taste acuity.

Olfactory bulbs also show significant atrophy with old age. In a population-based, cross-sectional study of adults aged 53 to 97, the prevalence of impaired olfaction by olfaction testing was 24.5% and increased with age to 62.5% of 80- to 97-year-olds (Murphy et al., 2002). Taste and olfactory changes together may account for the lessened interest in food shown by older adults.

POLYNEUROPATHY

Patients with polyneuropathy have impairments in balance and an increased risk for falls and falls causing injury (Richardson, 2002). Epidemiological data on polyneuropathy are relatively limited. In a study from Italy of subjects ages 55 and older, the prevalence of polyneuropathy was 11%. Diabetes mellitus was the most common risk factor (44% of patients with polyneuropathy). The next most common risk factors were alcoholism, nonalcoholic liver disease, and malignancy (Beghi and Monticelli, 1998). In a natural history study of type 2 diabetes mellitus, 42% of the diabetic population had nerve conduction abnormalities consistent with polyneuropathy after 10 years (Partanen et al., 1995). The prevalence of diabetes mellitus in older persons is increasing, and, therefore, the prevalence of polyneuropathy is likely to increase as well.

In chronic polyneuropathies, such as diabetes mellitus, symptoms usually begin in the lower extremities and sensory symptoms usually precede motor symptoms. In demyelinating polyneuropathies, such as Guillain-Barré syndrome, weakness rather than sensory loss is more typical. The physical examination should focus on the sensory examination, including pin prick, light touch, vibration, cold, and proprioception, and on muscle strength testing and appearance of muscle wasting. Extensive diagnostic testing is usually not necessary in a patient with mild symptoms and a known underlying diagnosis such as diabetes mellitus or alcohol abuse. In patients with no clear etiology, electrodiagnostic testing should be the initial diagnostic study (Dyck et al., 1996). Rutkove has described an algorithm for a diagnostic approach to polyneuropathy (Rutkove, 2002; see Fig. 13-3). Laboratory tests, which might include a complete blood count, erythrocyte sedimentation rate, thyroid-stimulating hormone, serum and urine protein electrophoresis, blood glucose, vitamin B_{12} level, antinuclear antibody, and urinalysis, should be directed by the electrodiagnostic testing results.

Treatment should address the underlying disease process and alleviation of symptoms. Avoidance of toxins, such as alcohol or drugs, is the most important step. In patients with diabetes, tight control may help maintain nerve function (see Chap. 12). In painful neuropathies, tricyclic antidepressants are effective, as is gabapentin. In patients with weakness, physical therapy evaluation is important and use of ankle–foot orthosis, splints, and walking-assistance devices can improve function. Proper foot and nail care is important in reducing risk for foot ulcers.

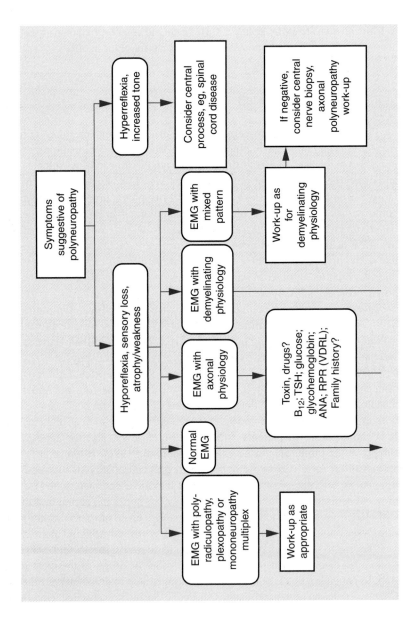

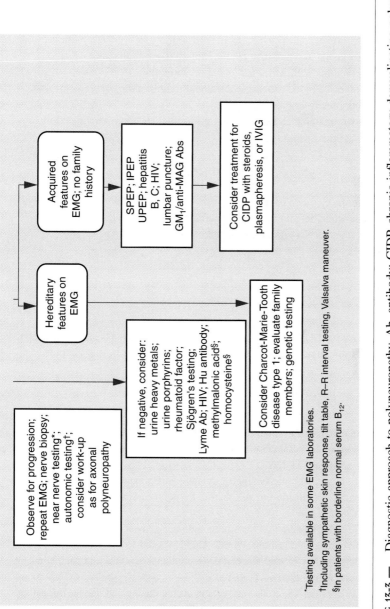

— FIGURE 13-3 — Diagnostic approach to polyneuropathy. Ab, antibody; CIDP, chronic inflammatory demyelinating polyneuropathy; EMG, electromyography; GM1, ganglioside antibodies; Hu, human; IPEP, immunoprotein electrophoresis; IVIG, intravenous immunoglobulin; MAG, myelin-associated glycoprotein; SPEP, serum protein electrophoresis; UPEP, urine protein electrophoresis. (From Rutkove, 2002.)

*Testing available in some EMG laboratories.
†Including sympathetic skin response, tilt table, R–R interval testing, Valsalva maneuver.
§In patients with borderline normal serum B_{12}.

EVIDENCE SUMMARY

Do's

- Screen for visual and auditory dysfunction in older adults.
- Refer all patients with AMD for visual rehabilitation.
- Initiate intensive blood glucose control and tight blood pressure control to reduce retinopathy in type 2 diabetes.
- Evaluate for treatable causes of hearing loss such as cerumen impaction and chronicotitis media.

Consider

- Cataract surgery when cataract progresses to interfering with activities.
- Glaucoma when defects in the peripheral visual field are present.
- AMD when central visual acuity is affected.

ACKNOWLEDGMENT

The authors wish to thank Dr. Douglas Noffsinger for his assistance in preparing material for an earlier version of the section on hearing in this chapter.

References

Anonymous. Ranibizumab (*Lucentis*) for macular degeneration. Med Lett. 2006;48:85-86.

Anand KB, Eschmann E. Systemic effects of ophthalmic medication in the elderly. *NY State J Med.* 1988;88:134-136.

Beghi E, Monticelli ML. Chronic symmetric symptomatic polyneuropathy in the elderly: a field screening investigation of risk factors for polyneuropathy in two Italian communities. *J Clin Epidemiol.* 1998;51:697-702.

Bogardus ST, Yueh B, Shekelle PG. Screening and management of adult hearing loss in primary care: clinical applications. *JAMA.* 2003;289:1986-1990.

Bourla DH, Young TA. Age-related macular degeneration: a practical approach to a challenging disease. *JAGS.* 2006;54:1130-1135.

Dyck PJ, Dyck PJB, Grant IA, et al. Ten steps in characterizing and diagnosing patients with peripheral neuropathy. *Neurology.* 1996;47:10-17.

Fine SL, Berger JW, Maguire MG, et al. Age-related macular degeneration. *N Engl J Med.* 2000;342:483-492.

Haines JL, Pericak-Vance MA. Rapid dissection of the genetic risk of age-related macular degeneration. *JAMA.* 2007;297:401-402.

Havlik RJ. Aging in the eighties, impaired senses for sound and light in persons age 65 years and over. *NCHS Advance Data*, 1986; 25.

Kini MM, Liebowitz HM, Colton T, et al. Prevalence of senile cataract, diabetic retinopathy, senile macular degeneration, and open-angle glaucoma in the Framingham Eye Study. *Am J Ophthalmol*. 1978;85:28-34.

Mohamed Q, Gillies MC, Wong TY. Management of diabetic retinopathy: a systematic review. *JAMA*. 2007;298:902-916.

Murphy C, Schubert CR, Cruickshanks KJ, et al. Prevalence of olfactory impairment in older adults. *JAMA*. 2002;288:2307-2312.

Partanen J, Niskonen L, Lehtinen J, et al. Natural history of peripheral neuropathy in patients with non-insulin dependent diabetes mellitus. *N Engl J Med*. 1995;89(333):89-94.

Peifer KJ, Rosen GP, Rubin AM. Tinnitus: etiology and management. *Clin Geriatr Med*. 1999;15:193-204.

Reuben DB, Walshk K, Moore AA, et al. Hearing loss in community-dwelling older persons: national prevalence data and identification using simple questions. *J Am Geriatr Soc*. 1998;46:1008-1011.

Richardson JK. Factors associated with falls in older patients with diffuse polyneuropathy. *J Am Geriatr Soc*. 2002;50:1767-1773.

Rutkove SB. Overview of polyneuropathy. *UpToDate 2002*. See www.uptodate.com. Last accessed August, 2008.

Schaumberg DA, Hankinson SE, Guo Q, et al. A prospective study of 2 major age-related macular degeneration susceptibility alleles and interactions with modifiable risk factors. *Arch Ophthalmol*. 2007;125:55-62.

Yueh B, Shapiro N, MacLean CH, et al. Screening and management of adult hearing loss in primary care: scientific review. *JAMA*. 2003;289:1976-1985.

Suggested Readings

Gottlieb JL. Age-related macular degeneration. *JAMA*. 2002;288:2233-2236.

Kollarits CR, Rubin AM, Goebel JA (eds). Visual and auditory challenges. *Clin Geriatr Med*. 1999;15:1-204.

Lavizzo-Mourey RJ, Siegler EL. Hearing impairment in the elderly. *J Gen Intern Med*. 1992;7:191-198.

Mulrow CD, Lichtenstein MJ. Screening for hearing impairment in the elderly: rationale and strategy. *J Gen Intern Med*. 1991;6:249-258.

Uhlmann RF, Rees TS, Psatz BM, et al. Validity and reliability of auditory screening tests in demented and non-demented older adults. *J Gen Intern Med*. 1989;4:90-96.

Weblinks

American Academy of Ophthalmology: http://www.aao.org/
American Glaucoma Society: http://www.glaucomaweb.org/

American Macular Degeneration Foundation: http://www.macular.org

Facts about Age-Related Macular Degeneration: http://www.nei.nih.gov/health/maculardegen/armd_facts.htm

"Learn about Glaucoma": http://www.glaucoma.org/learn/

Lighthouse for the Blind: http://www.lighthouse-sf.org/

Macular Degeneration Foundation: http://www.es.org

Macular Degeneration International: http://www.maculardegeneration.org

Macular Degeneration Network: http://www.macular-degeneration.org

Macular Degeneration Partnership: http://www.macd.net

American Academy of Audiology: http://www.audiology.org

Clinical Advisory: NIDCD/VA Clinical Trial Finding Can Benefit Millions with Hearing Loss: http://www.nlm.nih.gov/databases/alerts/hearing.html

Healthy Hearing http://www.healthyhearing.com

Hearing Aid Help http://www.hearingaidhelp.com/

Hearing Handicap Inventory for the Elderly Screening: http://teachhealthk-12.uthscsa.edu/curriculum/vision-hearing/pa06pdf/0608E-eng.pdf

CHAPTER 14

DRUG THERAPY

Geriatric patients are sometimes viewed as "walking chemistry sets" because they are frequently prescribed multiple drugs in complex dosage schedules. In some instances, this is justified because of the presence of multiple chronic medical conditions, the proven efficacy of an increasing number of drugs for these conditions, and practice guidelines that recommend their use. The nature of drug therapy in managing chronic disease has changed greatly. Many conditions can be better controlled, but at a cost. In many instances, however, complex drug regimens are unnecessary; they are costly and predispose to nonadherence and adverse drug reactions. Many older patients are prescribed multiple drugs, take over-the-counter drugs, and are then prescribed additional drugs to treat the side effects of medications they are already taking. This scenario can result in an upward spiral in the number of drugs being taken and commonly leads to polypharmacy.

Several important considerations, some pharmacological and others non-pharmacological, influence the safety and effectiveness of drug therapy in the geriatric population. This chapter focuses on these considerations and gives practical suggestions for prescribing drugs for older patients. Drug therapy for specific geriatric conditions is discussed in several other chapters throughout this text.

NONPHARMACOLOGICAL FACTORS INFLUENCING DRUG THERAPY

Discussions of geriatric pharmacology frequently center on age-related changes in drug pharmacokinetics and pharmacodynamics. Detailed reviews of these areas are provided in the Suggested Readings section at the end of the chapter. Although these changes are often of clinical importance, nonpharmacological factors can play an even greater role in the safety and effectiveness of drug therapy in the geriatric population. Several steps make drug therapy safe and effective (Fig. 14-1). Many factors can interfere with this scheme in the geriatric population, and, as can be seen, most of them come into play before pharmacological considerations arise.

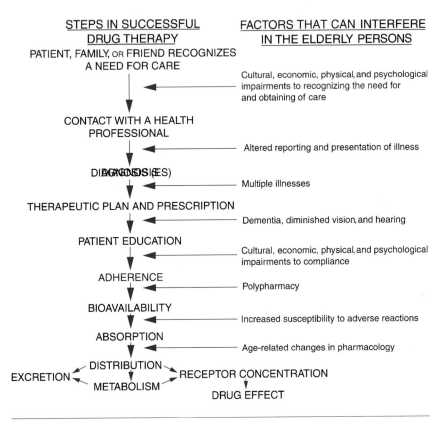

— FIGURE 14-1 — Factors that can interfere with successful drug therapy.

Effective drug therapy requires accurate diagnoses. Many older patients tend to underreport symptoms; complaints of other patients may be vague and multiple. Symptoms of physical diseases frequently overlap with symptoms of psychological illness. To add to this complexity, many diseases present with atypical symptoms. Consequently, making the correct diagnoses and prescribing the appropriate drugs are often difficult tasks in the geriatric population.

Health-care professionals tend to treat symptoms with drugs rather than to evaluate the symptoms thoroughly. Because older patients tend to have multiple problems and complaints and consult several health-care professionals, they often end up with prescriptions for several drugs. Moreover, older patients or their family members sometimes exert pressure on health-care professionals to prescribe medication, thus adding to the tendency for polypharmacy. This pressure is intensified by direct-to-consumer advertising of drugs.

Frequently, neither the patients nor the health-care providers have a clear picture of the total drug regimen. New patients undergoing initial geriatric assessment should be asked to empty their medicine cabinets and to bring all bottles to their first appointments. Simple medication records, such as the one shown in Fig. 14-2, carried by the patient and maintained as an integral part of the overall medical record, may help to eliminate some of the polypharmacy and noncompliance common in the geriatric population. Such records should be updated at each patient visit. Drug regimens should be simplified whenever possible and patients instructed to discard old medications. Incorporation of medication lists into electronic medical records with medication adjudication at each visit can be very helpful in maintaining an accurate medication list, reducing polypharmacy, and improving adherence. A good principle is to ask each time a new drug is added if one can be deleted.

Adherence plays a central role in the success of drug therapy in all age groups (see Fig. 14-1). In addition to the tendency for polypharmacy and complex dosage schedules, older patients face other potential barriers to adherence. The chronic nature of illness in the geriatric population can play a role in nonadherence. The consequences of these illnesses are often delayed (as opposed to the more dramatic effects of acute illnesses), and chronic illnesses necessitate ongoing prophylactic or suppressive rather than relatively short and

NAME _____ DOCTOR _____ PHONE: ( )_____

MEDICATION NAME	REASON FOR USE	DESCRIBE OR TAPE MEDICINE HERE	WHEN TO TAKE MEDICINE				SPECIAL NOTES

REMEMBER
BRING THIS CHART TO ALL DOCTOR APPOINTMENTS
INCLUDE ALL THE MEDICATIONS YOU ARE TAKING
DO NOT CHANGE THE WAY YOU TAKE THE MEDICATIONS WITHOUT CALLING THE DOCTOR
DO NOT SHARE MEDICATIONS
IF YOU HAVE ANY QUESTIONS, CALL THE DOCTOR

— FIGURE 14-2 — Example of a medication record.

time-limited courses of therapy. Adherence tends to be poor for these types of drug regimens. Diminished hearing, impaired vision, poor literacy, and poor short-term memory can interfere with patient education and adherence. Problems with transportation can make getting to a pharmacy difficult. Outpatient prescriptions are now covered by Medicare to some extent, but many older persons still have to pay for some of the costs of their drugs from a limited income. Even if the older person gets to the pharmacy, can afford the prescription, understands the instructions, and remembers when to take it, the use of childproof bottles and tamper-resistant packaging may hinder adherence in those with arthritic or weak hands.

Several strategies might improve adherence in the geriatric population (Table 14-1). As few drugs as possible should be prescribed; and the dosage schedule should be as simple as possible. Drugs should be given on the same dosage schedules whenever possible, and the administration should correspond to a daily routine in order to enhance the consistency of taking the drugs and compliance. For many drugs, once-daily dosing is available and should be prescribed when clinically appropriate. Relatives or other caregivers should be instructed in the drug regimen, and they, as well as others (eg, home health aides and pharmacists), should be enlisted to help the older patient comply. Specially

TABLE 14-1   STRATEGIES TO IMPROVE COMPLIANCE IN THE GERIATRIC POPULATION

1. Making drug regimens and instructions as simple as possible
   a. Use the same dosage schedule for all drugs whenever feasible (eg, once or twice per day)
   b. Time the doses in conjunction with a daily routine
2. Instruct relatives and caregivers on the drug regimen
3. Enlist others (eg, home health aides, pharmacists) to help ensure compliance
4. Make sure the older patient can get to a pharmacist (or vice versa), can afford the prescriptions, and can open the container
5. Use aids (such as special pillboxes and drug calendars) whenever appropriate
6. Perform careful medication adjudication and patient/family education at the time of every hospital discharge
7. Keep updated medication records (see Fig. 14-2) and review them at each visit
8. Review knowledge of and compliance with drug regimens regularly

designed pill dispensers, dosage calendars, and other innovative techniques can be useful. Geriatric patients and their health-care providers should keep an updated record of the drug regimen (see Fig. 14-2). For older patients who are hospitalized, medication adjudication and education should be performed at the time of discharge, as posthospital medication discrepancies are common in the older population and can have serious consequences (Coleman et al., 2005). Medication misuse can result, for example, in potentially unnecessary emergency room visits. Three medications: warfarin, insulin, and digoxin account for a substantial portion of these visits (Budnitz et al., 2007). Medications should be brought to appointments, and patients and families should show all medications to their physicians, particularly on initial visits to new primary care physicians or at a consultation with a specialist. Health-care professionals should regularly inquire about other medications being taken (prescribed by other physicians or purchased over the counter) and review their patients' knowledge of and compliance with the drug regimen.

ADVERSE DRUG REACTIONS AND INTERACTIONS

Primum non nocere ("first, do no harm"), a watchword phrase in the practice of medicine, is nowhere more applicable than when drugs are being prescribed for the geriatric population. Concerns are frequently heard about inappropriate prescribing of medications with serious side effects in older people. Although there have been several efforts to create guidelines, new standards are needed (O'Mahony and Gallagher, 2008). Adverse drug reactions are the most common forms of iatrogenic illness. The incidence of adverse drug reactions in hospitalized patients increases from approximately 10% in those between 40 and 50 years of age to 25% in those older than age 80 (Lazarou, Pomeranz, and Corey, 1998). They account for between 3% and 10% of hospital admissions of older patients each year, and result in several billion dollars in yearly health-care expenditures. Many drugs can produce distressing, and sometimes disabling or life-threatening, adverse reactions (Table 14-2). Psychotropic drugs and cardiovascular agents are common causes of serious adverse reactions in the geriatric population. In part, this is because of the narrow therapeutic to toxic ratio of many of these drugs. In some instances, age-related changes in pharmacology, such as diminished renal excretion and prolonged duration of action, predispose to adverse reactions. Some side effects can have a therapeutic benefit and may be key factors in drug selection (see below).

Because symptoms can be nonspecific or may mimic other illnesses, adverse drug reactions may be ignored or unrecognized. Patients and family members should be educated to recognize and report common and potentially serious adverse reactions. In some instances, another drug is prescribed to treat these

DRUG	COMMON ADVERSE REACTIONS
ANALGESICS (SEE CHAP. 10)	
Anti-inflammatory agents, aspirin	Gastric irritation and ulcers Chronic blood loss
Narcotics	Constipation
ANTIMICROBIALS	
Aminoglycosides	Renal failure Hearing loss
Other antimicrobials	Diarrhea
ANTIPARKINSONIAN DRUGS (SEE CHAP. 10)	
Dopaminergic agents	Nausea Delirium Hallucinations Postural hypotension
Anticholinergics	Dry mouth Constipation Urinary retention Delirium
CARDIOVASCULAR DRUGS (SEE CHAP. 11)	
Angiotensin-converting enzyme (ACE) inhibitors	Cough Impaired renal function
Antiarrhythmics	Pulmonary toxicity, bradycardia, hypotension (amiodarone) Diarrhea (quinidine) Urinary retention (disopyramide)
Anticoagulants	Bleeding complications
Antihypertensives	Hypotension
Calcium-channel blockers	Decreased myocardial contractility Edema Constipation
Diuretics	Dehydration Hyponatremia Hypokalemia Incontinence

TABLE 14-2   EXAMPLES OF COMMON AND POTENTIALLY SERIOUS
ADVERSE DRUG REACTIONS IN THE GERIATRIC POPULATION
(*Continued*)

DRUG	COMMON ADVERSE REACTIONS
CARDIOVASCULAR DRUGS (SEE CHAP. 11)	
Digoxin	Arrhythmias
	Nausea
	Anorexia
Nitrates	Hypotension
Statins	Myopathy, hepatotoxicity
HYPOGLYCEMIC AGENTS	
Insulin	Hypoglycemia
Oral agents	Edema (glitazones)
	Diarrhea (metformin)
LOWER URINARY TRACT DRUGS (SEE CHAP. 8)	
Antimuscarinics	Dry mouth, eyes
Oral agents	Constipation
	Esophageal reflux
α-Blockers	Postural hypotension
PSYCHOTROPIC DRUGS (SEE TABLES 14-8 AND 14-9)	
Antidepressants	(See Chap. 7)
Antipsychotics	Sedation
	Hypotension
	Extrapyramidal movement disorders
Cholinesterase inhibitors	Nausea, diarrhea
Lithium	Weakness
	Tremor
	Nausea
	Delirium
Sedative and hypnotic agents	Excessive sedation
	Delirium
	Gait disturbances and falls

TABLE 14-2   EXAMPLES OF COMMON AND POTENTIALLY SERIOUS
ADVERSE DRUG REACTIONS IN THE GERIATRIC POPULATION
(*Continued*)

OTHERS	
Alendronate, risedronate	Esophageal ulceration
Aminophylline, theophylline	Gastric irritation Tachyarrhythmias
Carbamazepine	Anemia Hyponatremia Neutropenia
Cimetidine	Mental status changes
Terbutaline	Tremor

symptoms, thus contributing to polypharmacy and increasing the likelihood of an adverse drug interaction. The problem of polypharmacy is exacerbated by visits to multiple physicians, who may prescribe still more drugs and the use of multiple pharmacies. Medication records kept by the patient (see Fig. 14-2), the physician's medical record, and the increasing use of electronic medical records should help to prevent unnecessary polypharmacy when many physicians are involved. Several drugs commonly prescribed for the geriatric population can interact with adverse consequences (Table 14-3). The more common types of potential adverse drug interactions are drug displacement from protein-binding sites by other highly protein-bound drugs, induction or suppression of the metabolism of other drugs, and additive effects of different drugs on blood pressure and mental function (mood, level of consciousness, etc.). Interactions among drugs metabolized by the cytochrome P-450 system in the liver are especially common. Because many older patients are treated with warfarin for atrial fibrillation or venous thrombosis, clinicians must be aware of the many potential drug–drug and drug–nutrient interactions with this medication (Holbrook et al., 2005). In addition to the potential to interact with other drugs, several drugs can interact adversely with underlying medical conditions in the geriatric population, creating "drug–patient" interactions (Table 14-4). A good example of this problem is the increased risk of hospitalization for congestive heart failure (CHF) among older patients taking diuretics who are told to take a nonsteroidal anti-inflammatory drug (Heerdink et al., 1998).

     Health-care professionals should have a thorough knowledge of the more common drug side effects, adverse reactions to drugs, and potential drug interactions

TABLE 14-3 EXAMPLES OF POTENTIALLY CLINICALLY IMPORTANT DRUG-DRUG INTERACTIONS

INTERACTION	EXAMPLES	POTENTIAL EFFECTS
Interference with drug absorption	Antacids interacting with digoxin, isoniazid, antipsychotics, enteral tube feedings, and liquid phenytoin; iron; and ciprofloxacin	Diminished drug effectiveness
Displacement from binding proteins	Warfarin, oral hypoglycemics, and other highly protein-bound drugs	Enhanced effects and increased risk of toxicity
Altered distribution	Digoxin and quinidine	Increased risk of toxicity
Altered metabolism	Antifungals, erythromycin, clarithromycin SSRIs, with antihistamines, calcium-channel blockers, and others[*]	Decreased metabolism, increased levels of toxicity
Altered excretion	Lithium and diuretics	Increased risk of toxicity and electrolyte imbalance
Pharmacological antagonism	Antimuscarinic drugs (for the bladder) and cholinesterase inhibitors	Decreased effectiveness
Pharmacological synergism	α-Blockers (for lower urinary tract symptoms in men) and antihypertensives	Increased risk of hypotension

*See Wilkinson, 2005.
SSRI, selective serotonin reuptake inhibitor.

TABLE 14-4 EXAMPLES OF POTENTIALLY CLINICALLY IMPORTANT DRUG–PATIENT INTERACTIONS

Drug	Patient Factors	Clinical Implications
Diuretics	Diabetes	Decreased glucose tolerance
	Poor nutritional status	Increased risk of dehydration and electrolyte imbalance
	Urinary frequency, urgency	Incontinence may result
Angiotensin-converting enzyme (ACE) inhibitors	Renovascular disease (severe)	Worsening renal function
β-Blockers	Stress incontinence	Precipitate incontinence (cough)
	Diabetes	Sympathetic response to hypoglycemia may be masked
	Chronic obstructive lung disease	Increased bronchospasm
	Congestive heart failure (CHF)	Decreased myocardial contractility
	Peripheral vascular disease	Increased claudication
Narcotic analgesics	Chronic constipation	Worsening symptoms, fecal impaction
Antimuscarinics, tricyclic antidepressants, antihistamines, and other drugs with anticholinergic effects	Constipation, glaucoma, prostatic hyperplasia, reflux esophagitis	Worsening of symptoms
Antipsychotics	Parkinsonism	Worsening of immobility
Psychotropics	Dementia	Further impairment of cognitive function
Nonsteroidal anti-inflammatory drugs	CHF, on diuretics	Increased risk of exacerbation of CHF

in the geriatric population. Electronic databases available on the World Wide Web or on personal digital assistants (PDAs) can be very helpful in this regard. Careful questioning about side effects should be an important part of reviewing the drug regimen at each visit. Many institutions use computers to detect potential adverse drug interactions and to prevent their occurrence. Software programs are available that can assist in identifying potential adverse drug interactions. Special attention should be given to the potential for any newly prescribed drug to interact with drugs already being taken or with underlying medical or psychological conditions.

AGING AND PHARMACOLOGY

Several age-related biological and physiological changes are relevant to drug pharmacology (Table 14-5). With the exception of changes in renal function, however, the effects of these age-related changes on dosages of specific

TABLE 14-5   AGE-RELATED CHANGES RELEVANT TO DRUG
             PHARMACOLOGY

Pharmacological Parameter	Age-Related Changes
Absorption	Decreases in absorptive surface splanchnic blood flow Increased gastric pH Altered gastrointestinal motility
Distribution	Decreases in total body water, lean body mass, serum albumin Increased fat Altered protein binding
Metabolism	Decreases in liver blood flow, enzyme activity, enzyme inducibility
Excretion	Decreases in renal blood flow, glomerular filtration rate, tubular secretory function
Tissue sensitivity	Alterations in receptor number, receptor affinity, second-messenger function, cellular and nuclear responses

drugs for individual patients are variable and difficult to predict. In general, an understanding of the physiological status of each patient (taking into account factors such as state of hydration, nutrition, and cardiac output) and how that status affects the pharmacology of a particular drug is more important to clinical efficacy than are age-related changes. Drug delivery systems, such as oral sustained-release preparations and skin patches, may be useful in designing strategies to account for the effect of aging changes on pharmacology and to make many drugs safer in the geriatric population. Given these caveats, the effects of aging on each pharmacological process are briefly discussed below.

Absorption

Several age-related changes can affect drug absorption (see Table 14-5). Most studies, however, have failed to document any clinically meaningful alterations in drug absorption with increasing age. Absorption, therefore, appears to be the pharmacological parameter least affected by increasing age.

Distribution

In contrast to absorption, clinically meaningful changes in drug distribution can occur with increasing age. Serum albumin, the major drug-binding protein, tends to decline, especially in hospitalized patients. Although the decline is numerically small, it can substantially increase the amount of free drug available for action. This effect is of particular relevance for highly protein-bound drugs, especially when they are used simultaneously and compete for protein-binding sites (see Table 14-3).

Age-related changes in body composition can prominently affect pharmacology by altering the volume of distribution (Vd). The elimination half-life of a drug varies with the ratio of Vd to drug clearance. Thus, even if the rate of clearance of a drug is unchanged with age, changes in Vd can affect a drug's half-life and duration of action.

Because total body water and lean body mass decline with increasing age, drugs that distribute in these body compartments, such as most antimicrobial agents, digoxin, lithium, and alcohol, may have a lower Vd and can, therefore, achieve higher concentrations from given amounts of drugs. On the other hand, drugs that distribute in body fat, such as many of the psychotropic agents, have a large Vd in the geriatric patients. The larger Vd will thus cause a prolongation of the half-life unless the clearance increases proportionately, which is unlikely to happen with increasing age.

Metabolism

The effects of aging on drug metabolism are complex and difficult to predict. They depend on the precise pathway of drug metabolism in the liver and on several other factors, such as gender and amount of smoking. The pharmacokinetics and elimination of drugs commonly used in the elderly are now readily available on the internet and several PDA-based programs.

There is some evidence that the first, or preparative, phase of drug metabolism, including oxidations, reductions, and hydrolyses, declines with increasing age, and that the decline is more prominent in men than in women. In contrast, the second phase of drug metabolism (biotransformation, including acetylation and glucuronidation) appears to be less affected by age. There is also evidence that the ability of environmental factors (most importantly smoking) to induce drug-metabolizing enzymes declines with age. Even when liver function is obviously impaired, as by intrinsic liver disease or right-sided CHF, the effects of aging on the metabolism of specific drugs cannot be precisely predicted. It is *not* safe to assume, however, that geriatric patients with normal liver function tests can metabolize drugs as efficiently as can younger individuals.

The cytochrome P-450 system in the liver has been extensively studied. More than 30 isoenzymes have been identified and classified into families and subfamilies. Genetic mutations in some of these enzymes, while relatively uncommon, can impair metabolism of specific drugs. Although aging may affect this system, the effects of commonly used drugs are probably more important (Wilkinson, 2005).

Excretion

Unlike metabolism, the effects of aging on renal functions are somewhat more predictable. The tendency for renal function to decline with increasing age can affect the pharmacokinetics of several drugs (and their active metabolites) that are eliminated predominantly by the kidney. These drugs are cleared from the body more slowly, their half-lives (and duration of action) are prolonged, and there is a tendency to accumulate to higher (and potentially toxic) drug concentrations in the steady state.

Several considerations are important in determining the effects of age on renal function and drug elimination:

1. There is wide interindividual variation in the rate of decline of renal function with increasing age. Thus, although renal function is said to decline by 50% between the ages of 20 and 90 years, this is an *average* decline. A 90-year-old individual may not have a creatinine clearance of only 50% of normal. Applying average declines to individual elderly patients can result in over- or underdosing.

2. Muscle mass declines with age; therefore, daily endogenous creatinine production declines. Because of this decline in creatinine production, serum creatinine may be normal at a time when renal function is substantially reduced. Serum creatinine, therefore, does not reflect renal function as accurately in elderly people as it does in younger persons.

TABLE 14-6   RENAL FUNCTION IN RELATION TO AGE*

Cockcroft and Gault equation

$$\text{Creatinine clearance} = \frac{(140 - \text{age}) \times \text{body weight (kg)}}{72 \times \text{serum creatinine level}} \quad (\times 0.85 \text{ for women})$$

---

*Several other factors can influence creatinine clearance (see text).
Data compiled from Cockcroft and Gault, 1976.

3. A number of factors can affect renal clearance of drugs and are often at least as important as age-related changes. State of hydration, cardiac output, and intrinsic renal disease should be considered in addition to age-related changes in renal function.

Several formulas and nomograms have been used to estimate renal function in relation to age. Table 14-6 shows one of the most widely used and accepted formulas. Another commonly used equation is the Modification of Diet in Renal Disease (MDRD) equation. MDRD calculators are readily available on the internet (eg, www.nephron.com/MDRD_GFR.cgi; accessed 12/31/07). These formulae are useful in *initial estimations* of creatinine clearance for the purpose of drug dosing in the geriatric population. Clinical factors (such as state of hydration and cardiac output), which vary over time, should be considered in determining drug dosages.

When drugs with narrow therapeutic to toxic ratios are being used, actual measurements of creatinine clearance and drug blood levels (when available) should be used.

Tissue Sensitivity

A proportion of the drug or its active metabolite will eventually reach its site of action. Age-related changes at this point—that is, responsiveness to given drug concentrations (without regard to pharmacokinetic changes)—are termed *pharmacodynamic changes*. Older persons are often said to be more sensitive to the effects of drugs. For some drugs, this appears to be true. For others, however, sensitivity to drug effects may decrease rather than increase with age. For example, older persons may be more sensitive to the sedative effects of given blood levels of benzodiazepines but less sensitive to the effects of drugs mediated by α-adrenergic receptors. There are several possible explanations for these changes (see Table 14-5). The effects of age-related pharmacodynamic changes on dosages of specific drugs for individual geriatric patients remain largely unknown.

GERIATRIC PRESCRIBING

General Principles

Several considerations make the development of specific recommendations for geriatric drug prescribing very difficult. These include the following:

1. Multiple interacting factors influence age-related changes in drug pharmacology.
2. There is wide interindividual variation in the rate of age-related changes in physiological parameters that affect drug pharmacology. Thus, precise predictions for individual older persons are difficult to make.
3. The clinical status of each patient (including such factors as state of nutrition and hydration, cardiac output, intrinsic renal and liver disease) must be considered in addition to the effects of aging.
4. As more research studies with newer drugs are carried out in well-defined groups of older subjects, more specific recommendations will be possible.

Adherence to several general principles can make drug therapy in the geriatric population safer and more effective (Table 14-7) (Holmes et al., 2006). Quality indicators for medication use (Shrank, Polinski, and Avorn, 2007) and new federal guidance to surveyors on drug therapy in nursing homes ("F-Tag 329"— http://www.ascp.com/resources/nhsurvey/upload/S&C-06-29.09-F329Instructor Guide.pdf; accessed 12/31/07) provide helpful information for geriatric prescribing practices. Because psychotropic drugs are so commonly used in the geriatric population, they are discussed in greater detail below.

GERIATRIC PSYCHOPHARMACOLOGY

Psychotropic drugs can be broadly categorized as antidepressants (discussed in detail in Chap. 7), antipsychotics (Table 14-8), and sedative/hypnotics (Table 14-9). These drugs are probably the most misused class of drugs in the geriatric population. Several studies show that more than half of nursing home residents are prescribed at least one psychotropic drug and that these prescriptions are changed frequently. Ironically, there is also evidence that antidepressants may be underused in nursing homes, where there is a high prevalence of depression. Other studies suggest that psychotropic drugs are commonly prescribed inappropriately in the nursing home setting. This is of special concern because of the frequency of adverse reactions to these drugs. Federal rules and regulations given in the Omnibus Budget Reconciliation Act of 1987 (OBRA 1987) contained specific guidelines on the use of psychotropic drugs in nursing homes. These guidelines, as

TABLE 14-7   GENERAL RECOMMENDATIONS FOR GERIATRIC PRESCRIBING

1. Evaluate geriatric patients thoroughly in order to identify all conditions that could (a) benefit from drug treatment; (b) be adversely affected by drug treatment; (c) influence the efficacy of drug treatment

2. Manage medical conditions without drugs as often as possible

3. Know the pharmacology of the drug(s) being prescribed

4. Consider how the clinical status of each patient could influence the pharmacology of the drug(s)

5. Avoid potential adverse drug interactions

6. For drugs or their active metabolites eliminated predominantly by the kidney, use a formula or nomogram to approximate age-related changes in renal function and adjust dosages accordingly

7. If there is a question about drug dosage, start with smaller doses and increase gradually

8. Drug blood concentrations can be helpful in monitoring several potentially toxic drugs used frequently in the geriatric population

9. Help to ensure adherence by paying attention to impaired intellectual function, diminished hearing, and poor vision when instructing patients and labeling prescriptions (and by using other techniques listed in Table 14-1)

10. Monitor older patients frequently for adherence, drug effectiveness, and adverse effects, and adjust drug therapy accordingly

well as the surveyor guidance for F-Tag 329, emphasize avoiding the use of frequent "as needed" dosing for nonspecific symptoms (eg, agitation, wandering) and the inappropriate use of these drugs as chemical restraints. The appropriate use of antipsychotics for psychosis and several behavioral symptoms associated with dementia must, however, be distinguished from their use as "chemical restraints."

Several considerations can be helpful in preventing the misuse of psychotropic drugs in the geriatric population:

1. Psychological symptoms (depression, anxiety, agitation, insomnia, paranoia, disruptive behavior) are often caused or exacerbated by medical conditions in geriatric patients. A thorough medical evaluation should therefore be done before symptoms are attributed to psychiatric conditions alone and psychotropic drugs are prescribed.

2. Reports of psychiatric symptoms, such as agitation, are often presented to physicians by family caregivers and nursing home personnel who are inexperienced in the description, interpretation, and differential diagnosis of

TABLE 14-8   EXAMPLES OF ANTIPSYCHOTIC DRUGS[*]

| | | | POTENTIAL FOR SIDE EFFECTS | |
DRUG	USUAL GERIATRIC DAILY DOSE RANGE (MG)	RELATIVE SEDATION	HYPOTENSION	EXTRAPYRAMIDAL EFFECTS[†]
Aripiprazole	2.5-20[‡]	Moderate	Moderate	Moderate
Haloperidol (Haldol)	0.25-5	Low	Low	Very high
Olanzapine (Zyprexa)	2.5-10	Low	Low	Low
Quetiapine (Seroquel)	12.5-150	Moderate	Moderate	Low
Risperidone (Risperdal)	0.25	Low	Low	Low
Ziprasidone (Geodon)	20-40	Low	Moderate	Low

[*]Other agents are also available. All of the second generation antipsychotics have been associated with increased mortality, and their efficacy in treating behavioral symptoms associated with dementia has been questioned (see text).
[†]Rigidity, bradykinesia, tremor, akathisia.
[‡]Geriatric dosage ranges not well studied.

TABLE 14-9 EXAMPLES OF HYPNOTICS APPROVED FOR INSOMNIA BY THE US FOOD AND DRUG ADMINISTRATION*

	DOSE (MG)	DURATION OF ACTION	HALF-LIFE[‡]
BENZODIAZEPINES[†]			
Lorazepam (Ativan)	0.5-2.5	Intermediate	10-20
Temazepam (Restoril)	7.5-30	Intermediate	8-15
BENZODIAZEPINE RECEPTOR AGONISTS			
Eszopiclone (Lunesta)	1-3	Intermediate	5-7
Zalpeon (Sonata)	5-20	Ultra short	1
Zolpidem (Ambien)	5-10	Short	3
Zolpidem extended release (Ambien CR)	6.5 or 12.5	Short	3[§]
MELATONIN RECEPTOR AGONIST			
Ramelteon	8	Short	2-5

*Other drugs are also approved. Effectiveness for short-term use in the elderly is questioned (Glass et al., 2005). Table is adapted from Silber, 2005.
[†]Long-acting benzodiazepines should not be used in geriatric patients.
[‡]Half-life includes active metabolites.
[§]Duration of action larger because of extended release preparation.
Table is adapted with permission from Silber MH. Clinical practice. Chronic insomnia. *N Engl J Med.* 2005;353:803-810.

these symptoms. "Agitation" or "disruptive behavior" may, in fact, have been a reasonable response to an inappropriate interaction or situation created by the caregiver. Psychotropic drugs should, therefore, be prescribed only after the physician has clarified what the symptoms are and what correctable factors might have precipitated them.

3. Psychological symptoms and signs, like physical symptoms and signs, can be nonspecific in the geriatric patient. Therefore, appropriate drug treatment often depends on an accurate psychiatric diagnosis. Psychiatrists and psychologists experienced with geriatric patients should be consulted, when available, in order to identify and help target psychotropic drug treatment to the major psychiatric problem(s).

4. Many nonpharmacological treatment modalities can either replace or be used in conjunction with psychotropic drugs in managing psychological symptoms. Behavioral modification, environmental manipulation, supportive psychotherapy, group therapy, recreational activities, and other related techniques can be useful in eliminating or diminishing the need for drug treatment (see Chap. 6).

5. Within each broad category of psychotropic drug, there are considerable differences among individual agents with regard to effects, side effects, and potential interactions with other drugs and medical conditions. Rational prescription of these drugs necessitates careful consideration of the characteristics of each drug in relation to the individual patient.

6. Because geriatric patients are, in general, more sensitive to the effects and side effects of psychotropic drugs, initial doses should be lower, increases should be gradual, and monitoring should be frequent.

7. Careful, ongoing assessment of the response of target symptoms and behaviors to psychotropic drugs is essential. In addition to reports from patients themselves, objective observations by trained and experienced professionals should be continuously evaluated in order to adjust psychotropic drug therapy.

All psychotropic drugs must be used judiciously in geriatric patients because of their potential side effects. The most common and potentially disabling side effects of psychotropic drugs fall into four general categories: changes in cognitive status (eg, sedation, delirium, dementia) and extrapyramidal, anticholinergic, and cardiovascular effects. Psychotropic drugs can contribute to cognitive impairment and are associated with hip fractures in the geriatric population.

Extrapyramidal side effects are most common with several older antipsychotic drugs but may occur with newer atypical antipsychotics (see Table 14-8). These effects—which include pseudoparkinsonism (rigidity, bradykinesia, tremor), akathisia (restlessness), and involuntary dystonic movements (such as tardive dyskinesia)—can be severe and may cause substantial disability. Rigidity and bradykinesia can lead to immobility and related complications. Akathisia can make the patient appear more anxious and agitated, and can lead to the inappropriate prescription of more medication. Tardive dyskinesia can cause permanent disability as a consequence of continuous orolingual movements and difficulty with eating. All of the second generation antipsychotics have been associated with an increase in mortality in older patients (Wang et al., 2005; Schneider, Dagerman, and Insel, 2005). Moreover, their efficacy in treating the behavioral symptoms associated with dementia has been questioned (Schneider et al., 2006). Thus, antipsychotics must be used judiciously in carefully selected patients with psychosis and related symptoms that pose a threat to themselves or others.

Insomnia, like agitation, can be the manifestation of depression or physical illness. It is a very common complaint in geriatric patients, and causes of sleep disorders such as sleep apnea and restless leg syndrome should be sought. Nonpharmacological measures (such as increasing activity during the day, diminishing nighttime noise, and ensuring cooler nighttime temperatures) are sometimes helpful. Several alternatives are available for drug treatment of insomnia (see Table 14-9). Melatonin, a naturally occurring hormone available over the counter, has gained increasing popularity as a hypnotic. Geriatric sleep disturbances are associated with changes in the melatonin cycle. Doses of 1 to 3 mg may improve the initiation and maintenance of sleep. The long-term effects of chronic hypnotic use in the geriatric population are unknown, but rebound insomnia can become a problem in patients who use hypnotics (especially benzodiazepine hypnotics and melatonin) regularly and then discontinue them. Whatever the indication, it is extremely important that after a hypnotic drug is prescribed the patient be closely monitored for the effects of the drug on the target symptoms and side effects, and that the drug regimen be adjusted accordingly.

When prescribed, optimal efficacy of psychotropic drugs necessitates consideration of characteristics of the drugs in relation to several clinical factors in each patient (Table 14-10). The antipsychotic agents should be reserved for treatment of psychoses (ie, paranoid states, delusions, and hallucinations), which are common in patients with severe symptoms that fail to respond to nonpharmacological interventions. Environmental and behavioral interventions should be attempted before psychotropic drugs are prescribed. There is no clear choice of one antipsychotic agent over another based on controlled clinical trials. In some situations, intermittent agitation, especially at night, is best treated by a short-acting benzodiazepine. When antipsychotics fail or cause side effects, and sedation is not desired, carbamazepine and valproic acid may be useful alternatives in some patients. Both of these drugs, however, have the potential for hematological and hepatic toxicity and must be used cautiously in the geriatric population. Periodic attempts to taper and discontinue the use of these drugs are required in nursing facilities, and can result in the successful removal of psychotropics for some patients.

A variety of nonpharmacological measures can be effective in geriatric patients with agitation or excessive anxiety. Specific behavioral and other nonpharmacological therapeutic approaches are discussed in some of the Suggested Readings at the end of this chapter (see also Chap. 6). These measures, however,

TABLE 14-10 CLINICAL CONSIDERATIONS IN PRESCRIBING PSYCHOTROPIC DRUGS

Clinical Indicator	Most Useful Types	Comments
Depression with psychomotor retardation	Less sedating antidepressant (eg, fluoxetine, paroxetine, sertraline)	See Chap. 7
Depression with insomnia and/or weight loss	Antidepressant with sedative and weight-gaining effects (eg, mirtazapine)	
Agitation without psychosis that occurs at night	Short-acting sedative (eg, lorazepam) or a hypnotic (see Table 14-9)	Should generally be used on an "as-needed" basis. Nonpharmacologic intervention may be more appropriate
Psychoses without prominent agitation (eg, delusions and hallucinations in patients with depression or dementia)	Less sedating antipsychotic (eg, risperidone, olanzapine)	Extrapyramidal effects may occur Risperidone may cause postural hypotension if not titrated slowly
Severe physical or verbal agitation poorly controlled by nonpharmacological intervention	More sedating antipsychotic (eg, quetiapine)	Akathisia can make patient appear more agitated
Insomnia	See Table 14-9	Underlying cause(s) should be sought; nonpharmacological interventions often helpful

are often unavailable, impractical, inappropriate, or unsuccessful. Patients with severe impairment of cognitive function can be especially difficult to manage with nonpharmacological measures alone, particularly when their physical and/or verbal agitation is interfering with their care (or the care of others around them). Thus, drug treatment of physical and/or verbal agitation is necessary in some patients.

EVIDENCE SUMMARY

Do's

- Simplify drug regimens as much as possible.
- "Start low and go slow," but increase doses to maximum if appropriate based on response.
- Carefully assess for drug effectiveness and side effects.
- Help ensure adherence by education, attention to out-of-pocket costs, and availability of caregiver's support for patients with cognitive impairment.
- Utilize the expertise and education available through pharmacists.
- Keep careful medication records and review them at each visit.

Don'ts

- Automatically prescribe all drugs that may be indicated in younger patients for older patients with multiple comorbidities.
- Use two drugs when one may be effective.
- Make drug regimens unnecessarily complicated.
- Use multiple psychotropic drugs, except in very limited circumstances.

Consider

- Drug–drug and drug–disease interactions when prescribing for older patients.
- Using specially designed pillboxes or technologic approaches (eg, devices that help monitor adherence) for selected patients.

References

Budnitz DS, Shehab N, Kegler SR, et al. Medication use leading to emergency department visits for adverse drug events in older adults. *Ann Intern Med.* 2007;147:755-765.

Cockcroft DW, Gault MH. Predictions of creatinine clearance from serum creatinine. *Nephron.* 1976;16:31-41.

Coleman EA, Smith JD, Raha D, et al. Posthospital medication discrepancies. *Arch Intern Med.* 2005;165:1842-1847.

Gill SS, Bronskill SE, Normand S-LT, et al. Antipsychotic drug use and mortality in older adults with dementia. *Ann Intern Med.* 2007;146:775-786.

Glass J, Lanctot KL, Herrmann N, et al. Sedative-hypnotics increase adverse effects more than they improve sleep quality in older persons with insomnia. *BMJ.* 2005; 331:1169-1172.

Heerdink ER, Leufkens HG, Herings RMC, et al. NSAIDs associated with increased risk of congestive heart failure in elderly patients taking diuretics. *Arch Intern Med.* 1998;158:1108-1112.

Holbrook AM, Pereira JA, Labiris R, et al. Systematic overview of warfarin and its drug and food interactions. *Arch Intern Med.* 2005;165:1095-1106.

Holmes HM, Hayley DC, Alexander GC, et al. Reconsidering medication appropriateness for patients late in life. *Arch Intern Med.* 2006;166:605-609.

Lazarou J, Pomeranz BH, Corey PN. Incidence of adverse drug reactions in hospitalized patients: a meta-analysis of prospective studies. *JAMA.* 1998;279:1200-1205.

O'Mahony D, Gallagher PF. Inappropriate prescribing in the older population: need for new criteria. *Age Ageing.* 2008;37:138-141.

Schneider LS, Dagerman KS, Insel P. Risk of death with atypical antipsychotic drug treatment for dementia: meta-analysis of randomized placebo-controlled trials. *JAMA.* 2005;294:1934-1943.

Schneider LS, Tariot PN, Dagerman KS, et al. Effectiveness of atypical antipsychotic drugs in patients with Alzheimer's disease. *N Engl J Med.* 2006;355:1525-1538.

Shrank WH, Polinski JM, Avorn J. Quality indicators for medication use in vulnerable elders. *J Am Geriatr Soc.* 2007;55:S373-S382.

Silber MH. Chronic insomnia. *N Engl J Med.* 2005;353:803-810.

Wang PS, Schneeweiss S, Avorn J, et al. Risk of death in elderly users of conventional vs. atypical antipsychotic medications. *N Engl J Med.* 2005;353:2335-2341.

Wilkinson GR. Drug metabolism and variability among patients in drug response. *N Engl J Med.* 2005;352:2211-2221.

Suggested Readings

Anonymous. Drugs that may cause psychiatric symptoms. *Med Lett.* 2002;44:59-62.

Bain KT. Management of chronic insomnia in elderly persons. *Am J Geriatr Pharmacother.* 2006;4:168-192.

Board of Directors of the American Association for Geriatric Psychiatry, Clinical Practice Committee of the American Geriatrics Society, and Committee on Long-Term Care and Treatment for the Elderly. Psychotherapeutic medications in the nursing home. *J Am Geriatr Soc.* 1992;40:946-949.

Bowie MW, Slattum PW. Pharmacodynamics in older adults: a review. *Am J Geriatr Pharmacother.* 2007;5:263-303.

Carlson DL, Fleming KC, Smith GE, et al. Management of dementia-related behavioral disturbances: a nonpharmacologic approach. *Mayo Clin Proc.* 1995;70:1108-1115.

McCall WV. Diagnosis and management of insomnia in older people. *J Am Geriatr Soc.* 2005;53:S272-S277.

Selma TP, Beizer JL, Higbee MD. *Geriatric Dosage Handbook.* 12th ed. Hudson, OH: Lexi-Comp; 2007.

Wilkinson GR. Drug metabolism and variability among patients in drug response. *N Engl J Med.* 2005;352:2211-2221.

CHAPTER 15

HEALTH SERVICES

Geriatrics can be thought of as the intersection of chronic disease care and gerontology. The latter refers largely to the contents of this book: the syndromes associated with aging, the atypical presentations of disease, and the difficulties of managing multiple, simultaneous, interactive problems. Health care for older persons consists largely of addressing the problems associated with chronic illness. However, medical care continues to be practiced as though it consisted of a series of discrete encounters. What is needed is a systematic approach to chronic care that encourages clinicians to recognize the overall course expected for each patient and to manage treatment within those parameters. Chapter 4 traces a number of strategies designed to improve the management of chronic disease.

Care for frail older persons has been impeded by an artificial dichotomy between medical and social interventions. This separation has been enhanced by the funding policies, such as the auspices of Medicare and Medicaid, but it also reflects the philosophies of the dominant professions. A prerequisite for effective coordination is shared goals. Until the differences in goals are reconciled, there is little hope for integrated care.

Medical practice has been driven by what may be termed a therapeutic model. The basic expectation from medical care is that it will make a difference. The difference may not always be reflected in an improvement in the patient's status. Indeed, for many chronically ill patients decline is inevitable, but good care should at least delay that decline. Because many patients do get worse over time, it may be difficult for clinicians to see the effects of their care. The invisibility of this benefit makes it particularly hard to create a strong case for investing in such care.

Appreciating the benefits of good care in the context of decline in function over time may require a comparison between what happens and what would have occurred in the absence of that care. In effect, the yield from good care is the difference between what is observed and what is reasonable to expect; but without the expected value, the benefit may be hard to appreciate. Figure 15-1 provides a theoretical model of these two curves. Both trajectories show decline, but the slope associated with better care is less acute. The area between them represents the effects of good care. Unfortunately, that benefit is invisible unless specific steps are taken to demonstrate the difference between the observed and expected course. Appreciating the need to make this benefit visible is essential to make the political and social case for a greater investment in chronic disease and long-term care. Without such evidence, people simply see decline and view this area as not worth investing in.

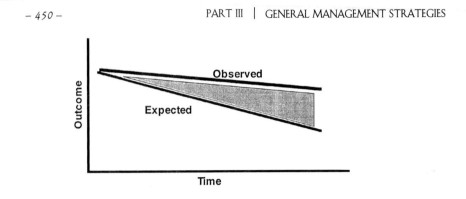

— FIGURE 15-1 —   Theoretical model of observed versus expected clinical course. The area between the observed and expected outcomes represents the benefits of good care. Thus a patient's condition may deteriorate and still be considered as an indication of good care if the rate of deterioration is less than expected.

The alternative model, usually associated with social services, is compensatory care. Under this concept, a person is assessed to determine deficits and a plan of care is developed to address the identified deficits. Good care is defined as providing services that meet the profile of dependencies and thereby allow the client to enjoy as normal a lifestyle as possible without incurring any adverse consequences.

Although these two approaches seem at odds, they could be compatible. Providing needed services should enhance functioning or at least slow its decline. Care for the frail older patient requires a synthesis of medical and social attention. One thing is certain. If the medical and social systems are to work together harmoniously, they must share a common set of goals. The first step in collaboration is to identify the common ground to assure both elements are working in the same direction.

The medical care system has not facilitated that interaction. The new developments in managed care could provide a framework for achieving this coordination, but the track record so far does not suggest that the incentives are yet in place to produce this effect. A few notable programs have been able to merge funding and services for this frail population. Probably the best example of creative integration is seen in the Program of All-inclusive Care of the Elderly (PACE), which uses pooled capitated funding from Medicare and Medicaid to provide integrated health and social services to older persons who are deemed to be eligible for nursing home care but who are still living in the community (Kane, 1999; Eng et al., 1997). Whether managed care will achieve its potential as a vehicle for improving coordination of care for older persons remains to be seen. In any event, care for older persons will require such integration and eventually some reconciliation must be achieved about what constitutes the desired goals of such care.

Geriatric care thus implies team care. This concept implies trust in other disciplines with special skills and training to undertake the tasks for which they have the requisite skills. However, these colleagues must not be expected to operate alone. Good communication and coordination will avoid duplication of effort and lead to a better overall outcome. To play a useful role on the health-care team, physicians need to appreciate what other health professions can do and know how and when to call on their skills. Efficient team care does not involve extensive meetings. Rather, information can be communicated by various means. However, good team care will not arise spontaneously. Just as sports teams spend long hours practicing to work collectively, so too must health-care teams develop a knowledge and trust of each other's inputs. They need a common language and common playbook. Effective teamwork thus requires an investment of effort. Thus, careful thought must be given to when such an investment is justified.

The nature of health care has changed over the past several decades. Figure 15-2 contrasts the patterns of health-care expenditures between 1980 and 2005. There has been a proportionately sharp decrease in the use of hospitals and

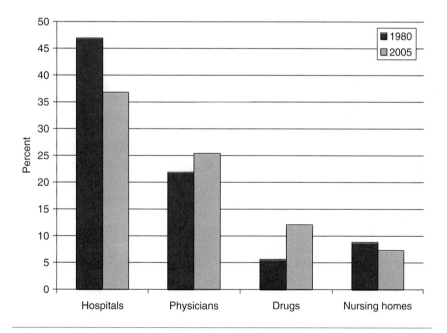

— FIGURE 15-2 —   Distribution of personal health expenditures, 1980 and 2005. (From: Health Care Financing Review, 2007 Statistical Supplement. http:// www.cms. hhs.gov/MedicareMedicaidStatSupp/downloads/07Fig1.1.pdf. Accessed July 2008.)

a marked increase in expenditures on drugs. The costs of physician care have risen and the use of nursing homes has declined. It is important to recall, however, that spending on health care in 1980 was about $215.3 billion, compared to $1661.4 billion in 2005.

PUBLIC PROGRAMS

The physician caring for elderly patients must have at least a working acquaintance with the major programs that support older people. We are accustomed to thinking about care of older people in association with Medicare. In fact, at least three parts (called *Titles*) of the Social Security Act provide important benefits for the elderly: Title XVIII (Medicare), Title XIX (Medicaid), and Social Services Block Grants (formerly Title XX). Medicare was designed to address health care, particularly acute-care hospital services. The Medicare program is in flux. Changes in the payment system have been introduced to counter what some saw as abuses (certainly expansions) of the previous system. The transitions are still in flux. Medicare was intended to deal with long-term care only to the extent that long-term care can supplant more expensive hospital care, leaving the major funding for long-term care to Medicaid. However, the funding demarcation between acute- and long-term care services became blurred. The imposition of a prospective payment for hospitals created a new market for what became post-acute care (PAC), care that was formerly provided in hospitals but could now be delivered and billed separately by nursing homes, rehabilitation units, or home health care. Especially with regard to home health care, Medicare began to cover more care that would be considered long term. In 1993, approximately 60% of home health-care visits under Medicare were delivered to persons who have received such care for at least 6 months, well beyond the traditional designation of acute care (Welch, Wennberg, and Welch, 1996). As a result, a new prospective payment system was introduced for home health care under Medicare. This approach caps the amounts paid and links them to patient characteristics. Long bouts of services are discouraged. The prospective payment approach was eventually applied to each type of PAC, but each was based on a separate calculation. Thus, three silos were created, different approaches to providing similar services. Work is now underway to find a way to recognize this interchangeability and create a single approach to funding.

This distinction in programmatic responsibility between Medicare and Medicaid is a very important one. Whereas Medicare is an insurance-type program to which persons are entitled after contributing a certain amount, Medicaid is a welfare program, eligibility for which depends on a combination of need and poverty. Thus, to become eligible for Medicaid, a person must not only prove illness but also exhaustion of personal resources—hardly a situation conducive to restoring autonomy.

The pattern of coverage is quite different for the various services covered. Figures 15-3 and 15-4 trace spending on health care for elderly persons by

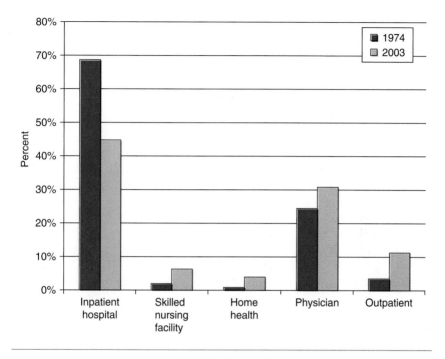

— FIGURE 15-3 — Medicare expenditures by type of service, 1974 and 2003. (From: http://www.cms.hhs.gov/MedicareMedicaidStatSupp/LT/, Table 131. Accessed 4/14/08.)

Medicare and Medicaid, respectively. Medicare is a major payer of hospital and physician care but pays for only a small portion of nursing home care, whereas just the reverse applies to Medicaid. (Medicare has played a larger role in nursing home and home health care as the role of PAC grew, but new funding priorities have attempted to reduce that role.)

Medicare

Eligibility for Medicare differs for each of its two major parts. Part A (Hospital Services Insurance) is available to all who are eligible for Social Security, usually by virtue of paying the Social Security tax for a sufficient number of quarters. This program is supported by a special payroll tax, which goes into the Medicare Trust Fund. Part B (Medical Services Insurance) is offered for a monthly premium, paid by the individual but heavily subsidized by the government (which pays approximately 70% of the cost from general tax revenues). Almost everyone older than age 65 is automatically covered by Part A. (Federal, state, and local government

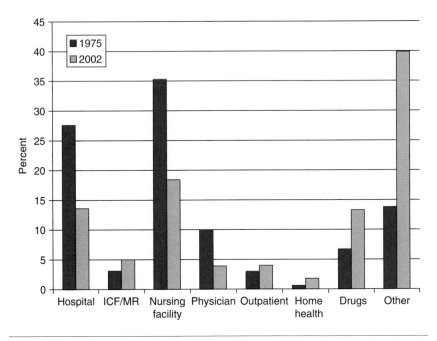

— FIGURE 15-4 —   Medicaid expenditures by type of service, 1975 and 2002. (From: http://www.cms.hhs.gov/MedicareMedicaidStatSupp/LT/, Table 101. Accessed 9/23/07.)

employees are exceptions; until recently they were not covered by social security and had their own pension and medical programs.) The introduction of prospective payment for hospitals under Medicare created a new set of complications. Hospitals are paid a fixed amount per admission according to the diagnosis-related group (DRG), to which the patient is assigned on the basis of the admitting diagnosis. The rates for DRGs are, in turn, based on expected lengths of stay and intensity of care for each condition. The incentives in such an approach run almost directly contrary to most of the goals of geriatrics. Whereas geriatrics addresses the functional result of multiple interacting problems, DRGs encourage concentration on a single problem. Extra time required to make an appropriate discharge plan is discouraged. Use of ancillary personnel, such as social workers, is similarly discouraged. As a result of DRGs, hospital lengths of stay have decreased, leading to the phenomenon of "quicker and sicker" discharges. Many of these former hospital patients are now cared for through home health and nursing homes. In effect, Medicare is paying for care twice: It pays for the hospital stay regardless of length and then pays for the posthospital care. The rapid rise in this latter sector has led Medicare to search for solutions. Different types of Medicare prospective payment for the different types of posthospital care have been established. Nursing homes are paid on a per-diem basis, whereas home health agencies and rehabilitation units are paid on a per-episode basis. A more effective solution would be to combine the payment for hospital and posthospital care into a single-bundled payment, although some fear that such a step would place too much control in the hands of hospitals. The Balanced Budget Act of 1997 (BBA) included a small step in this direction. For selected DRGs, hospital discharges to PAC are treated as transfers. Hospitals receive a lower payment than the usual DRG payment if the length of stay is less than the median.

Up until recently, the payment system was even more paradoxical. The DRG payment was higher for patients with complications, even if those complications arose from treatment during the hospitalization. That approach has been modified to exclude iatrogenic complications, creating a better business case for involving geriatricians in the care of frail patients.

The payment systems now in effect create much confusion for Medicare beneficiaries. Although hospitals are paid a fixed amount per case, the patients continue to pay under a system of deductibles and co-payments.

Managed care is aggressively being pursued as an option to traditional fee-for-service care. Under that arrangement, the managed care organizations receive a fixed monthly payment from Medicare in exchange for providing at least the range of services covered by Medicare. Although many managed care companies were initially attracted to this business because of the generous rates offered, subsequent reductions have made the business less attractive and many are exiting the program, leaving beneficiaries to scramble for alternative coverage, especially for the so-called Medigap policies that pay for deductibles and co-payments.

The pricing system used by Medicare basically reflects the prices paid for fee-for-service care in each county. Managed care organizations are paid a fixed amount calculated on the basis of the average amount Medicare paid for its beneficiaries in that county. This adjusted average per capita cost (AAPCC) varies widely from one location to another. Newer approaches to calculating Medicare-managed care premiums use prior utilization and other factors in what is called hierarchical clinical conditions (HCC). The BBA called for a shift to national pricing. In an effort to attract more providers into managed care, the BBA broadened the definition of what kinds of organizations can provide managed care to Medicare beneficiaries, removing many of the restrictions (especially financial surety bonding) that left managed care largely in the hands of insurance companies. Unlike managed care enrollees in the rest of the population, who are locked into health plans for a year, Medicare beneficiaries have the right to disenroll at any time. There is some evidence to suggest that Medicare beneficiaries may move in and out of managed care as they use up available benefits. The future of managed care as a Medicare venue is still unclear. The current administration continues to back this approach despite the number of managed care companies exiting from the market. In 2005, Medicare Advantage (the name for managed care under Medicare) covered 15.4% of Medicare beneficiaries.

The likelihood of managed care achieving its potential symbiosis with geriatrics appears dim. Ideally, managed care could provide an environment where many of the principles of geriatrics could be implemented to the benefit of all; on the other hand, the performance to date suggests that managed care for Medicare beneficiaries has so far responded more to the incentives from favorable selection (recruiting healthy patients and getting paid average rates), discounted purchasing of services, and barriers to access than to the potential benefits from increased efficiency derived from a geriatric philosophy (Kane, 1998).

Although Medicare does pay for authorized posthospital services in nursing homes and through home health care, the payment for physicians does not encourage their active participation. For example, while a physician would be paid a regular consultation visit fee for daily rounds on a Medicare patient in a hospital, if the patient is discharged to a nursing home the following day, both the rate of physician reimbursement for a visit and the number of visits per week considered customary decrease dramatically. Although physician home visits are still a rarity, payment for these services has increased substantially in recent years. There are now physician groups that have made a business out of nursing home care and home health care. An interesting model of Medicare-managed care directed specifically at nursing home residents is Evercare, which makes active use of nurse practitioners to increase the primary care attention residents receive. They have shown that it is possible to reduce the use of hospital care by this means (Kane et al., 2003).

Many Medicare beneficiaries have also purchased so-called Medigap insurance. This insurance comes in a variety of forms (federal law now dictates the various components); most of this insurance covers only the gaps up to the ceilings established by Medicare (ie, it pays deductibles and coinsurance but generally does not cover the difference between billed charges and allowable charges). An increasing number of policies cover at least some drug costs. In some cases, older persons may have purchased multiple Medigap policies under the erroneous assumption they were buying more coverage.

Medicare coverage is important but not sufficient for three basic reasons: (1) To control use, it mandates deductible and co-payment charges for both Parts A and B. (2) It sets physician's fees by a complicated formula called the Resource-Based Relative Value Scale (RBRVS). The RBRVS is designed to pay physicians more closely according to the value of their services as determined both within a specialty and across specialties. Theoretically, both the value of the services provided and the investment in training are considered in setting the rates. This new payment approach was intended to increase the payment for primary care relative to surgical specialties, but early reports suggest that, ironically, many geriatric assessment services have been reimbursed at a level lower than before its introduction. Under Medicare Part B, physicians are generally paid less than they would usually bill for the service. (Some physicians opt to bill the patient directly for the difference but a number of states have mandated that physicians accept "assignment" of Medicare fees, that is, they accept the fee [plus the 20% co-payment] as payment in full.) (3) The program does not cover several services essential to patient functioning, such as eyeglasses, hearing aids, and many preventive services (although the benefits for the latter are expanding). Medicare specifically excludes services designed to provide "custodial care"—the very services often most critical to long-term care. (However, as noted above, the boundary between acute- and long-term care exclusions seems to be eroding.)

A major expansion of the Medicare program occurred in 2005 with the passage of the Medicare Modernization Act, which included Part D coverage of drugs. This legislation also provides substantial incentives to Medicare Advantage providers and creates a new class of managed care coverage, Special Needs Plans. These are groups of beneficiaries presumed to be at high risk and hence eligible for higher premiums.

The coverage of prescription drugs involves a complicated formula, often referred to as the "doughnut hole," because of the odd design of benefits. Basically, the patient pays a deductible ($275 in 2008). Then the drug plan pays 75% of the yearly drug costs from $275 to $2,510, and the plan pays the other 75% of these costs. Then the patient pays 100% of the next $3,216.25 in drug costs and after that a coinsurance amount (like 5% of the drug cost) or a co-payment (like $2.25 or $5.60 for each prescription) for the rest of the calendar year after the patient has spent $4,050 out of pocket. The patient's plan pays the rest. Part D is administered by a series of drug management firms that offer a confusing array of plans. From a basic plan that covers the Part D pattern to more inclusive coverage that eliminates the doughnut hole. Of course, the premium cost rises as the coverage expands. Plans are required to cover at least two drugs in each identified category but the choice of drugs is left to them. Medicare beneficiaries must scramble to find the most affordable plan that covers the drugs they need, but even then there is no guarantee that those drugs will continue to be covered.

As a result of these three factors, a substantial amount of the medical bill is left to the individual. Today, elderly persons' out-of-pocket costs for health care represent more than 20% of their income, a figure comparable to before the passage of Medicare. In general, out-of-pocket costs are less for those in managed care.

Medicaid

Medicaid, in contrast to Medicare, is a welfare program designed to serve the poor. It is a state-run program to which the federal government contributes (50%-78% of the costs, depending on the state's capita income). In some states, persons can be covered as medically indigent even if their income is above the poverty level if their medical expenses would impoverish them. As a welfare program, Medicaid has no deductibles or coinsurance (although current proposals call for modest charges to discourage excess use). It is, however, a welfare program cast in the medical model.

It is important to appreciate that the shape of the Medicaid expenditures for older people is determined largely by the gaps in Medicare. Medicaid serves primarily two distinct groups: mothers and young children under Aid to Families with Dependent Children and elderly persons eligible for Old Age Assistance. The other major route to eligibility for older people is the medically needy program, whereby eligibility is conferred when medical costs—usually nursing homes—exceed a fixed fraction of a person's income. Medicaid has been described as a universal health program that had a deductible of all of your assets and a co-pay of all of your income. The numerically larger group made up of mothers and children use less care per capita. They use some hospital care around birth and for the small group of severely ill children. A large portion of the Medicaid dollar goes to the services needed by the elderly enrollees, most of whom are also eligible for Medicare, but the services needed are not covered by Medicare, namely nursing home care and community-based long-term care. (Most states automatically enroll eligible Medicaid recipients in Medicare Part B.)

Medicaid is the major source of nursing home payments. It requires physicians to certify a patient's physical limitations in order to gain the patient admittance to a nursing home. In some cases physicians may have to invent medical justifications for primarily social reasons (ie, lack of social supports necessary to remain in the community).

Medicaid is thus important in shaping nursing home policies. It pays about half of the nursing costs but covers almost 70% of the residents. The discrepancy is explained by the policies that require residents to expend their own resources first. Thus Social Security payments, private pensions, and the like are used as primary sources of payment, and Medicaid picks up the remainder. However, it does not directly pay for most physician care in the nursing home; that is covered by Medicare. Medicaid would pay the deductibles and co-payments and those services not covered under Medicare.

Medicaid also supports home- and community-based long-term care services (HCBS). In some states personal care is included as mandatory Medicaid service, but in many states HCBS is offered as a waivered service. Under this arrangement, the federal government allows states to use money that would otherwise have gone to nursing homes to fund HCBS. The waiver allows states to offer the service in only specific areas and to limit the numbers of persons enrolled in the program. In theory, these funds are supposed to be offset by concomitant savings in nursing home care.

Whereas going on Medicaid was once seen as a great social embarrassment, associated with accepting public charity, there appears to be a growing sense among many older persons that they are entitled to receive Medicaid help when their health-care expenses, especially their long-term care costs, are high. The stigma appears to be displaced by the idea that they paid taxes for many years and are now entitled to reap the rewards. As a result of this shift in sentiment, at least in the states with generous levels of Medicaid eligibility, there is a burgeoning industry of financial advisers to assist older persons in preparing to become Medicaid eligible. Because eligibility is usually based on both income and assets, such a step necessitates advance planning. Usually state laws require that assets transferred within two or more years of applying for Medicaid funds are considered to still be owned. (The situation is more complicated in the case of a married couple, where provisions have been made to allow the spouse to retain part of the family's assets.) This requirement means that older persons contemplating becoming eligible for Medicaid must be willing to divest themselves of their assets at least several years in advance of the time they expect to need such help. This step places them in a very dependent position, financially and psychologically. Much has been made of the "divestiture phenomenon" whereby older people scheme to divest themselves of their assets in order to qualify for Medicaid, but there is no good evidence about the scale of the phenomenon.

There is also growing enthusiasm for promoting various forms of private long-term care insurance. This coverage, in effect, protects the assets of those who might otherwise be marginally eligible for Medicaid or who simply want to preserve an inheritance for their heirs. Like any insurance linked to age-related events but to a greater degree, long-term care insurance is quite affordable when purchased at a young age (when the likelihood of needing it is very low) but becomes quite expensive as the buyer reaches age 75 or older. Thus, those most likely to consider buying it would have to pay a premium close to the average cost of long-term care itself. Only a small number of young persons have shown any interest in purchasing such coverage, especially when companies are not anxious to add it to their employee benefit packages as a free benefit. Although economic projections suggest that private long-term care insurance is not likely to save substantial money for the Medicaid program, several states have developed programs to encourage individuals to purchase the insurance by offering linked Medicaid benefits.

Other Programs

The third part of the Social Security legislation pertinent to older persons is Title XX, now administered as Social Services Block Grants. This is also a welfare program targeted especially to those on categorical welfare programs such as Aid to Families with Dependent Children and, more germane, Supplemental Security Income. The latter is a federal program, which, as the name implies, supplements Social Security benefits to provide a minimum income. Title XX funds are administered through state and local agencies, which have a substantial amount of flexibility in how they allocate the available money across a variety of stipulated services. The state also has the option of broadening the eligibility criteria to include those just above the poverty line.

Another relevant federal program is Title III of the Older Americans Act. This program is available to all persons over the age of 60 regardless of income. The single largest component goes to support nutrition through congregate meal programs where elderly persons can get a subsidized hot meal, but it also provides meals-on-wheels (home-delivered meals) and a wide variety of other services. Some services duplicate or supplement those covered under Social Security programs; others are unique.

Table 15-1 summarizes these four programs and their current scope. It is important to appreciate that this summary attempts to condense and simplify a complex and ever-changing set of rules and regulations. Physicians should be familiar with the broad scope and limitations of these programs but will have to rely on others, especially social workers, who are familiar with the operating details.

LONG-TERM CARE

A proportion of older patients require substantial long-term care. There is no uniform definition for long-term care, but the following description of the term highlights the important aspects: "A range of services that addresses the health, personal care, and social needs of individuals who lack some capacity for self-care. Services may be continuous or intermittent but are delivered for sustained periods to individuals who have a demonstrated need, usually measured by some index of functional incapacity." This statement emphasizes the common thread of most discussions of long-term care: the dependence of an individual on the services of another for a substantial period. The definition is carefully vague about who provides those services or what they are. Figure 15-5 illustrates the diverse sources of care for frail older people. Over two-thirds live in the community. Of these the majority rely solely on unpaid care, and another large group use a mixture of paid and unpaid care. A little more than 20% are in nursing homes, and another 8% are in some other form of residential care. Long-term care is certainly not the exclusive purview of the medical profession; in fact, most of the long-term care in this country is not provided by professionals at all, but by a host of individuals loosely referred to as *informal support*. These persons may be family, friends, or neighbors.

Informal care has been and remains the backbone of long-term care. In many instances, the family (and often nonrelatives) is the first line of support. The ideal program would keep older people at home, relying on family care and bolstering their efforts with more formal assistance to provide professional services and occasional respite care. More than 80% of all the care given in the community comes from informal sources. (In truth, the proportion is higher because much of the formal care is made possible by a substrate of informal care.) Surprisingly, this figure seems to remain fairly constant in countries with more generous provision of formal long-term care. Many observers have questioned whether the informal care role, which is largely performed by women, can be sustained as

TABLE 15-1   SUMMARY OF MAJOR FEDERAL PROGRAMS FOR ELDERLY PATIENTS

Program	Eligible Population	Services Covered	Deductibles and Co-payments
Medicare (Title XVIII of the Social Security Act) Part A: Hospital Services Insurance	All persons eligible for social security and others with chronic disabilities, such as end-stage renal disease, plus voluntary enrollees age 65+ years	Per benefit period, "reasonable cost" (DRG-based) for 90 days of hospital care plus 60 lifetime reserve days; 100 days of skilled nursing facility (SNF); home health visits (see text); hospice care*	Full coverage for hospital care after a deductible of about 1 day for days 2-60; then one-quarter day co-pay for days 61-90. Can use "lifetime reserve" days thereafter. 20 SNF days fully covered; one 8-day co-pay for days 21-100
Part B: Supplemental Medical Insurance	All those covered under Part A who elect coverage; participants pay a monthly premium	80% of "reasonable cost" for physicians' services; supplies and services related to physician services; outpatient, physical, and speech therapy; diagnostic tests and radiographs; mammograms; surgical dressings; prosthetics; ambulance	Deductible and 20% co-payment (no co-pay after a limit reached)

– 461 –

TABLE 15-1   SUMMARY OF MAJOR FEDERAL PROGRAMS FOR ELDERLY PATIENTS (*Continued*)

Program	Eligible Population	Services Covered	Deductibles and Co-payments
Medicaid (Title XIX of the Social Security Act)	Persons receiving Supplemental Security Income (SSI) (such as welfare) or receiving SSI and state supplement or meeting lower eligibility standards used for medical assistance criteria in 1972 or eligible for SSI or were in institutions and eligible for Medicaid in 1973; medically needy, who do not qualify for SSI but have high medical expenses are eligible for Medicaid in some states; eligibility criteria vary from state to state	Mandatory services for categorically needy: Inpatient hospital services; outpatient services; SNF; limited home health care; laboratory tests and radiographs; family planning; early and periodic screening, diagnosis, and treatment for children through age 20 Optional services vary from state to state: Dental care; therapies; drugs; intermediate-care facilities; extended home health care; private duty nurse; eyeglasses; prostheses; personal-care services; medical transportation and home health care services (states can limit the amount and duration of services)	None, once patient spends down to eligibility level Spend-down based on income and assets

Program	Eligibility	Services	Payment
Social Services Block Grant (Title XX of the Social Security Act)	All recipients of TANF and SSI; optionally, those earning up to 115% of state median income and residents of specific geographic areas	Day care; substitute care; protective services; counseling; home-based services; employment, education, and training; health-related services; information and referral; transportation; day services; family planning; legal services; home-delivered and congregate meals	Fees are charged to those with family incomes > 80% of state's median income
Title III of the Older Americans Act	All persons age 60 and older; low-income, minority, and isolated older persons are special targets	Homemaker; home-delivered meals; home health aides; transportation; legal services; counseling; information and referral plus 19 others (50% of funds must go to those listed)	Some payment may be requested

*Certified hospice providers are paid a preset amount when a patient who is certified as terminal opts for this benefit in lieu of regular Medicare.

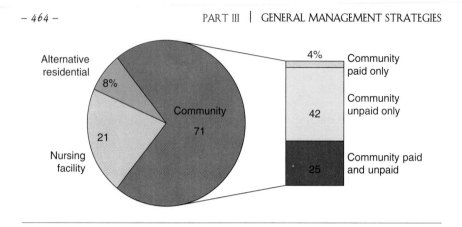

— FIGURE 15-5 —   Sources of care for frail older persons. (From: 1999 National Long-Term Care Survey, 2002 Medicare Current Beneficiary Survey, and 2005 CMS Minimum Data Set.)

more women enter the labor force and are already managing several roles. Despite dire predictions about its inevitable collapse, there is yet no evidence of serious decline in informal care. It is important to bear in mind that as the age of frailty rises, the "children" of these frail older people may themselves be in their seventh and eighth decades.

The best estimates suggest that about 15% of the elderly population need the help of another person to manage their daily lives. The good news is that the prevalence of disability among older persons has declined about 1% per year over the last several decades, as shown in Fig. 15-6. At the same time, the proportion of persons who have difficulty performing one or more activity of daily living (ADL) or instrumental ADL (IADL) increases with age, from approximately 6.5% at age 65 to 69 to 27% at age 80 to 84, and over 80% at age 95+ (see Fig. 15-7). The sum effect of the relative decline in disability and the substantial growth in the elderly population will produce major increase in the numbers of disabled persons (Cutler, 2001). That forecast is shown in Fig. 15-8. Recall that for each person in a nursing home today, there are between one and three equally disabled persons living in the community. Thus, the first instincts are not always the best. Physicians have been trained to respond to the dependent elderly person by thinking of admission to a nursing home. Nursing home placement should be the *last* resort, not the first. Physicians should consider the importance of maximizing both quality of care and quality of life. For many frail older persons, the personal price of living in a nursing home is too high. Many would prefer to remain in the community, even if it means taking the risk of getting less care, which is not necessarily the case.

Current practice is trying to shift the balance between institutional care and home- and community-based services to emphasize use of the latter (Kane et al., 1998).

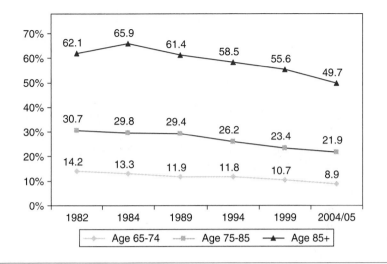

— FIGURE 15-6 — Change in prevalence of chronic disability (impairment in ADLs or IADLs) by age group, 1982-2004. (Data compiled from Manton, Gu, and Lamb, 2006.)

The waiver programs noted earlier are designed to do just that. The tide is turning; the use of nursing homes is declining. Another major factor that has reduced the use of nursing homes has been assisted living. This concept has taken on a variety of meanings as it has been actively marketed.

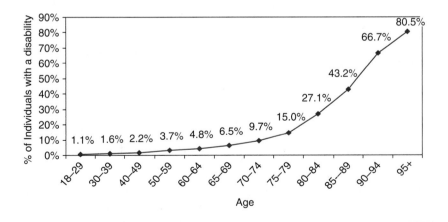

— FIGURE 15-7 — Prevalence of disability by age. (From: 1999 National Long Term Care Survey and the 1994 National Health Interview Survey Disability Supplement.)

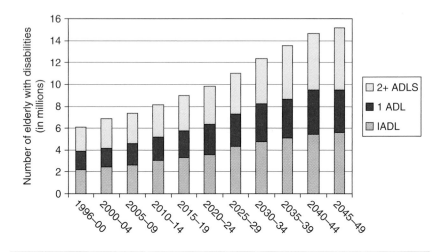

— FIGURE 15-8 —   Projected growth in numbers of older persons with disabilities, 1996-2050. (From: The Lewin Group based on the Long-Term Care Financing Model.)

Why then does our system rely so heavily on the nursing home? Several reasons can be posited. First, nursing homes are available; there are more nursing home beds than acute-care hospital beds in this country. Nonetheless, there is usually a waiting list to get in, especially into a relatively good home. (That situation is beginning to change, however. With the growth in alternatives, especially assisted living, we are seeing for the first time substantial numbers of empty nursing home beds.) Second, nursing home care is cheap; it runs around $100 a day in most states, while a hospital day costs at least $1000, and even a good hotel room costs more than $100. Finally, and related to the first two points, the nursing home comes as an already assembled package of services. The programs to cover long-term care services have become a complex maze of eligibility and regulations, which has not encouraged anyone to develop innovative alternatives. The pressure for faster discharge from hospitals has created a new industry of post-acute nursing home care. Although changes in Medicare payment have dampened some of the enthusiasm, this sector is still vital.

There have been periodic efforts to develop alternatives to nursing home care. Some were the results of deliberate public policies; others arose as new marketing efforts. For a period of time, great effort was expended trying to find less-expensive ways of caring for people needing long-term care in the community. The upshot of these efforts was the recognition that community care is preferable in many cases, but not always cheaper. A major difficulty in controlling the cost of this care is the potential for widespread use. Because a large number of dependent older persons live in the community, a dependency-based eligibility system will include many people who would not opt for a nursing home. This need to control entry has stimulated great interest in case management. The continuing need to improve community care has led to some innovations, including Medicaid waiver programs that allow use of nursing home funds for community care if the total long-term care budget is kept constant. As a result, there has been uneven development of community programs in different parts of the country.

The earlier emphasis on seeking community-based alternatives to nursing home care has shifted to some extent to developing other mechanisms for providing the combined housing and service functions. Among these are assisted living and adult foster care. Assisted living, in effect, renders the recipient first and foremost a tenant, who has control over her singly occupied living space (eg, a lock on the door and determination about waking and retiring times). In addition to single occupancy, the client's autonomy is reinforced by providing modest cooking and refrigeration facilities, which allow the person to function independently without relying exclusively on the services of the institution and even to entertain modestly (Kane, 2001). However, as assisted living became a more desirable product, it began to lose its identity. A variety of providers surfaced, many of whom offered very different services under that name. Today, it is hard to know just what one is getting when assisted living is cited.

Adult foster care homes are usually limited to a small number of clients in any home (usually no more than five). Single rooms are not required; the situation is more analogous to individuals taking clients into their own homes, with small numbers of flexibly deployed nonprofessional staff. Recent trends suggest that the historic growth in nursing home use is changing. The last few years have witnessed a decline in nursing home occupancy. At least some of this effect undoubtedly comes from the growing availability of other residential models, which consumers find more attractive.

At the same time, there is concern that a preoccupation with a search for alternatives to nursing homes may distract efforts from the sorely needed work to improve the quality of nursing home care. Even in the best situation, a substantial number of older persons will continue to need such care. One scenario for the future holds that the form of nursing homes will change. Many of the residents currently cared for in nursing homes will be treated in more flexible situations, like assisted living, which emphasize living arrangements with nursing and other services brought to the residents on a more individualized basis. Those patients needing more intensive care will be treated in more medically oriented facilities. Figure 15-9 shows the various payment sources for covering long-term care costs. Medicaid and out-of-pocket payments cover about three-fourths of the costs.

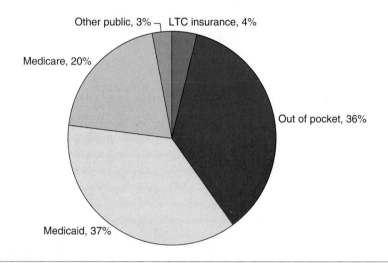

— FIGURE 15-9 — Sources of long-term care payments, 2006 ($150.8 billion). (From: The Lewin Group based on the Long-Term Care Financing Model.)

THE NURSING HOME

Despite its frequent vilification, the nursing home is an important part of the health-care delivery system for frail older persons. Virtually without planning, it has emerged as the touchstone of long-term care. Given its origins as the stepchild of the almshouse and the hospital, it is not surprising that it has enjoyed a poor reputation. Since the passage of the Medicaid legislation in 1965, the nursing home industry has gone through growth and transformation. As a reaction to scandals during the early years, nursing homes are heavily regulated.

Today's nursing homes operate under two different principles, which compli- cate any attempt to describe them. For one group of clients admitted from hospitals for rehabilitation, they function as Medicare posthospital care providers, responsi- ble for administering rehabilitative and restorative services to get these persons back into community living as soon as possible. For another stream of clients (often supported by Medicaid), they provide long-term care, which may last a lifetime.

Seen from one vantage point, the term *nursing home* is a misnomer. Although these institutions are better staffed and run than in the past, they remain generally somber places that offer their residents neither a great deal of real nursing care nor a very homelike environment.

Most nursing home residents are required to share their rooms. There is little privacy and few opportunities to retain control over even small parts of one's life. Fire regulations often prevent residents from bringing personal furniture into the homes. The nursing home is not a miniature hospital. Nursing homes are smaller and less well-staffed than hospitals. Whereas a hospital has a ratio of greater than three staff for each bed, the nursing home has only about a sixth of that number, and most of those staff are aides. Whereas the distinction whereby nursing homes were certified as being capable of caring for patients with different needs based on these levels has been abandoned, the distinction between nursing home care and that provided in purely residential facilities with little or no nursing component has been retained. But even here the boundaries are blurred. Some forms of assisted living seek to serve a population that heavily overlaps the long-term care groups served by nursing homes.

Admission to a nursing home is very much a function of age. Figure 15-10 illustrates two separate trends in the nursing home utilization picture. (1) There is a sharp rise in the rate of nursing home use with each decade after age 65, such that only about 1% of people age 65 to 74 are in nursing homes, but 4% of those age 74 to 85 and 14% of those age 85 or more are in nursing homes. (2) At the same time, the proportion of older persons in nursing homes has decreased substantially from 1973 to 2004. The greatest change has been seen in the oldest group. Much of this shift can be traced to the use of alternative residential settings. Figure 15-11 contrasts the patterns of institutional care use in 1985 and 2004. Especially among those 85+ there was substantial use of alternative residential settings.

Table 15-2 shows the dynamic nature of long-term care today. A cohort of persons turning 65 can expect, on an average, to require 3 years of care. Of those who actually use care, the span will be about 4.3 years. Overall, the care will be divided between community care (1.9 years) and facility-based care (1.1 years).

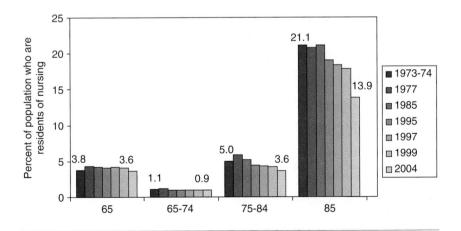

— FIGURE 15-10 —   Change in the rate of nursing home use by age group, 1973-2004. (From: 1973-1974, 1997, 1985, 1995, 1997, 1999, and 2004 National Nursing Home Survey.)

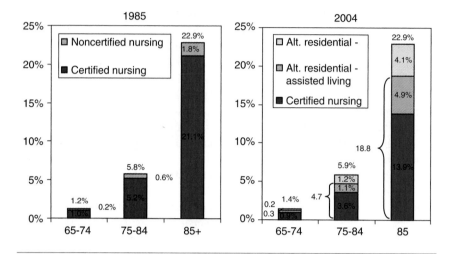

— FIGURE 15-11 — Use of different types of institutional long-term care by age group, 1985 and 2004. (From: 1985 and 2004 National Nursing Home Survey and 2002 Medicare Current Beneficiary Survey.)

TABLE 15-2   REMAINING LIFETIME USE OF LONG-TERM SUPPORTIVE SERVICES (LTSS) BY PEOPLE TURNING 65 IN 2005

TYPE OF CARE	AVG. YEARS OF CARE	% OF PEOPLE USING	AVG. YEARS OF CARE AMONG USERS
All LTSS need	3.0	69	4.3
At home			
Informal care only	1.4	59	2.4
Formal care	0.5	42	1.2
Any care at home	1.9	65	2.9
In facilities			
Nursing facilities	0.8	35	2.3
Assisted living	0.3	13	2.3
Any care in facilities	1.1	37	3.0

Reproduced with permission from Kemper P, Komisar HL, Alecxih L. Long-term care over an uncertain future: what can current retirees expect? *Inquiry*. 2005/2006; Winter 42(4):335-350.

For the actual users the split between community and institutional care is about even, as is the split between time in assisted living and in a nursing home.

The other factor that may complicate forecasts is the growing number of people who are suffering from diseases that reflect lifestyle choices. As shown in Fig. 15-12, the risk of nursing home use rises sharply with the presence of conditions like hypertension and diabetes. Moreover, both are exacerbated by a lack of physical activity.

The residents in nursing homes are distinguishable from older persons living in the community on several basic parameters. As shown in Table 15-3, in addition to being older, they are more likely to be white, female, unmarried, and have multiple chronic problems.

Nursing home users appear to have become more disabled in the last several years. Some attribute this change to the impact of DRGs, but the trend had begun well in advance of that change. The contemporary nursing home user is older and more disabled than in the past.

Any effort to describe the nursing home resident population must recognize that the nursing home plays multiple roles. It caters to a wide variety of clientele. At least five distinct groups of residents can be identified.

1. Those actively recuperating or being rehabilitated. These are largely persons discharged from hospitals and are expected to have a short course in the nursing home before returning home. This care has been called "subacute" or "transitional." The evidence of the nursing home's capacity to provide effective care of this type is mixed (Kramer et al., 1997; Kane et al., 1996).
2. Those with substantial physical dependencies. These residents need regular and usually frequent assistance during the day. Their care could be managed in the community with sufficient formal and informal support.

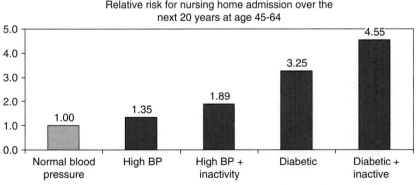

— FIGURE 15-12 —   Relative likelihood of using a nursing home as function of potentially changeable lifestyle disease. (Data compiled from Valiyeva E et al., 2006.)

TABLE 15-3   COMPARISON OF NURSING HOME RESIDENTS AND THE
NONINSTITUTIONALIZED POPULATION AGE 65, 1995

	PERCENT OF NURSING HOME RESIDENTS[*]	PERCENT OF NONINSTITUTIONALIZED POPULATION[†]
Age (years)		
65-74	17.5	55.9
75-84	42.3	33.2
85+	40.2	10.8
Sex		
Male	24.7	40.8
Female	75.3	59.2
Race		
White	89.5	89.6
Black	8.5	8.1
Other	2	2.3
Marital status		
Married	16.5	56.9
Widowed	66	33.2
Divorced and/or separated	5.5	5.7
Never married/single	11.1	4.2
Unknown	0.8	—

[*]From Dey, 1997.
[†]From US Census Bureau, 1996.

3. Those with primarily severe cognitive losses. These people present special management problems because of their behavior and their propensity to wander. Some favor separate facilities for them, primarily to remove them from the environment of those who are cognitively intact. There is no evidence of improvement in the outcomes of demented residents from these "special care units" (Phillips, Sloane, and Hawes, 1997).

4. Those receiving terminal care. This hospice care is directed toward making the person as comfortable as possible. Palliative care is provided, but no heroic efforts are undertaken.

5. Those in a permanent vegetative state. This group is distinguished by its inability to relate to the environment. Care is primarily directed toward avoiding complications (eg, decubitus ulcers).

For those who are sensitive to their environments and likely to be in the nursing home for some time (ie, groups 2 and 4), quality-of-life issues will be at least as salient as traditional technical quality-of-care issues (Kane, 2001).

Especially in the wake of changing hospital practice and the rise of "subacute care," great care must be exercised in using nursing home data because of the differences in the characteristics of those entering or leaving and those residing at any point in time. The latter are more likely to have chronic problems such as dementia, whereas the former will have problems that are either rehabilitable or fatal (eg, hip fracture and cancer). This distinction makes it tricky to talk about nursing home patients and may explain the often contradictory data presented.

The problem with data about nursing home residents is made more confusing when different approaches to sampling are used. The characteristics of discharges are different from those of a cross-section of residents. The former have shorter lengths of stay, whereas the latter have a preponderance of dementia.

Payment for nursing home care has been increasingly based on measures that reflect the costs of providing that care. Although this type of payment is often called "prospective reimbursement," it is important to recognize that it is quite different from that used with hospitals. Nursing home prospective payment is calculated on a daily rate basis in contrast to the episode basis used for hospitals. Hence as a person's status changes, so does the payment. Medicare payments now use a daily prospective payment rate based on case mix and many states are adapting a corresponding approach for Medicaid payments, although the specific systems may use fewer categories. This form of case-mix reimbursement is largely driven by the costs of the nursing personnel, who provide that care. The costs are usually calculated by estimating these costs based on a set of observed times spent by different types of personnel (nurses' aides, LPNs, and RNs) for different classes of residents. In some cases, the time spent is self-reported by the staff; in other instances, it is based on observations. These data are then used to construct models that relate the cost of professional time to the characteristics of the clients. This approach has two major problems.

1. The models generally rely on looking at what kind of care is being given rather than what sort of care is actually needed; the care is not related to outcomes obtained nor is it based on any models of especially good care.
2. The logic behind this approach to estimating payments is inherently perverse. If carried to its logical extreme, this system of payment rewards nursing homes for residents becoming more dependent instead of more independent.

The most commonly used case-mix system is the resource utilization groups (RUGs). Since its development for use in New York, it has been revised several times and is now linked to a form of the Minimum Data Set (MDS), which is the mandated assessment approach for nursing home care. Figure 15-13 illustrates the RUGs-III approach to classifying nursing home residents according to

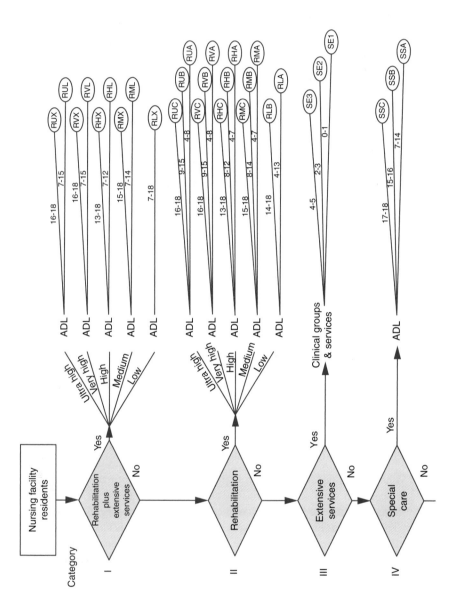

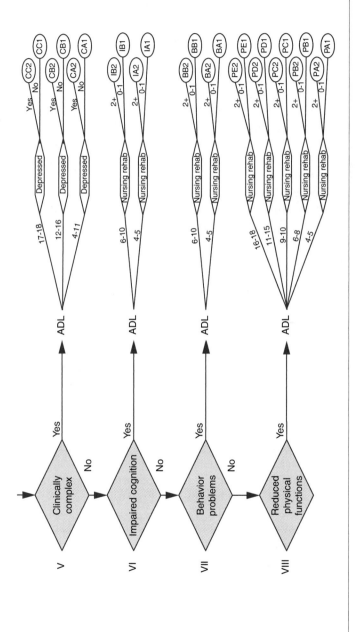

—FIGURE 15-13 — The resource utilization group (RUG-III) case-mix classification system. RUGs are generated from items in the Minimum Data Set (MDS) and used as a basis for case-mix reimbursement. (Courtesy of Meyers and Stauffer, LC.)

groups that imply different levels of staffing needs. This approach has been used by some Medicaid programs and is the basis for Medicare skilled nursing facility payments.

The physician's role in nursing home care is discussed in greater detail in Chap. 16. Suffice it to say here that the nursing home has not been an attractive place for physicians to practice. However, conditions are changing. The physician can play a critical role in setting the tone for the care of patients in the nursing home. Physicians' expectations of professional performance and their advocacy of their patients' needs can be very influential in shaping staff behavior.

New types of personnel can be used effectively to deliver primary care to nursing home patients. Nurse practitioners and physician assistants deliver high-quality care in this setting (Kane et al., 2003). Medicare regulations covering Part B were altered to allow greater use of physician assistants and nurse practitioners. Similarly, clinical pharmacists are very helpful for simplifying drug regimens and avoiding potential drug interactions.

A managed care program directed specifically at nursing home patients points to the art of the possible. Building on the prior successes of using nurse practitioners as key figures to provide primary care to nursing home residents, the Evercare program has developed Medicare-managed care risk contracts specifically for long-stay nursing home patients. Under this arrangement, Evercare is responsible for all the residents' Medicare costs (both Part A and Part B) but not their nursing home costs. The underlying concept is that by providing more aggressive primary care, they can prevent hospital admissions.

Evercare places nurse practitioners in each participating nursing home to work with the residents' own physicians. The nurse practitioners provide closer follow-up and work closely with the nursing home staff to identify problems early. In some cases, Evercare will pay the nursing home extra to increase nursing attention for patients in order to treat that person in the nursing home rather than admitting the patient to a hospital. The theory is that the savings from avoided or shortened hospital stays will offset the added costs of more attentive primary care provided by the nurse practitioners. The apparent success of the Evercare model has spawned similar approaches.

A study by the Institute of Medicine pointed to the need for reforms, many of which were incorporated into Omnibus Budget Reconciliation Act of 1987 (OBRA 1987). The implementation of the OBRA 1987 regulations has produced a number of changes in the way nursing homes are operated. In addition to the standardized assessment mandated in the MDS (described in Chap. 16), the emphasis in regulation has shifted more toward addressing the outcomes of patient care; but some increases in process measures have also been introduced. For example, guidelines for the use of psychoactive drugs have been mandated. All residents admitted and already living in the nursing home must be screened to determine if they are there primarily because of chronic mental illness. If so, a specific plan of care must be developed with appropriate participation from mental health professionals.

Those residents who do not require skilled care are supposed to be transferred to more appropriate care settings. More training is mandated for nurses' aides and the staffing requirements overall have been upgraded.

Data elements from the MDS have been used to create a series of quality indicators, which are antedated to reflect potential areas of poor care in need of further exploration by state surveyors (Zimmerman et al., 1995). In a move to foster informed consumer choice, some of these quality indicators are now being posted on Web sites to provide consumers and their families with better information about the quality of nursing home care.

New models of nursing home care are being developed despite regulatory constraints on creativity. In some settings, large institutions are being converted into smaller living communities, where residents exert more control over their lives. The Eden Alternative has provided a model for how to humanize nursing home care. The Wellspring Movement is trying to pursue a quality improvement agenda by empowering nursing home staff to take greater responsibility for identifying ways to improve care. Although both are attractive concepts, neither has yet been shown to produce dramatic improvements in residents' quality of care or quality of life.

ASSISTED LIVING

A new form of chronic care is emerging. "Assisted living" describes a form of care for many of those persons who currently require nursing home care. It is designed to provide services to persons as they require them, in a setting that more closely resembles a person's home. In effect, service recipients need not lose their personhood and their autonomy to get care. Residents still live in institutional settings that house many people within the same facility, thus maximizing efficiency of service delivery. They use common facilities, such as a dining room, but they also retain their privacy. Basically, each resident is treated as a tenant and has control over a living unit. At a minimum, each individually occupied dwelling unit contains space for living and sleeping, a bathroom, and at least minimal cooking facilities. (The stove can be disconnected for those for whom it might pose a serious danger.) Each unit can be locked by the occupant.

Under this approach, control is shifted toward empowering the recipient of care. In contrast to the situation in a nursing home, where residents are expected to conform to the norms of the institution, in an assisted living facility individualized care is stressed. As the tenant, the resident has control over the use of her space: care providers must be invited in; care plans must be accepted by the resident. These shifts, while subtle at one level, are fundamental at another. They imply a dramatically altered approach to care, some of which is tangible and some of which is not. The lore of nursing homes is laden with evidence of learned helplessness and enforced dependency. This approach to care is aimed at maximizing a resident's sense of self and independence as much as possible.

Especially for those chronically impaired persons who have retained an appreciation of their environment, such a philosophy of care makes great sense. Examples of such care are becoming more prevalent. Assisted living has been able to serve quite disabled persons, although most recipients are less impaired. The majority of assisted living exists as a privately paid service. Medicaid in most states has been slow to cover this service, and where it has, it covers only the services component, leaving Social Security and welfare payments to address the room and board costs.

The costs of assisted living are usually much less than comparable nursing home care. One reason that assisted living is less expensive and more flexible is that it has thus far been spared the heavy regulatory mantle laid on nursing homes. Staffing patterns are not as intense or as professionally dictated. Staff performs multiple functions. If it is regulated in the same way, it will inevitably come to resemble nursing home care.

Once again, the form of care is determined by society's willingness to accept some risks. At a minimum, those who receive the care should have an opportunity to choose what kind of care they want to get.

At the same time, assisted living has come under criticisms reminiscent of those addressed at nursing homes in years past. With growth has come great variation. It is no longer clear just what is being offered by whom. Some standardized taxonomy is needed to allow consumers to make more informed choices. Concerns about quality are frequently expressed, especially with regard to the management of the more frail and medically complex residents.

HOME CARE

As already noted, we have developed a backward system of long-term care in this country that focuses on the nursing home. We tend to speak of the nursing home and alternatives to it, when we should begin with the premise that elderly people belong at home and want to be cared for at home. Institutional care will be needed in some cases, when the strain on caregivers is too great, but it should not be the resource of first resort. Our system has not evolved that way, and the resources available for home care are meager, but not so underdeveloped as to be ignored. Even today, most communities have at least some home care services, and more are likely to develop.

Home care involves at least two basic types of care: home health services; and homemaking and chore services. As shown in Table 15-4, different programs provide one or both types. Most elderly people treated at home require homemaking more than home health services.

Sometimes the differences between the two are purely arbitrary. If we consider that the homemaker replaces or supplements a family member, many of the tasks involved are extensions of home nursing (eg, supervising medication or giving baths). The definitions have emerged to fit the regulations governing a

TABLE 15-4 HOME CARE PROVIDED UNDER VARIOUS FEDERAL PROGRAMS

	MEDICARE	MEDICAID	TITLE XX
Eligibility criteria	Must be homebound; need skilled care; need and expect benefit in a reasonable period; need certification by physician	State can use homebound criterion; not limited to skilled care; need certification by physician	Vary from state to state
Payment to provider	Final costs per episode based on functional status, case needs, and diagnoses	Varies with state	Three modes of payment possible: (1) direct provision by government agency; (2) contract with private agency; (3) independent provider
Services covered	Home health services, skilled nursing, physical, or speech therapy as primary services; secondary services (social worker and home health aide) available *only* if primary service is provided; position of occupational therapy in service hierarchy ambiguous*	Limited home health care mandatory; expanded home care optional; personal care in home optional	Wide variety of home services allowed, including home health aide, homemaker, chore worker, meal services

*Occupational therapy is considered an "extended" secondary service, which may continue if needed after primary services are discontinued.

particular program. The physician will usually find that the home health agency is familiar with these regulations and how to deal with them.

The major problem at present is getting services. In response to political pressures, Medicare broadened its long-term care benefit (including waiving the former requirement that a person have a prior hospital stay of at least 3 days) and moved the program from Part B to Part A, thereby removing the co-payment requirement. The subsequent enormous growth in home health care under Medicare has led to instituting prospective payment and making revisions in coverage that move part of the program back under Part B. (Home health care not related to a prior 3-day hospital stay, or visits after the 100th visit if related to a stay, will be covered under Part B.) Medicare-covered home health care had been growing annually until the imposition of prospective payment in 1997.

Despite the growth in use, some still maintain that the criteria for eligibility for these services severely restrict their use. To get home health services for a patient, a physician must certify that the patient is homebound and that intermittent skilled care is likely to produce a benefit in a reasonable time. Thus, a large number of dependent older persons who need continuing home nursing but are "custodial" are ineligible unless the physician misrepresents their situation. *Skilled service* is defined as a skilled service offered by a nurse, a physical therapist, or a speech therapist.

If one of these establishing services is present, the patient may also receive the skilled services of an occupational therapist or medical social worker and/or the services of a home health aide if required by the plan. Medicare has begun to allow home health agencies to continue to serve clients who need case management, thus permitting some cases to remain open longer than the "intermittent" rule might otherwise imply. All reimbursed services must be given by a certified home health agency. (To be certified, the agency needs to offer nursing plus at least one of the five other services.) The requirement for using a certified agency greatly increases the costs of the services, although the assumption is that this certification assures at least a minimal level of professional oversight. A recurring question is how much administrative overhead is affordable as the pressure on the long-term care dollar grows.

Medicare-certified home health agencies are required to complete an OASIS (Outcome and Assessment Information Set) form at several stages of care to track outcomes and need for care. This recording burden has proven onerous for many agencies.

Medicaid funds can be used to provide home health care to persons eligible for nursing home care. Until recently, Medicaid funds have not been widely used for home care. In fact, until 1980, one state (New York) accounted for almost 95% of the Medicaid moneys spent on home health care. (It is still by far the largest user of Medicaid home care.) Home care under Medicaid must have a physician's authorization, but the patient need not be homebound, and the care need not be "skilled." All agencies delivering home care under Medicaid must meet Medicare certification standards, but if no organized home health agencies exist in a region, a registered nurse may be reimbursed for the services. Home care can be provided under two auspices under Medicaid. It is a mandated service and it can be part of a waivered service package (ie, services authorized in lieu of nursing home care). In practice, states have often modeled their Medicaid home care benefits after the medically oriented Medicare benefit and thus restricted its use. Under Medicaid, the nursing care is a required component of home health services, and the state has the option to provide physical, occupational, and speech therapy; medical social services; and personal-care services. Medicaid allows homemaking assistance on a more generous basis than does Medicare. Personal-care services must be prescribed by a physician and supervised by a registered nurse. These services may not be delivered by persons related to the patient.

Recent changes in legislation have broadened the permissible use of Medicaid moneys to support a wide variety of long-term care services in an effort to reduce nursing home costs. A number of states have received waivers to develop this broader package of services in lieu of nursing home care, but most of these waivered services are limited in the numbers of "slots" they are allowed. The waivers require some evidence of budget neutrality. The assumption is that as more care is provided in the community, fewer people will use nursing homes.

Despite the growth of home care under Medicaid and the growing numbers of alternative waiver programs, the large bulk of Medicaid long-term care funds continue to flow to nursing homes. However, the relative dominance of spending on nursing home care varies widely from state to state. An analysis of 1996 data showed that only 18% of Medicaid long-term care expenditures go to home- and community-based services; the proportion ranges from 44% (Oregon) to 0.05% (Pennsylvania). Nationally, total monthly expenditure on home- and community-based services per person aged 65+ was $247, with a range from $4137 (Alaska) to $16 (Tennessee). Nursing home Medicaid expenditures per person aged 65+ likewise varied widely, from $2163 in New York to $343 in Nevada, with a national average of $893 (Ladd, Kane, and Kane, 1999).

The bulk of support for homemaking services, however, continues to rest with Title III and Title XX. Title XX provides at least four methods of payment: local public agencies can provide the service directly; they can contract with agency providers (perhaps using competitive bidding); they can purchase services from agencies at negotiated prices; or they can permit the recipient to enter into agreement with independent providers, who do not work for an agency. It is possible to have all these arrangements operating in the same community.

This provision for independent vendors has prompted controversy because maintaining standards is difficult in the absence of any supervisory system or institutional responsibility. Under Title XX, an employment category known as *chore worker* has emerged; although performing functions similar to the home health aide and the homemaker, chore workers do not need to be tightly supervised and cannot be reimbursed under Medicare or Medicaid.

Persons eligible for cash assistance from the state, and other persons with low incomes and unmet service needs, are eligible for Title XX as long as 50% of a state's annual federal allotment is expended on those receiving cash assistance.

Fees are charged to those whose family income exceeds 80% of the state's median income for a family of four.

Home services are one of four priority items under Title III of the Older Americans Act. Although the dollar volume is low, this source is important because means testing (whereby eligibility is set by income) is prohibited for programs under the Older Americans Act, making it possible to target a group that cannot afford private care but is ineligible for Title XX or Medicaid. Generally speaking, the Area Agency on Aging subcontracts for home care services rather than providing them directly. The usual pattern is that Administration on Aging dollars permit existing agencies to develop or expand a home care component. Services vary from area to area but can include personal care, homemaker service, chore service, and service for heavier jobs (eg, minor home repairs or renovations, insect eradication, gardening, and painting). The provisions for assistance under the Area Agency on Aging are sharply limited by their constrained budgets and the competing demands for programs.

The extent of services under these several programs is still limited at present, although enthusiasm for in-home care is growing. The total sum of public dollars spent on home care remains only a fraction of that devoted to nursing homes.

OTHER SERVICES

A number of other modes of care can be tapped on behalf of elderly patients. Table 15-5 lists some of these services. However, despite their growing availability, they are still not widely used. The most frequently used service in that set is the senior center, a service designed for the well elderly person.

TABLE 15-5   EXAMPLES OF COMMUNITY LONG-TERM CARE
PROGRAMS

Home care (home nursing and homemaking)	Caregiver support
Adult day care	Congregate housing
Adult foster care	Home repairs
Assisted living	Meals (congregate and in-home)
Geriatric assessment	
Hospice/terminal care	Respite care
Telephone reassurance	Emergency alarms

Day care can fulfill a number of needs. Most day care programs provide some combination of recreational and restorative activity. In contrast to senior centers, which are usually sponsored by recreational departments and targeted at the well elderly, day care programs serve persons with limited functional ability. Some are for cognitively impaired persons. The programs provide supervised activities, which may improve basic ADL skills and social skills. At the very least, they provide an important respite for the primary caregiver and thus may make the critical difference for allowing an impaired older person to remain at home. To increase efficiency, most programs serve any given client fewer than 5 days a week, usually 2 or 3 days.

Other forms of day care can include a larger medical component. Some areas have developed day hospitals for seniors, where virtually all the services of the hospital are available on an ambulatory basis. Emphasis is usually placed on rehabilitation, especially occupational and physical therapy. The adult day health center is an intermediate model, which combines day care with nursing, physical therapy, and perhaps social work. Such sites can also be used for periodic ambulatory care clinics.

A problem common to all day-care programs is transportation. It is hard to arrange, expensive, and time consuming. Special vans are usually needed, and, to avoid excessive travel times, services are usually confined to very limited areas.

In many communities, a variety of services exist to help seniors: ombudsmen, peer counselors, mental health clinics, transportation, congregate meal sites, and meals-on-wheels—just to name a few. Availability varies greatly from place to place. Good sources of information are the social work department in a hospital and the Area Agency on Aging.

The physician cannot be expected to know all the resources available for geriatric patients and will have to rely on other professionals to make appropriate arrangements to take advantage of them. But a physician should have a good sense of what can be done in general and what needs to be done for any particular patient. Often knowing what is needed but not locally available can lead to its development, particularly if responsible professionals take an active role on behalf of their patients.

There is growing interest in providing older people and their families with better information with which to make more informed decisions about long-term care choices. Most states have developed some form of web-based information system that provides information about LTC options. Medicare provides online information about the quality of nursing homes (Nursing Home Compare) and home healthy agencies (Home Health Compare), as well as comparative reports on hospital quality indicators (Hospital Compare).

CASE MANAGEMENT

The growing interest in the plethora of community long-term care services has sparked some concerns about the need to control use. A frequent answer is *case management.* This term has been widely and variably used. Some people refer to case management as "political pixie dust." Because whenever the legislature finds itself proposing a long-term care program that will be hard to implement, they call for case management to make it work as desired. The basic components of case management are assessment, prescription, authorization, coordination, and monitoring. Much of the confusion about the effectiveness of case management can be traced to the confusion about just what is being described. Table 15-6 distinguishes several different types of case management.

Of these five variants of case management, eligibility management may be the most common. It is hardly likely to affect care directly. Disease management and chronic care coordination are closely related to the activities of primary care and hence may lead to some concern about role overlap between the case manager and the primary care physician. Disease management is often conducted independently of primary care by an organization contracted by insurance companies. By contrast, chronic care coordination is closely linked to and integrated with primary care, it is the basis for proactive primary care. It is possible for physicians to serve as case managers, but most do not have the interest or the resources to perform this task. It is usually more efficient to look to other disciplines to perform this function but to recognize the important role of the physician in the overall care of the long-term care patient. Where a full range of geriatric services is available, case management is usually included.

Regardless of discipline, the case manager faces some difficult tasks. There is often a discrepancy between responsibility and authority. It is very different to prescribe, authorize, or mandate.

Case managers may or may not have the purchasing authority to pay for services they feel are necessary. Case managers may easily find themselves in the same bind as physicians. Specifically, they are expected to serve simultaneously as patient advocates and gatekeepers. The two roles are incompatible. For everyone's peace of mind, it is important to clarify at the outset who is the principal client. Because many decisions involve advocating on behalf of one group over another, this distinction is critical. It is very different to work on behalf of a client to obtain all the resources you believe they need than it is to work to distribute a fixed pool of resources to those who will best use them.

Another frequently heard concern about case management is the need to affix responsibility. On the one hand, the easiest way to do this is to give the case manager a budget and expect the case manager to work within it to achieve the most possible. However, some have expressed anxieties that the person charged with authorizing services should be at arm's length from those providing them. Specific concerns are heard about hospital discharge planners' decisions as to when to refer patients to services owned or operated by the hospital. There is a real potential for client skimming. Similarly, if the case manager works for a care-giving agency, there is the risk that agency may get a disproportionate share of the choicest clients. On the other hand, even when case managers are separated from direct care, they are not immune to pressure from the purveyors, just as the physician is pursued by the drug companies.

TABLE 15-6 VARIATIONS IN CASE MANAGEMENT

TYPE OF CASE MANAGEMENT	CASE MANAGER	COMPONENTS
Eligibility management	Social worker or nurse	Assessment to see if client reaches threshold for eligibility Care plan Implementations Cursory monitoring for change in status that would affect eligibility
Care coordination	Social worker or nurse	Structured assessment to identify needs Care plan addressing each need Arrange services to meet each need Follow up to assure services are delivered Reassess periodically and adjust care plan
Utilization management	Usually a nurse	Identify high-volume/high-cost cases Work with high users to change clinical course Monitor intensively Counsel to encourage compliance Seek ways to prevent problems Flag charts to alert clinicians
Disease management	Usually a nurse, possibly MD	Focus on a single disease Provide reminders Counseling Monitoring Usually not coordinated with primary care

TABLE 15-6   VARIATIONS IN CASE MANAGEMENT (*Continued*)

TYPE OF CASE MANAGEMENT	CASE MANAGER	COMPONENTS
Chronic care coordination	Nurse or nurse practitioner	Establish expected clinical course Monitor salient parameter for each condition followed Patients can do most of the monitoring Communicate with clinicians by phone, web Intervene when actual course differs from expected course Indication for active intervention See clients primarily when their condition changes significantly Can monitor many conditions simultaneously Can address function as well as diseases

Case management has also become a mainstay of managed care. In this context, cases are usually identified on the basis of some risk indicators—either a record of heavy use of services or the presence of risk factors that imply such a pattern in the future. While some case management within managed care is patient centered, operating on the premise that closer care can stave off costly problems, much of it revolves primarily around utilization controls.

Several states utilized a program called "cash and counseling." Modeled after successful programs in California and Europe, disabled seniors can receive direct cash payments for care, which they can, in turn, use to purchase services, including from relatives. The preliminary reports have been enthusiastic. Clients have been able to purchase more care for less money with no evidence of untoward effects. In general, these clients are on the low end of the disability spectrum, but the program shows promise. It is, after all, simply creating a situation analogous to what people would do with their own funds. There is still some uneasiness about just how much discretion such programs should allow, many still require limited choices of vendors and evidence that the funds were used for the intended purposes. Nonetheless, these efforts represent a new direction of giving frail older clients more leeway in how to obtain services.

References

Cutler DM. Declining disability among the elderly. *Health Aff (Millwood)*. 2001;20(6):11-27.

Dey AN. *Characteristics of Elderly Nursing Home Residents: Data from the 1995 National Nursing Home Survey. Advance Data from Vital and Health Statistics.* Hyattsville, MD: National Center for Health Statistics; 1997.

Eng C, Pedulla J, Eleazer GP, et al. Program of All-inclusive Care for the Elderly (PACE): an innovative model of integrated geriatric care and financing. *J Am Geriatr Soc.* 1997;45:223-232.

Kane RA. Long-term care and a good quality of life: bringing them closer together. *Gerontologist.* 2001;41(3):293-304.

Kane RL. Managed care as a vehicle for delivering more effective chronic care for older persons. *J Am Geriatr Soc.* 1998;46:1034-1039.

Kane RL. Setting the PACE in chronic care. *Contemp Gerontol.* 1999;6(2):47-50.

Kane RL, Chen Q, Blewett LA, et al. Do rehabilitative nursing homes improve the outcomes of care? *J Am Geriatr Soc.* 1996;44:545-554.

Kane RL, Keckhafer G, Flood S, et al. The effect of Evercare on hospital use. *J Am Geriatr Soc.* 2003;51(10):1427-1434.

Kramer AM, Steiner JF, Schlenker RE, et al. Outcomes and costs after hip fracture and stroke: a comparison of rehabilitation settings. *JAMA.* 1997;277:396-404.

Ladd RC, Kane RL, Kane RA. *State LTC Profiles Report, 1996.* Minneapolis, MN: University of Minnesota School of Public Health; 1999.

Manton KG, Gu X, and Lamb VL. Change in chronic disability from 1982 to 2004/2005 as measured by long-term changes in function and health in the US elderly population. *PNAS.* 2006;103(48):18374-18379 at http://www.pnas.org/cgi/content/full/103/48/18374. Accessed November 2007.

Phillips CD, Sloane PD, Hawes C, et al. Effects of residence in Alzheimer disease special care units on functional outcomes. *JAMA.* 1997;278:1340-1344.

Valiyeva E, et al. Lifestyle-related risk factors and risk of future nursing home admission. *Arch Intern Med.* May 8, 2006;166:985-990.

Welch HG, Wennberg DE, Welch WP. The use of Medicare home health services. *N Engl J Med.* 1996;335:324-329.

Zimmerman DR, Karon SL, Arling G, et al. Development and testing of nursing home quality indicators. *Health Care Fin Rev.* 1995;16(4):107-127.

Suggested Readings

Boult C, Boult L, Pacala JT. Systems of care for older populations of the future. *J Am Geriatr Soc.* 1998;46:499-505.

Kane RA, Kane RL, Ladd R. *The Heart of Long-term Care*. New York: Oxford University Press; 1998.

Kane RA, Wilson KB. *Assisted Living in the United States: A New Paradigm for Residential Care for Older Persons?* Washington, DC: American Association of Retired Persons; 1993.

Kosecoff J, Kahn KL, Rogers WH, et al. Prospective payment system and impairment at discharge. The "quicker-and-sicker" story revisited. *JAMA*. 1990;264:1980-1983.

Lachs MS, Ruchlin HS. Is managed care good or bad for geriatric medicine? *J Am Geriatr Soc*. 1997;45:1123-1127.

Morgan RO, Virnig BA, DeVito CA, et al. The Medicare–HMO revolving door—the healthy go in and the sick go out. *N Engl J Med*. 1997;337:169-175.

Wunderlich GS, Kohler P (eds). *Improving the Quality of Long-term Care. Report of the Institute of Medicine*. Washington, DC: National Academy Press; 2001.

CHAPTER 16

NURSING HOME CARE

The focus of this chapter is the clinical care of nursing home residents. Some of the basic demographic and economic aspects of nursing home care are discussed in Chaps. 2 and 15. Many older people who would have otherwise been in nursing homes are now residing in assisted living facilities. Management of older people with multiple medical problems and geriatric conditions in this setting is challenging. Chapter 15 and the Suggested Readings at the end of this chapter provide more information on this level of care.

The poor quality of care provided in many nursing homes has been recognized for decades (Vladek, 1980). Since the Institute of Medicine issued its critical report in 1986 (Institute of Medicine, 1986) and the mandating of the Resident Assessment Instrument in 1987, the overall quality of care has improved. A more recent report from the Institute of Medicine, however, indicates a need for further improvements in care quality (Institute of Medicine, 2000).

Despite the logistical, economic, and attitudinal barriers that can foster inadequate medical care in the nursing home, many straightforward principles and strategies can improve the quality of medical care for nursing home residents. Fundamental to achieving these improvements is a clear perspective on the goals of nursing home care, which differ in many respects from the goals of medical care in other settings and patient populations.

THE GOALS OF NURSING HOME CARE

The modern nursing home serves multiple roles. Table 16-1 lists the key goals of nursing home care. While the prevention, identification, and treatment of chronic, subacute, and acute medical conditions are important, most of these goals focus on the functional independence, autonomy, quality of life, comfort, and dignity of the residents. Physicians and other clinicians who care for nursing home residents must consider these goals while the more traditional goals of medical care are being addressed.

The heterogeneity of the nursing home population results in a diversity of goals for nursing home care. Nursing home residents can be subgrouped into five basic types (Fig. 16-1). While it is not always possible to isolate these different

TABLE 16-1   GOALS OF NURSING HOME CARE

1. Provide a safe and supportive environment for chronically ill and dependent people

2. Restore and maintain the highest possible level of functional independence

3. Preserve individual autonomy

4. Maximize quality of life, perceived well-being, and life satisfaction

5. Provide comfort and dignity for terminally ill patients and their loved ones

6. Stabilize and delay progression, whenever possible, of chronic medical conditions

7. Prevent acute medical and iatrogenic illnesses, and identify and treat them rapidly when they do occur

types of residents geographically, and although residents often overlap or change between the types described, subgrouping nursing home residents in this manner will help the physician and interdisciplinary team to focus the care-planning process on the most critical and realistic goals for individual residents.

The underlying social contract implied by nursing home admission is quite different for each of these groups. In some cases, access to treatment takes precedence over the living environment; in other circumstances, the environment may be the most critical element of care. Those admitted to a nursing home with the intent of active treatment and discharge home may be willing to accept a living

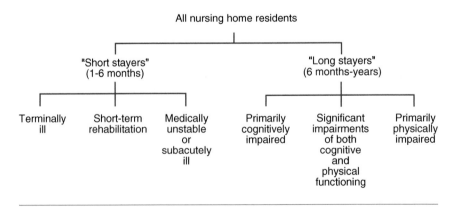

— FIGURE 16-1 —   Basic types of nursing home patients.

situation akin to that of a hospital in the expectation that the benefit they receive from treatment will offset any discomfort or inconvenience. For terminally ill persons under the hospice model, the living environment is made as flexible and supportive as possible. Efforts are directed toward making these patients comfortable and permitting them to enjoy, to the extent possible, their last days.

There has been a trend to separate the cognitively impaired from those who are primarily physically impaired. Special care units (SCUs) for the cognitively impaired are present in many nursing homes, where care can be coordinated to maximize attention to the behavioral aspects of dementia care and to minimize the use of psychoactive drugs and restraints while maintaining a safe environment. Some see SCUs as a way of achieving better results. Others view them as controlled environments in which demented residents can be treated more humanely by staff who have chosen to concentrate on such care. Still others see the primary gain from SCUs as removing otherwise disruptive patients from the environment of those still alert enough to resent the intrusion. No strong data, however, demonstrate major improvements in outcomes of patients treated on these units.

CLINICAL ASPECTS OF CARE FOR NURSING HOME RESIDENTS

In addition to the different goals for care in the nursing home, several factors make the assessment and treatment of nursing home residents different from those in other settings (Table 16-2). Many of these factors relate to the process of care and are discussed in the following section. (For a more complete discussion of medical care in the nursing home, see the Suggested Readings section.) A fundamental difference in the nursing home care is that medical evaluation and treatment must be complemented by an assessment and care-planning process involving staff from multiple disciplines. The integral involvement of nurses' aides in the development and implementation of care plans is crucial to high-quality nursing home care. Data on medical conditions and their treatment are integrated with assessments of the functional, mental, and behavioral status of the resident in order to develop a comprehensive database and individualized plan of care.

Medical evaluation and clinical decision making for nursing home residents are complicated for several reasons. Unless the physician has cared for the resident before nursing home admission, it may be difficult to obtain a comprehensive medical database. Residents may be unable to relate their medical histories accurately or to describe their symptoms, and medical records are frequently unavailable or incomplete, especially for residents who have been transferred between nursing homes and acute-care hospitals. When acute changes in status occur, initial assessments are often performed by nursing home staff with limited skills and are transmitted to physicians by telephone. Even when the diagnoses are known or strongly suspected, many diagnostic and therapeutic procedures among nursing home

TABLE 16-2   FACTORS THAT DISTINGUISH ASSESSMENT AND
TREATMENT IN THE NURSING HOME DIFFERENT
FROM THAT IN OTHER SETTINGS

1. The goals of care are often different (see Table 16-1)
2. Specific clinical disorders are prevalent among nursing home residents (see Table 16-3)
3. The approach to health maintenance and prevention differs (see Table 16-6)
4. Mental and functional status are just as important, if not more so, than medical diagnoses
5. Assessment must be interdisciplinary, including:
   a. Nursing
   b. Psychosocial
   c. Rehabilitation
   d. Nutritional
   e. Other (eg, dental, pharmacy, podiatry, audiology, ophthalmology)
6. Sources of information are variable:
   a. Residents often cannot give a precise history
   b. Family members and nurses' aides with limited assessment skills may provide the most important information
   c. Information is often obtained over the telephone
7. Administrative procedures for record keeping in both nursing homes and acute-care hospitals can result in inadequate and disjointed information
8. Clinical decision making is complicated for several reasons:
   a. Many diagnostic and therapeutic procedures are expensive, unavailable, or difficult to obtain and involve higher risks of iatrogenic illness and discomfort than are warranted by the potential outcome
   b. The potential long-term benefits of "tight" control of certain chronic illnesses (eg, diabetes mellitus, congestive heart failure, hypertension) may be outweighed by the risks of iatrogenic illness in many very old and functionally disabled residents
   c. Many residents are not capable (or are questionably capable) of participating in medical decision making, and their personal preferences based on previous decisions are often unknown (see Table 16-7)
9. The appropriate site for and intensity of treatment are often difficult decisions involving medical, emotional, ethical, economic, and legal considerations that may be in conflict with each other in the nursing home setting
10. Logistic considerations, resource constraints, and restrictive reimbursement policies may limit the ability of and incentives for physicians to carry out optimal medical care of nursing home residents

residents are associated with an unacceptably high risk-benefit ratio. For example, an imaging study may require sedation with its attendant risks; nitrates and other cardiovascular drugs may precipitate syncope or disabling falls in frail ambulatory residents with baseline postural hypotension; and adequate control of blood sugar may be extremely difficult to achieve without a high risk for hypoglycemia among cognitively impaired diabetic residents with marginal or fluctuating nutritional intake, who may not recognize or complain of hypoglycemic symptoms.

Further compounding these difficulties is the inability of many nursing home residents to participate effectively in important decisions regarding their medical care. Their previously expressed wishes are often not known, and an appropriate or legal surrogate decision maker has often not been appointed. These issues are discussed further on in this chapter and in Chap. 17.

Table 16-3 lists the most commonly encountered clinical disorders in the nursing home population. They represent a broad spectrum of chronic medical illnesses; neurological, psychiatric, and behavioral disorders; and problems that are especially prevalent in frail older adults (eg, incontinence, falls, nutritional disorders, chronic pain syndromes). Although the incidence of iatrogenic illnesses has not been systematically studied in nursing homes, it is likely to be as high as or higher than that in acute-care hospitals. The management of many of the conditions listed in Table 16-3 is discussed in some detail in other chapters of this text (for specific conditions, see Table of Contents and Index).

TABLE 16-3   COMMON CLINICAL DISORDERS IN THE NURSING HOME POPULATION

Medical conditions
    Congestive heart failure
    Degenerative joint disease
    Diabetes mellitus
    Obstructive lung disease
    Renal failure
    Infections
        Lower respiratory tract
        Urinary tract
        Skin (pressure sores, vascular ulcers)
        Conjunctivitis
        Gastroenteritis
    Gastrointestinal disorders
        Reflux esophagitis
        Constipation
        Diarrhea

TABLE 16-3   COMMON CLINICAL DISORDERS IN THE NURSING
HOME POPULATION (*Continued*)

Malignancies

Neuropsychiatric conditions
  Dementia
  Behavioral disorders associated with dementia
    Wandering
    Agitation
    Aggression
    Depression

Neurological disorders other than dementia
  Stroke
  Parkinsonism
  Multiple sclerosis
  Brain or spinal cord injury

Functional disabilities necessitating rehabilitation
  Stroke
  Hip fracture
  Joint replacement
  Amputation

Geriatric problems
  Delirium
  Incontinence
  Gait disturbances, instability, falls
  Malnutrition, feeding difficulties, dehydration
  Pressure sores
  Insomnia

Chronic pain: musculoskeletal conditions, neuropathies, malignancy

Iatrogenic disorders
  Adverse drug reactions
  Falls
  Nosocomial infections
  Induced disabilities
  Restraints and immobility, catheters, unnecessary help with basic
    activities of daily living

Death and dying, palliative care

In addition to the numerous factors already mentioned that render the medical assessment and treatment of these conditions different, the process of care in nursing homes also differs substantially from that in acute-care hospitals, clinics, and home care settings.

PROCESS OF CARE IN THE NURSING HOME

The process of care in nursing homes is strongly influenced by numerous state and federal regulations, the highly interdisciplinary nature of nursing home residents' problems, and the training and skills of the staff that delivers most of the hands-on care. Federal rules and regulations contained in the Omnibus Budget Reconciliation Act of 1987 (OBRA, 1987) and implemented in 1991 place heavy emphasis on assessment and care planning as a means of achieving the highest practicable level of functioning for each resident and the use of the Resident Assessment Instrument (http://www.hpm.umn.edu/nhregsPlus/CMS_RAI_manual/cms_rai_manual.pdf; accessed 7/23/08). Detailed guidance for state and federal surveyors has been developed for several clinical care areas, such as unnecessary drugs and urinary incontinence. Failure to adhere to the clinical recommendations contained in the regulations and related guidance to surveyors can result in citations and, in some instances, financial penalties for the nursing home. Increasingly, failure to appropriately manage medical conditions in the nursing home puts the facility and physician at risk for lawsuits (Stevenson and Studdert, 2003).

Physician involvement in nursing home care and the nature of medical assessment and treatment offered to nursing home residents are often limited by logistic and economic factors. Few physicians have offices based either inside the nursing home or in close proximity to the facility. Many physicians who do visit nursing homes care for relatively small numbers of residents, often in several different facilities. Many nursing homes, therefore, have numerous physicians who make rounds once or twice per month, who are not generally present to evaluate acute changes in resident status, and who attempt to assess these changes over the telephone. In some areas, practice patterns are shifting to a model of physician-nurse practitioner practices caring for large numbers of residents in several nursing homes. Such physician-nurse practitioner teams have been shown to improve care and reduce hospitalization rates (Ackerman and Kemle, 1998; Reuben et al., 1999; Kane et al., 2003; Konetzka et al., 2008). Many nursing homes do not have ready availability of laboratory, radiologic, and pharmacy services with the capability of rapid response, further compounding the logistics of evaluating and treating acute changes in medical status. Thus, nursing home residents are often sent to hospital emergency rooms, where they are evaluated by personnel who are generally not familiar with their baseline status and who frequently lack training and interest in the care of frail and dependent elderly patients.

Medicare and Medicaid reimbursement policies may also dictate certain patterns of nursing home care. While physicians are required to visit nursing home residents only every 30 to 60 days, many residents require more frequent assessment and monitoring of treatment—especially with the shorter acute-care hospital stays brought about by the prospective payment system. While Medicare reimbursement for physician visits in nursing homes has improved, reimbursement for a routine visit is generally inadequate for the time that is required to provide good medical care in the nursing home, including travel to and from the facility; assessment and treatment planning for residents with multiple problems; communication with members of the interdisciplinary team and the resident's family; and proper documentation in the medical record. Activities often essential to good care in the nursing home, such as attendance at interdisciplinary conferences, family meetings, complex assessments of decision-making capacity, and counseling residents and surrogate decision makers on treatment plans in the event of terminal illness, are generally not reimbursable at all. Medicare intermediaries sometimes restrict reimbursement for rehabilitative services for residents not covered under Part A skilled care, thus limiting the treatment options for many residents. Although Medicaid programs vary considerably, many provide minimal coverage for ancillary services that are critical for optimum medical care, and may restrict reimbursement for several types of drugs that may be especially helpful for nursing home residents.

Amid these logistic and economic constraints, expectations for the care of nursing home residents are high. Table 16-4 outlines the various types of assessment generally recommended for the optimal care of nursing home residents. Physicians are responsible for completing an initial assessment within one week of admission and for arranging for monthly visits thereafter for the next 90 days. More frequent visits are generally necessary for residents admitted on a Medicare Part A skilled nursing benefit. Licensed nurses assess new residents as soon as they are admitted, on a daily basis, and generally summarize the status of each resident weekly. The nationally mandated Minimum Data Set (MDS) must be completed within 14 days of admission and updated when a major change in status occurs; several sections must be routinely updated on a quarterly basis.

The extent of involvement of other disciplines in the assessment and care-planning process varies depending on the residents' problems, the availability of various professionals, and state regulations. Representatives from nursing, social services, dietary management, activities, and rehabilitation therapy (physical and/or occupational) participate in an interdisciplinary care-planning meeting. Residents are generally discussed at this meeting within 2 weeks of admission and quarterly thereafter. The product of these meetings is an interdisciplinary care plan that separately lists interdisciplinary problems (eg, restricted mobility, incontinence, wandering, diminished food intake, poor social interaction), goals for the resident related to the problem, approaches to achieving these goals, target dates for achieving the goals, and assignment of responsibilities for working toward the goals among

TABLE 16-4   IMPORTANT ASPECTS OF VARIOUS TYPES OF ASSESSMENT IN THE NURSING HOME

TYPE OF ASSESSMENT	TIMING	MAJOR OBJECTIVES	IMPORTANT ASPECTS
Medical initial	Within 72 h to one week after admission	Verify medical diagnoses Document baseline physical findings, mental and functional status, vital signs, and skin condition Attempt to identify potentially remediable, previously unrecognized medical conditions Get to know the resident and family (if this is a new resident) Establish goals for the admission and a medical treatment plan	A thorough review of medical records and physical examinations is necessary Relevant medical diagnoses and baseline findings should be clearly and concisely documented in the patient's record Medication lists should be carefully reviewed and only essential medications continued Request for specific types of assessment and input from other disciplines should be made A database should be established (see example in Fig. 16-2)
Periodic	Monthly or every other month	Monitor progress of active medical conditions Update medical orders Communicate with patient and nursing home staff	Progress notes should include clinical data relevant to active medical conditions and focus on changes in status Unnecessary medications, orders for care, and laboratory tests should be discontinued

TABLE 16-4 IMPORTANT ASPECTS OF VARIOUS TYPES OF ASSESSMENT IN THE NURSING HOME (*Continued*)

TYPE OF ASSESSMENT	TIMING	MAJOR OBJECTIVES	IMPORTANT ASPECTS
			Mental, functional, and psychosocial status should be reviewed with nursing home staff and changes from baseline noted
			The medical problem list should be updated
As needed	When acute changes in status occur	Identify and treat causes of acute changes	Onsite clinical assessment by the physician (or nurse practitioner or physician's assistant), as opposed to telephonic consultations, will result in more accurate diagnoses, more appropriate treatment, and fewer unnecessary emergency room visits and hospitalization
			Vital signs, food and fluid intake, and mental status often provide essential information
			Infection, dehydration, and adverse drug effects should be at the top of the differential diagnosis for acute changes in status

Major reassessment	Annual	Identify and document any significant changes in status and new potentially remediable conditions	Targeted physical examination and assessment of mental, functional, and psychosocial status and selected laboratory tests should be done (see Table 16-6)
Nursing	On admission, and then routinely with monitoring of daily and weekly progress; complete Minimum Data Set (MDS) within 14 days, update when major change in status occurs and annually; update selected sections quarterly	Identify biopsychosocial and functional status, strengths and weaknesses Develop an individualized care plan Document baseline data for ongoing assessments	Particular attention should be given to emotional state, personal preferences, and sensory function Careful observation during the first few days of admission is important to detect effects of relocation Potential problems related to other disciplines should be recorded and communicated to appropriate members of the interdisciplinary care team
Psychosocial	Within 1-2 weeks of admission and as needed thereafter	Identify any potentially serious psychosocial signs and symptoms and refer to mental health professional if appropriate Determine past social history, family relationships, and social resources Become familiar with personal preferences regarding living arrangements	Getting to know the family and their preferences and concerns is critical to good nursing home care Relevant psychosocial data should be communicated to the interdisciplinary team Discharge potential should be assessed

TABLE 16-4 IMPORTANT ASPECTS OF VARIOUS TYPES OF ASSESSMENT IN THE NURSING HOME (*Continued*)

Type of Assessment	Timing	Major Objectives	Important Aspects
Rehabilitation (physical and occupational therapy)	Within days of admission and daily or weekly thereafter (depending on the rehabilitation program)	Determine functional status as it relates to basic activities of daily living Identify specific goals and time frame for improving specific areas of function Monitor progress toward goals Assess progress in relation to potential discharge	Small gains in functional status can improve chances for discharge as well as quality of life Not all residents have areas in which they can reasonably be expected to improve; strategies to maintain function should be developed for these residents Assessment of and recommendation for modifying the environment can be critically important for improving function and discharge planning
Nutritional	Within days of admission and then periodically thereafter	Determine nutritional status and needs Identify dietary preferences Plan an appropriate diet	Restrictive diets may not be medically necessary and can be unappetizing Weight loss should be identified and reported to nursing and medical staff

Interdisciplinary care plan	Within 1-2 weeks of admission and every 3 months thereafter	Identify interdisciplinary problems Establish goals and treatment plans Determine when maximum progress toward goals has been reached	Each discipline should prepare specific plans for communication to other team members based on their own assessment
Capacity for medical decision making*	Within days of admission and then whenever changes in status occur	Determine which types of medical decisions the resident is capable of participating in A resident who is still capable of making decisions independently should be encouraged to identify a surrogate decision maker in the event the resident later loses this decision-making capacity If the resident lacks capacity for many or all decisions, appropriate surrogate decision makers should be identified (if not already done)	Residents with varying degrees of dementia may still be capable of participating in many decisions regarding their medical care Attention should be given to potentially reversible factors that can interfere with decision-making capacity (eg, depression, fear, delirium, metabolic and drug effects) Concerns of the family and health professional should be considered, but the resident's desires should be paramount The resident's capacity may fluctuate over time because of physical and emotional conditions

TABLE 16-4   IMPORTANT ASPECTS OF VARIOUS TYPES OF ASSESSMENT IN THE NURSING HOME (*Continued*)

TYPE OF ASSESSMENT	TIMING	MAJOR OBJECTIVES	IMPORTANT ASPECTS
Preferences regarding treatment intensity* and nursing homeroutines	Within days of admission and periodically thereafter	Determine residents' wishes as to the intensity of treatment they would want in the event of acute or chronic progressive illness	Attempt to identify specific procedures the resident would or would not want This assessment is often made by ascertaining the resident's prior-expressed wishes (if known), or through surrogate decision makers (legal guardian, durable power of attorney for health care, family)

*See Table 16-7 and Chap. 17.

the various disciplines. These care plans are an important force in driving nursing staff behavior and expectations and should be reviewed by the primary physician.

The MDS is intended to assist nursing home staff in identifying important clinical problems and to trigger the use of Resident Assessment Protocols (RAPs), which have been developed for 18 common clinical conditions. The MDS and the RAPs are critical tools for developing individual care plans. The interdisciplinary care-planning process serves as a cornerstone for resident management in many facilities, but is a difficult and time-consuming process that requires leadership and tremendous interdisciplinary (and interpersonal) cooperation.

Staffing limitations in relation to the amount of time and effort required makes intensive interdisciplinary care planning and teamwork unrealistic in many nursing homes. Although physicians are seldom directly involved in the care-planning meetings in most facilities, they are generally required to review and sign the care plan, and may find the team's perspective very valuable in planning subsequent medical care.

Implementation of the OBRA 1987 regulations primarily affects the activities of the nursing home staff. But some aspects of these regulations have a direct bearing on physicians who are caring for nursing home residents. Several of the RAPs require involvement of the physician, nurse practitioner, or physician assistant in the evaluation and management of common geriatric conditions seen in nursing home residents (eg, delirium, incontinence). The RAPs do not directly address many common medical conditions (eg, congestive heart failure, arthritis, infections) that must be identified and managed outside the MDS/RAP paradigm. Perhaps the most direct effect on physicians relates to the specifications around the use of psychoactive medications. OBRA 1987 defines criteria for appropriate use of these medications, and requires the documentation of specific diagnoses as well as the quantitative documentation of the response of target behavioral symptoms to these drugs. The appropriate use of antipsychotics for patients with dementia and psychosis must be distinguished from the use of drugs as "chemical restraints." Psychoactive medications can no longer be used simply as a means to control symptoms of aggressive or disruptive behavior (ie, as "chemical restraints"), or on a continued as-needed basis. These rules have stimulated a rethinking of psychoactive drug use among nursing home residents; especially given the recently recognized risks of these drugs (see Chap. 14). New guidance to surveyors on Federal Tag 329 ("F-Tag 329") provides detailed information on expectations regarding psychotropic and other drug use (www.ascp.com/resources/nhsurvey/upload/S&C-06-29.09-F329InstructorGuide.pdf; accessed 12/30/07). Physician attention is also directed to the use of physical restraints. In keeping with changing attitudes about such care, the use of these restraints is generally discouraged. Restraints can be applied only upon a physician's order and only after documenting that less restrictive measures are not effective. Physical restraints can be safely removed from most residents (Evans et al., 1997). While not all residents can be free of restraints at all times, a restraint-free environment is an appropriate goal in the nursing home setting.

The general pressure for better documentation of care and assessments should provide a welcome improvement in the quality of care for nursing home residents. Federal and state regulations, as well as evolving guidance to surveyors, will inevitably mean that physicians will be asked to make more detailed clinical notes, especially with respect to indicating the underlying reasons for their actions.

STRATEGIES TO IMPROVE MEDICAL CARE IN NURSING HOMES

Several strategies might improve the process of medical care delivered to nursing home residents. Four strategies are briefly described: (1) the use of improved documentation practices; (2) a systematic approach to screening, health maintenance, and preventive practices for the frail, dependent nursing home population; (3) the use of nurse practitioners or physicians' assistants; and (4) use of practice guidelines and related quality improvement activities.

In addition to these strategies, strong leadership of a medical director who is appropriately trained and dedicated to improving the facilities' quality of medical care is essential in order to develop, implement, and monitor policies and procedures for medical services. The role of the medical director in nursing homes is discussed in detail elsewhere (see the Suggested Readings), and certification through the American Medical Directors Association should be encouraged. The medical director should set standards for medical care and serve as an example to the medical staff by caring for some of the residents in the facility. He/she should also be involved in various committees (eg, quality, infection control), and should try to involve interested medical staff in these committees, as well as in educational efforts through formal in-service presentations, teaching rounds, and appropriate documentation procedures.

The federal government's approach to improving the quality of care in nursing homes is based on the OBRA 1987 rules, and the MDS and RAPs in particular. The survey and certification process and guidance to surveyors is used to monitor and enforce these rules. The Center for Medicare and Medicaid Services (CMS) also supports Quality Improvement Organizations (QIO) in each state to assist nursing homes in improving quality. There is some evidence that the QIO program has been effective (Rollow et al., 2006). The QIO support web site contains resources for quality improvement (www. qualitynet.org).

Computerized MDS data are now used to generate selected quality indicators and to identify outlier facilities that may require targeted evaluation. These data are available on Medicare's "Nursing Home Compare" web site (www.medicare.gov/ NHcompare). While some data suggest that various aspects of nursing home care have improved since the implementation of the OBRA 1987 rules and regulations, many caveats about these data have been voiced (Ouslander, 1997). For several conditions, the validity of MDS-derived quality indicators has been questioned (see, eg, Simmons et al., 2003). Other approaches to improving quality will be necessary to complement the OBRA rules and regulations (Kane, 1998; Mor, 2006). Quality indicators, developed through literature review and expert consensus, are one example of a promising approach to improving medical and overall care in the nursing home setting (Saliba and Schnelle, 2002; Saliba et al., 2004; Saliba et al,. 2005).

Documentation Practices

Nursing home residents often have multiple coexisting medical problems and long previous medical histories. Residents often cannot relate their medical histories, and their previous medical records are frequently unavailable or incomplete. There is also a danger in perpetuating old diagnoses that are inaccurate. This is especially true for psychiatric diagnoses, but may also occur for other medical diagnoses such as congestive heart failure and stroke. Thus, it is difficult and sometimes impossible to obtain a comprehensive medical database. The effort should, however, be invested and not wasted. Critical aspects of the medical database should be recorded on one page or face sheet of the medical record. Figure 16-2 shows an example of a format for a face sheet. Additional standardized documentation should contain social information, such as individuals to contact at critical times and information about the resident's treatment status in the event of acute illness. These data are essential to the care of the resident and should be readily available in one place in the record, so that when emergencies arise, when medical consultants see the resident, or when members of the interdisciplinary team need an overall perspective, they are easy to locate. The face sheet should be copied and sent to the hospital or other health-care facilities to which the resident might be transferred. Time and effort is required in order to keep the face sheet updated. For facilities with access to computers and/or word processing, incorporating the face sheet into a database should be relatively easy and facilitate its rapid completion and periodic updating.

Medical documentation in progress notes for routine visits and assessments of acute changes is frequently scanty and/or illegible. Statements such as "stable" or "no change" are too frequently the only documentation for routine visits. While time constraints may preclude extensive notes, certain standard information should be documented. The SOAP (*s*ubjective, *o*bjective, *a*ssessment, *p*lan) format for charting routine notes is especially appropriate for nursing home residents (Table 16-5). Simple forms, flow sheets, or databases with word-processing capabilities can be used to enable physicians to efficiently produce legible, concise, yet comprehensive progress notes. Another tool for documenting change in residents over time is the benchmark approach using flow sheets (see Chap. 4).

MEDICAL FACE SHEET

ACTIVE MEDICAL PROBLEMS

1. _____
2. _____
3. _____
4. _____
5. _____
6. _____
7. _____
8. _____

NEUROPSYCHIATRIC STATUS

A. Dementia   ___ Absent   ___ Present
   If present:

   ___ Alzheimer   ___ Mixed
   ___ Multi-infarct   ___ Uncertain/Other

B. Psychiatric/behavioral disorders

   1. _____
   2. _____

C. Usual mental status
   ___ Alert, oriented, follows simple instructions
   ___ Alert, *disoriented*, but *can* follow simple directions
   ___ Alert, *disoriented*, *cannot* follow simple directions
   ___ Not alert (lethargic, comatose)

D. Most recent Mini Mental State Score
   ___/30 (Date ___ / ___ / ___)

PAST HISTORY

A. Acute hospitalizations since admission to JHA

   Diagnoses   Month/Year

   1. _____   __ / __
   2. _____   __ / __
   3. _____   __ / __
   4. _____   __ / __

FUNCTIONAL STATUS

B. Major surgical procedures *before* admission to JHA

Procedure   Year

1. _____ _____

2. _____ _____

3. _____ _____

4. _____ _____

C. Allergies

1. _____

2. _____

A. Ambulation
___ Unassisted
___ With cane
___ With walker
___ Unable
Transfer: ___ Ind ___ Dep

B. Continence
          Cont   Inc
Urine   ___   ___
Stool   ___   ___

C. Basic ADL
          Ind   Dep
Bathing   ___   ___
Dressing   ___   ___
Grooming   ___   ___
Feeding   ___   ___

D. Vision
___ Adequate for regular print
___ Impaired-can see large print
___ Highly impaired-but can get around
___ Severely impaired-has difficulty getting around

E. Hearing
___ Adequate
___ Minimal difficulty
___ Hears only w/amplifier
___ Highly impaired-no useful hearing

TREATMENT STATUS   (See treatment Status Sheet Note Date ___ / ___ / ___)

___ Full code   ___ DNR   ___ DNR, do no hospitalize   ___ No tube feeding

This form completed by _____   Date ___ / ___ / ___

— FIGURE 16-2 — Example of a face sheet for a nursing home record.

TABLE 16-5   SOAP FORMAT FOR MEDICAL PROGRESS NOTES ON
NURSING HOME RESIDENTS

Subjective	New complaints
	Symptoms related to active medical conditions
Objective	General appearance and mood
	Weight
	Vital signs
	Physical findings relevant to new complaints and active medical conditions
	Laboratory data
	Reports from nursing staff
	Progress in rehabilitative therapy (if applicable)
	Reports of other interdisciplinary team members
	Consultant reports
Assessment	Presumptive diagnosis(es) for new complaints or changes in status
	Stability of active medical conditions
	Responses to psychotropic medications (if applicable)
Plans	Changes in medications or diet
	Nursing interventions (eg, monitoring of vital signs, skin care)
	Assessments by other disciplines
	Consultants
	Laboratory studies
	Discharge planning (if relevant)

Another area in which medical documentation is often inadequate relates to the residents' decision-making capacity and treatment preferences. These issues are discussed briefly at the end of this chapter as well as in Chap. 17. In addition to placing critical information in a standardized format in readily accessible locations, it is essential that physicians thoroughly and legibly document all discussions they have had with the resident, family, or legal guardians; they must also document any durable power of attorney for health care about these issues. Failure to do so may result not only in poor communication and inappropriate treatment, but also in substantial legal liability. Notes about these issues should not be removed from the medical record and are probably best kept on a separate page behind the face sheet.

All of these recommendations can and should be incorporated into electronic medical records as nursing homes increasingly begin to utilize health information technology.

Screening, Health Maintenance, and Preventive Practices

A second approach to improving medical care in nursing homes is the development and implementation of selected screening, health maintenance, and preventive practices. Table 16-6 lists examples of such practices. With few exceptions, the efficacy of these practices has not been well studied in the nursing home setting. In addition, not all the practices listed in Table 16-6 are relevant for every nursing home resident. For example, some of the annual screening examinations are inappropriate for short-stayers or for many long-staying residents with end-stage dementia (see Fig. 16-1). Thus, the practices outlined in Table 16-6 must be tailored to the specific nursing home population, as well as for the individual resident, and must be creatively incorporated into routine care procedures as much as possible in order to be time-efficient, cost-effective, and reimbursable by Medicare.

Nurse Practitioners and Physician Assistants

A third strategy that may help to improve medical care in nursing homes is the use of nurse practitioners and physician assistants. This approach appears to be cost-effective in both managed care and fee-for-service settings (Burl et al., 1998; Ackerman and Kemle, 1998; Reuben et al., 1999; Kane et al., 2004), and these health professionals may be especially helpful in carrying out specific functions in the nursing home setting. Physician assistants and nurse practitioners can bill for services under fee-for-service Medicare; moreover, several states will reimburse their services, and individual facilities and/or physician groups can hire them on a salaried basis. Evercare is a managed care program for long-stay nursing home residents that uses a nurse practitioner-based model of care and is available in several states. Nurse practitioners may have a especially helpful perspective in interacting with nursing staff about the nonmedical aspects of care for nursing home residents. Nurse practitioners and physician's assistants can be very helpful in implementing some of the screening, monitoring, and preventive practices outlined in Table 16-6, and in communicating with interdisciplinary staff, families, and residents at times when the physician is not in the facility. One of the most appropriate roles for nurse practitioners and physicians' assistants is in the initial assessment of acute or subacute changes in resident status. They can perform a focused history and physical examination, and can order appropriate diagnostic studies. Several algorithms have been developed for this purpose, one of which is shown in Fig. 16-3. The use of a similar algorithm for pneumonia resulted in reduced hospitalizations and related costs in 22 Canadian nursing homes (Loeb et al., 2006). This strategy enables the onsite assessment of acute change, the detection and treatment of new problems early in their course, more appropriate utilization of acute-care hospital emergency rooms, and the rapid identification of residents who need to be hospitalized.

TABLE 16-6   SCREENING, HEALTH MAINTENANCE, AND PREVENTIVE PRACTICES IN THE NURSING HOME

PRACTICE	RECOMMENDED FREQUENCY*	COMMENT
		SCREENING
History and physical examination	Yearly	Focused examination including rectal, breast, and, in some women, pelvic examination
Weight	Monthly	Generally required
		Persistent weight loss should prompt a search for treatable medical, psychiatric, and functional conditions
Functional status assessment, including gait and mental status testing and screening for depression†	Yearly	Functional status assessed periodically by nursing staff using the Minimum Data Set (MDS)
		Systematic global functional assessment done at least yearly using MDS to detect potentially treatable conditions (or prevent complications) such as early dementia, depression, gait disturbances, urinary incontinence
Visual screening	Yearly	Assess acuity, intraocular pressure, identify correctable problems
Auditory	Yearly	Identify correctable problems
Dental	Yearly	Assess status of any remaining teeth, fit of dentures, and identify any pathology
Podiatry	Yearly	More frequently in diabetics and residents with peripheral vascular disease
		Identify correctable problems and ensure appropriateness of shoes

Tuberculosis	On admission and yearly (may vary by state)	All residents and staff should be tested. Booster testing recommended for nursing home residents (see text)
Laboratory tests Stool for occult blood Complete blood count Fasting glucose Electrolytes Renal function tests Albumin, calcium, phosphorus Thyroid function tests (including thyroid-stimulating hormone level)	Yearly	These tests have reasonable yield in the nursing home population

MONITORING IN SELECTED RESIDENTS

All residents Vital signs, including weight	Monthly	More often if unstable or subacutely ill
Diabetes Fasting and postprandial glucose, glycosylated hemoglobin (Hgb A1C)	Every 1-2 months when stable (fasting) Every 4-6 months (Hgb A1C)	Fingerstick tests may be useful, but should not be overused for stable residents
Residents on diuretics or with renal insufficiency (creatinine > 2 or blood urea nitrogen [BUN] > 35): electrolytes, BUN, creatinine	Every 2-3 months	Nursing home residents are more prone to dehydration, azotemia, hyponatremia, and hypokalemia

TABLE 16-6   SCREENING, HEALTH MAINTENANCE, AND PREVENTIVE PRACTICES IN THE NURSING HOME
(*Continued*)

PRACTICE	RECOMMENDED FREQUENCY*	COMMENT
Anemic residents who are on iron replacement or who have hemoglobin < 10: hemoglobin/hematocrit	Monthly until stable, then every 2-3 months	Iron replacement and/or erythropoietin should be discontinued once hemoglobin value stabilizes
Blood level of drug for residents on specific drugs, for example: Carbamazepine Digoxin Dilantin Lithium	Every 3-6 months	More frequently if drug treatment has just been initiated
PREVENTION		
Influenza vaccine	Yearly	All residents and staff with close resident contact should be vaccinated
Oseltamivir, Zanamivir	Within 24-48 hours of outbreak of suspected influenza	Residents and staff should be treated throughout outbreak
Zoster vaccination	Once	Selected residents

Pneumococcal/pneumonia bacteremia Pneumococcal vaccine	Once	
Tetanus booster	Every 10 years, or every 5 years with tetanus-prone wounds	Many older people have not received primary vaccinations; they require tetanus toxoid, 250-500 units of tetanus immune globulin, and completion of the immunization series with toxoid injection 4-6 weeks later and then 6-12 months after the second injection
Tuberculosis Isoniazid 300 mg/day for 9-12 months	Skin-test conversion in selected residents	Residents with abnormal chest film (more than granuloma), diabetes, end-stage renal disease, hematological malignancies, steroid or immunosuppressive therapy, or malnutrition should be treated
Antimicrobial prophylaxis for residents at risk‡	Generally recommended for dental procedures, genitourinary procedures, and most operative procedures	Chronically catheterized residents should not be treated with continuous prophylaxis
Body positioning and range of motion for immobile residents	Ongoing	Frequent turning of very immobile residents is necessary to prevent pressure sores Semiupright position is necessary for residents with swallowing disorders or enteral feeding to help prevent aspiration Range of motion to immobile limbs and joints is necessary to prevent contractures

TABLE 16-6   SCREENING, HEALTH MAINTENANCE, AND PREVENTIVE PRACTICES IN THE NURSING HOME
(*Continued*)

PRACTICE	RECOMMENDED FREQUENCY*	COMMENT
Infection-control procedures and surveillance	Ongoing	Policies and protocols should be in effect in all nursing homes Surveillance of all infections should be continuous to identify outbreaks and resistance patterns
Environmental safety	Ongoing	Appropriate lighting, colors, and the removal of hazards for falling are essential in order to prevent accidents Routine monitoring of potential safety hazards and accidents may lead to alterations that may prevent further accidents

*Frequency may vary depending on resident's condition. Not all recommendations are relevant to every resident.
†The MDS can be supplemented by various standardized tools (see Chap. 3).
‡See The Medical Letter, 2006.

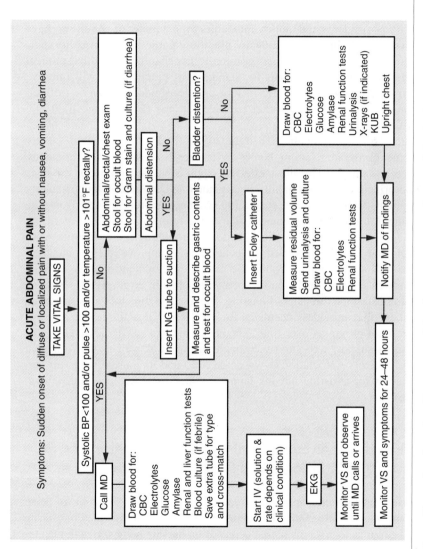

— FIGURE 16-3 — Example of an algorithm protocol for the management of acute abdominal pain in the nursing home by a nurse practitioner or physician's assistant. CBC, complete blood cell count; EKG, electrocardiogram; IV, intravenous; KUB, kidneys, ureters, bladder; MD, medical doctor; NG, nasogastric; VS, vital signs.

Clinical Practice Guidelines and Quality Improvement Activities

Several clinical practice guidelines relevant to nursing home care have been developed by the American Medical Directors Association (AMDA). In addition, the 18 RAPs contain basic approaches to common conditions among nursing home residents and quality indicators for a number of conditions have been developed (Saliba et al., 2004). While these guidelines and quality indicators are largely based on expert opinion rather than on controlled clinical trials, they are helpful as a basis for standards of practice that will improve care. Implementation and maintenance of practice guidelines can be difficult in nursing homes, as it is in other practice settings (Schnelle et al., 1997; Saliba et al., 2005).

Clinical practice guidelines can be useful tools in an overall quality improvement program. Nursing homes are required to have an ongoing quality assurance committee. The most effective approaches are probably the ones based on principles of total quality management (TQM) or continuous quality improvement (CQI) (Schnelle et al., 1993). These approaches use front-line staff to monitor objective outcomes (such as the frequency of falls, severity of incontinence, adverse drug reactions, and skin problems) and to identify work processes that can be modified to continuously improve these outcomes. Effective CQI activities will require the further development of software such as that which is used for incontinence care (Schnelle et al., 1995). Nursing home administrators, directors of nursing, and medical directors must create an environment that provides incentives for ongoing CQI activities in order to maintain these programs over time. The above-mentioned Medicare QIO program and its support web site (www.qualitynet.org), as well as the American Medical Directors Association (www.amda.com) and its journal have substantial resources for assisting nursing home providers with quality improvement initiatives.

SUBACUTE CARE AND THE NURSING HOME— ACUTE-CARE HOSPITAL INTERFACE

The increasing acuity of nursing home residents, a high incidence of acute conditions (Alessi et al., 2003), and the need for high levels of skilled post-acute care will continue to place increased demands on nursing homes. Health maintenance organizations (HMOs) commonly admit patients with acute but relatively stable conditions (eg, deep vein thrombosis, cellulitis) directly to nursing homes without an acute hospital stay. As a result, nursing homes are providing more and more high-level skilled care. The term *subacute care* has many connotations; for the purposes of this chapter, it refers to skilled care reimbursed by Medicare Part

A (or by a capitated system) in a free-standing nursing home. Subacute care is also discussed in Chap. 15, and more detail is provided in the Suggested Readings.

Caring for subacutely ill patients in a free-standing nursing home intensifies many of the challenges already alluded to in this chapter (see Table 16-2). This level of care requires greater involvement of physicians, nurse practitioners, and physician assistants; nursing staff trained for more acute patients; ready availability of ancillary services such as laboratory, x-ray, physical, and respiratory therapy; and more intensive discharge planning. Moreover, Medicare reimbursement for Part A services is "bundled," so that nursing homes will be at financial risk for services that are ordered by medical staff, including drugs, laboratory tests, x-rays, and therapies. This reimbursement structure requires close cooperation between physicians and nursing home administrators in order to make this form of subacute care economically viable.

As a result of the increasing acuity and frailty of the nursing home resident population, transfer back and forth between the nursing home and one or more acute-care hospitals is common. The major reasons for transfer include infection and the need for parenteral antimicrobials and hydration as well as acute cardiovascular conditions. Transfer to an acute-care hospital is often a disruptive process for a chronically or subacutely ill nursing home resident. In addition to the effects of the acute illness, nursing home residents are subject to acute mental status changes and a myriad of potential iatrogenic problems. Probably the most prevalent of these iatrogenic problems are related to immobility, including deconditioning, difficulty regaining ambulation and/or transfer capabilities, incontinence, polypharmacy, and the development of pressure sores.

Because of the risks of acute-care hospitalization, the decision to transfer a resident to the emergency room or hospitalize a resident must carefully balance a number of factors. A variety of medical, administrative, logistic, economic, and ethical issues can influence decisions to hospitalize nursing home residents. Decisions regarding hospitalization often boil down to the capabilities of the physician and the nursing home staff to provide services in the nursing home, the preferences of the resident and the family, and the logistic and administrative arrangements for acute hospital care. If, for example, the nursing home staff has been trained and has the personnel to institute intravenous therapy without detracting from the care of the other residents, or if it has arranged for an outside agency to oversee intravenous therapy and there is a nurse practitioner or physician's assistant to perform follow-up assessments, the resident with an acute infection who is otherwise medically stable may best be managed in the nursing home. Hypodermoclysis may be helpful in preventing some acute-care transfers (Remington and Hultman, 2007). Better advance care planning and advance directive use can also help to avoid unnecessary hospitalization of severely impaired nursing home residents (Molloy et al., 2000).

ETHICAL ISSUES IN NURSING HOME

Ethical issues arise as much or more in the day-to-day care of nursing home residents as in the care of patients in any other setting. These issues are also discussed in Chap. 17. Table 16-7 outlines several common ethical dilemmas that

TABLE 16-7   COMMON ETHICAL ISSUES IN THE NURSING HOME*

ETHICAL ISSUE	EXAMPLES
Preservation of autonomy	Choices in many areas are limited in most nursing homes (eg, mealtimes, sleeping hours) Families, physicians, and nursing home staff tend to be paternalistic
Decision-making capacity	Many nursing home residents are incapable or are questionably capable of participating in decisions about their care There are no standard methods of assessing decision-making capacity in this population
Surrogate decision making	Many nursing home residents have not clearly stated their preferences or appointed a surrogate before becoming unable to decide for themselves Family members may be in conflict, have hidden agendas, or be incapable of or unwilling to make decisions
Quality of life	This concept is often entered into decision making, but it is difficult to measure, especially among those with dementia Ageist biases can influence perceptions of nursing home residents' quality of life
Intensity of treatment	A range of options must be considered, including cardiopulmonary resuscitation and mechanical ventilation, hospitalization, treatment of specific conditions (eg, infection) in the nursing home without hospitalization, enteral feeding, comfort, or supportive care only

*See also Chap. 17.

occur in the nursing home. Although most attention has been directed toward those marginally able to express their preferences, important daily ethical dilemmas also face those who are capable of decision making. These more subtle problems are easily overlooked. Physicians, nurse practitioners, and physicians' assistants providing primary care must serve as strong advocates for the autonomy and quality of life for nursing homes residents.

Nursing homes do care for an extraordinarily high concentration of individuals who are unable or are questionably capable of participating in decisions concerning their current and future health care. Among these same individuals, severe functional disabilities and terminal illnesses are prevalent. Thus, questions regarding individual autonomy, decision-making capacity, surrogate decision makers, and the intensity of treatment that should be given at the end of life arise on a daily basis. These questions are both troublesome and complex, but must be dealt with in a straightforward and systematic manner in order to provide optimal medical care to nursing home residents within the context of ethical principles and state and federal laws. Nursing homes should be encouraged to develop their own ethics committees or to participate in a local existing committee in another facility. Ethics committees can be helpful in educating staff; developing, implementing, and monitoring policies and procedures; and in providing consultation in difficult cases. Some practical methods of approaching ethical issues are discussed in Chap. 17. References on end-of-life and hospice care in nursing homes are provided in the Suggested Readings.

References

Ackerman RJ, Kemle KA. The effect of a physician assistant on the hospitalization of nursing home residents. *J Am Geriatr Soc*. 1998;46:610-614.

Alessi CA, Ouslander JG, Maldague S, et al. Incidence and costs of acute medical conditions in long-stay incontinent nursing home residents. *J Am Med Dir Assoc*. 2003; 4:S5-S18.

Burl JB, Bonner A, Rao M, et al. Geriatric nurse practitioners in long-term care: demonstration of effectiveness in managed care. *J Am Geriatr Soc*. 1998;46:506-510.

Evans LK, Strumpf NE, Allen-Taylor SL, et al. A clinical trial to reduce restraints in nursing homes. *J Am Geriatr Soc*. 1997;45:675-681.

Institute of Medicine. *Improving the Quality of Care in Nursing Homes*. Washington, DC: National Academy Press; 1986.

Institute of Medicine. *Improving the Quality of Nursing Home Care*. Washington, DC: National Academy Press; 2000.

Kane RL. Assuring quality in nursing home care. *J Am Geriatr Soc*. 1998;46:232-237.

Kane RL, Keckhafer G, Flood S, et al. The effect of Evercare on hospital use. *J Am Geriatr Soc*. 2003;51:1427-1434.

Konetzka RT, Spector W, Limcangco RM. Reducing hospitalizations from long-term care settings. *Med Care Res Rev.* 2008;65:40-66.

Kramer AJ, Steiner JF, Schlenker RE, et al. Outcomes and costs after hip fracture and stroke: a comparison of rehabilitation settings. *JAMA.* 1997;277(5):396-404.

Loeb M, Carusone SC, Goeree R, et al. Effect of a clinical pathway to reduce hospitalizations in nursing home residents with pneumonia: a randomized controlled trial. *JAMA.* 2006;295:2503-2510.

The Medical Letter. Antimicrobial prophylaxis for surgery. *Med Lett.* December, 2006;52: 83-88.

Molloy DW, Guyatt GH, Russo R, et al. Systematic implementation of an advance directive program in nursing homes: a randomized controlled trial. *JAMA.* 2000;283: 1437-1444.

Mor V. Defining and measuring quality outcomes in long-term care. *J Am Med Dir Assoc.* 2006;7:532-540.

Ouslander JG. The Resident Assessment Instrument (RAI): promise and pitfalls. *J Am Geriatr Soc.* 1997;45:975-976.

Remington R, Hultman T. Hypodermoclysis to treat dehydration: a review of the evidence. *J Am Geriatr Soc.* 2007;55:2051-2055.

Reuben D, Buchanan J, Farley D, et al. Primary care of long-stay nursing home residents: a comparison of 3 HMO programs with fee-for-service care. *J Am Geriatr Soc.* 1999;47:131-138.

Rollow W, Lied TR, McGann P, et al. Assessment of the medicare quality improvement organization program. *Ann Intern Med.* 2006;145:342-353.

Saliba D, Schnelle JF. Indicators of the quality of nursing home residential care. *J Am Geriatr Soc.* 2002;50:1421-1430.

Saliba D, Solomon D, Rubenstein L, et al. Quality indicators for the management of medical conditions in nursing home residents. *J Am Med Dir Assoc.* 2004;5:297-309.

Saliba D, Solomon D, Rubenstein L, et al. Feasibility of quality indicators for the management of geriatric syndromes in nursing home residents. *J Am Med Dir Assoc.* 2005;6:S50-S59.

Schnelle J, Ouslander JG, Cruise PA, et al. Policy with technology: a barrier to improving nursing home care. *Gerontologist.* 1997;37(4):527-532.

Schnelle JF, McNees P, Crook V, et al. The use of a computer-based model to implement an incontinence management program. *Gerontologist.* 1995;36:656-665.

Schnelle JF, Ouslander JG, Osterweil D, et al. Total quality management: administrative and clinical applications in nursing homes. *J Am Geriatr Soc.* 1993;41:1259-1266.

Simmons SF, Garcia ET, Cadogan MP, et al. The minimum data set weight-loss quality indicator: does it reflect differences in care processes related to weight loss? *J Am Geriatr Soc.* 2003;51:1410-1418.

Stevenson DG, Studdert DM. The rise of nursing home litigation: findings from a national survey of attorneys. *Health Aff.* 2003;22:219-229.

Vladek B. *Unloving Care: The Nursing Home Tragedy.* New York, NY: Basic Books; 1980.

Suggested Readings

Nursing Home Care (General)

American Geriatrics Society. Assisted living facilities: American Geriatrics Society Position Paper AGS Health Care Systems Committee. *J Am Geriatr Soc.* 2005;53: 536-537.

Casarett D, Karlawish J, Morales K, et al. Improving the use of hospice services in nursing homes. *JAMA.* 2005;294:211-217.

Dobkin BH. Rehabilitation after stroke. *N Engl J Med.* 2005;352:1677-1684.

Harvell J. Subacute care: its role and the assurance of quality. *Annu Rev Gerontol Geriatr.* 1996;16:37-59.

Levenson SA. *Subacute and Transitional Care Handbook.* St. Louis, MO: Beverly Cracom; 1996.

Oliver DP, Porock D, Zweig S. End-of-life are in US nursing homes: a review of the evidence. *J Am Med Dir Assoc.* 2005;6:S21-S30.

Ouslander J, Osterweil D. Physician evaluation and management of nursing home residents. *Ann Intern Med.* 1994;121:584-592.

Ouslander J, Osterweil D, Morley J. *Medical Care in the Nursing Home.* 2nd ed. New York, NY: McGraw-Hill; 1996.

Osterweil D (ed). Medical Directors Role in Nursing Home Quality Improvement: An Educational Symposium of The New York Medical Directors Association. *J Am Med Dir Assoc.* 2007; (3):Supple 1-41.

Reddy M, Gill SS, Rochon PA. Preventing pressure ulcers: a systematic review. *JAMA.* 2006;296:974-984.

Saliba D, Rubenstein LV, Simon B, et al. Adherence to pressure ulcer prevention guidelines: implications for nursing home quality. *J Am Geriatr Soc.* 2003;51:56-62.

Smith RL, Osterweil D. The medical director in hospital-based transitional care units. *Med Dir Long-term Care.* 1995;11:373-389.

Stefanacci RG, Podrazik PM. Assisted living facilities: optimizing outcomes. *J Am Geriatr Soc.* 2005;53:538-540.

Selected Web Sites (Accessed 3/16/08)

http://www.medicare.gov/nhcompare/home.asp
http://www.healthinaging.org/agingintheknow/chapters_ch_trial.asp?ch=15
http://www.ahcancal.org/Pages/Default.aspx
http://www.aahsa.org/
http://www.nadona.org/
http://www.amda.com/

CHAPTER 17

ETHICAL ISSUES IN THE CARE OF OLDER PERSONS

Ethics is a fundamental part of geriatrics. Ethics, or the provision of ethical care, refers to a framework or guideline for determining what is morally good (ie, right) or bad (ie, wrong). Ethical problems arise when there is conflict about what is the "right" thing to do. This can and does occur when decisions need to be made around whether or not a medical intervention should be implemented and whether or not the intervention is futile. The answers to ethical questions are not straightforward and they involve a complex integration of thoughts, feelings, beliefs, and evidence-based data. Ageism can play a strong role in these decisions. Acknowledging and acting on the wishes of the older individual are a critical component of ethical care.

While ethical dilemmas are central to the practice of medicine itself, the dependent nature of the older adult and the imminence of death raise special concerns. Discussions of ethics and aging seem to focus on the roles of autonomy and cost containment, since a significant portion of the cost of delivering health care is incurred at the end of life.

There have been significant initiatives (eg, federal laws) intended to encourage health-care facilities and providers, including attending physicians, to discuss with older persons their preferences in an advance directive (AD). An AD, sometimes called a living will or health-care power of attorney, addresses how older individuals would wish to be treated in the event that they are too incapacitated to express their wishes. This advocacy has been viewed as sparing unnecessary suffering and is believed to improve the quality of end-of-life care. However, making these judgments at a time of relatively good health may cause older persons to overweigh fears of disability. It is important to distinguish ADs from end-of-life decisions, when a person has actually had an opportunity to experience what life would be like under these conditions. Moreover, the availability of palliative care and hospice care alternatives provide a range of options that can be discussed with patients. Advance care planning is the process that leads up to the development of the AD.

Popular belief may exaggerate older people's enthusiasm for dying. People aged 74 years and older were less likely than younger participants to want their health-care providers to make a decision to end their life when faced with a terminal illness (Catt et al., 2005). Although they believed death was easier to face for older people, they did not believe that younger people deserved more consideration than older people when dying, or that they should have priority for hospice care (Catt et al., 2005). Education, social class, hospice knowledge, and anxiety about death had little influence on overall attitudes.

A number of obstacles influence the development of ADs for older adults. These include being willing to discuss death and make end-of-life decisions, and/or having trouble predicting what their future treatment preferences might be in any given situation (Fagerlin and Schneider, 2004; Puchalski et al., 2000). Health-care providers, therefore, play a vital role in helping older adults to engage in the development of ADs and in evaluating the geriatric patients' current capacity to give direction about care. Specifically such direction includes withholding or withdrawing life-sustaining procedures, making clinical decisions that work for their proxy decision maker in the absence of an AD, or in setting some guidelines around determining medical futility with regard to clinical interventions. Mechanisms that facilitate the development of AD include specifically eliciting the older individuals' preferences for medical treatments under a variety of conditions (Emanuel and Emanuel, 1989; Resnick and Andrews, 2002), and encouraging older individuals to specify a proxy and discuss their end-of-life care preferences (Aging with Dignity: Five Wishes, 2007; Resnick and Andrews, 2002).

The issues affecting life-and-death decisions attract the greatest attention: Should one withhold or withdraw treatment? Should a "do not resuscitate" order be entered in the medical record? What about tube feeding? These are each important and taxing questions posed in the context of real people. However, they arise much less often than do the less-heralded ethical dilemmas that confront clinicians each day as they decide about discharge from hospital; arrange placement in a nursing home; make decisions about screening for diseases such as breast, prostate, or bowel cancer; or recommend therapies. Consideration of the ethics of geriatric care must address the full spectrum of these issues.

Some key points are worthy of special consideration:

- Ethics and law are separate, but overlapping. Ethical guidance may come from a variety of sources, such as national and state professional societies, local and national standards of practice, and other sources. However, health-care professional licensing boards commonly include among licensing standards and grounds for disciplinary action references to "unethical" conduct. Sometimes these may be based on an external standard incorporated by reference into local law, and in other states there may be a specific code of ethics incorporated into the licensing regulations.

Health-care providers are advised to consider this in the states in which they practice.

- In the area of end-of-life care, state law typically governs. A health-care decisions act or similar law may set out the obligations of health-care providers, health-care facilities, patients, and persons who may be authorized to act as proxies for an incapacitated individual. Those statutes, and the regulations or interpretations of agencies and attorneys general can affect the expectations imposed on health-care providers. Case law may reflect "common law" principles that guide expectations and conduct of health-care providers. Any general reading, including in a chapter such as this, should be measured against applicable state law.

- Many health-care facilities have "ethics committees," which are interdisciplinary committees empowered to bring together involved staff, independent advisors from various disciplines, and involved family members, to provide ethical guidance. Depending on state law, there may be legal protection for health-care providers following the recommendations of such committees.

- Informed consent is a routine and fundamental part of provider–patient interactions. A patient who makes an informed decision about health care makes a decision and gives direction that has a continuing effect. For example, a competent individual who refuses otherwise-needed dialysis despite knowing the consequences does not surrender his or her right to reconsider that decision once they suffer the consequences lack of dialysis brings and become unconscious.

- Patients can express their wishes about future health care in several ways. For example, geriatric patients not presently faced with a decision about artificial feeding via a tube may give direction about their future wishes, should that need arise. This may be done in a written form. In some states, state law permits an AD to be made verbally and may subsequently require such directives to be documented in a particular way. For example, these documents may require one or more physician determinations of a particular kind. Specifically, it may be necessary to include a determination of whether the patient was competent at the time an AD was signed, whether the patient is presently competent at the time someone wishes to invoke the document because the patient is incapacitated, and whether the patient is in a particular condition, such as terminal illness, a vegetative state, or some other condition the effect of which is to permit, or not permit, health care to be given, withheld, or withdrawn, even when it is life sustaining.

- State law may set out a process by which, in the absence of an AD from the patient, an individual may act as a surrogate, proxy, or similar title, making health-care decisions for others. This may require a physician determination of competency and evidence that the patient is in a particular clinical condition (eg, terminal).

- State guardianship laws authorize a court to appoint someone as guardian of the person. This is typically based on physician certification of incapacity.
- State law may recognize that health-care providers are not only ethically obligated to furnish care, they may also be empowered to refuse to furnish care that is medically futile and therefore not provided for ethical reasons.

AUTONOMY AND BENEFICENCE

Table 17-1 provides a framework for discussing ethical issues. The ethics of medicine is based on four principles: autonomy, beneficence, nonmaleficence, and justice, which are geared toward maximizing benefits over harm

TABLE 17-1 MAJOR ETHICAL PRINCIPLES

Goal of Ethical Care
Avoiding or minimizing harms and maximizing benefits. The concern and focus should be on preserving and respecting personhood. This is done through recognition of wants, collaboration, play, validating, facilitation, and giving. At the same time, ethics must recognize and deal with competition between organizational/community interests vs. individual interests

Autonomy
Refers to one's right to control one's destiny, that is, to exert one's will. The principal issue revolves around whether the older adult is able to assess the situation and make a rational decision independently

Beneficence
Refers to the duty to do good for others, and specifically to avoid harm in the process

Nonmaleficence
Involves doing no harm and avoiding negligence that leads to harm. Lastly, justice focuses on fairness in the treatment of others

Justice
Justice focuses on nondiscrimination and the duty to treat individuals fairly; not to discriminate on the basis of irrelevant characteristics. This involves a duty to distribute resources fairly, nonarbitrarily, and noncapriciously

Fidelity
Duty to keep promises

and doing the greatest good for the greatest number. *Autonomy* refers to one's right to control one's destiny, that is, to exert one's will. Obviously, there are limits to how freely such control can be expressed, but for geriatric purposes the principal issue revolves around whether the patient is able to assess the situation and make a rational decision independently. This raises the second concept, *beneficence*, which refers to the duty to do good for others, to help them directly, and to avoid harm. *Nonmaleficence* involves doing no harm and avoiding negligence that leads to harm. Lastly, *justice* focuses on fairness in the treatment of others.

The principles of autonomy and beneficence (doing good and putting others' interests first) conflict when others act in the "best interests" of the older individual. Providers can sometimes become paternalistic and undermine the personal autonomy of the individual. If acting in the older individuals' "best interests" is consistent with the greater good of the community, then overriding autonomy is justified.

The challenge then comes down to several fundamental issues:

1. Is the patient capable of understanding the dilemma?
2. Is the patient able to express a preference?
3. Has the patient received accurate information about the benefits and risks?
4. Are there clear options? Have they been made clear?
5. What happens when the patient's preferences are contrary to the preferences of their family or the physician?

COMPETENCE AND INFORMED CONSENT

In the case of older adults, much of the concern is directed toward the issue of understanding and expressing opinions. The two most extreme cases are the comatose patient, who clearly cannot communicate, and the aphasic patient, who may be unable to communicate effectively. In the former case, we must look for other ways to preserve autonomy. In the latter, we must be very careful to assess and separate areas of communication from reasoning.

There is an important difference between the concepts of competence and decision-making capability. The former is a legal term that refers to a person's ability to act reasonably after understanding the nature of the situation being faced. Someone not competent to act on his or her own behalf requires an agent to act *for* them.

In the case of dementia, persons may or may not be capable of understanding and interpreting complex situations and of making a rational decision. Intellectual deficits are spotty. A person may get lost easily or forget things but still be able to make decisions. The presence of a formal diagnosis of dementia, even by type, may not be a sufficient indicator of the individual's ability to comprehend and express a meaningful preference. Just as it is wrong to infantilize such patients by directing questions to others who are quicker to respond, so, too, might it be inappropriate to prejudge their ability to participate in decisions about their own care.

Determining cognitive ability and decision-making capacity is not easy. One must distinguish memory from understanding. Decisional capacity is predicated on four elements: (1) Understanding or the ability to comprehend the disclosed information about the nature and purpose of the study, the procedures involved, as well as the risks and benefits of participating versus not participating; (2) Appreciation of the significance of the disclosed information and the potential risks and benefits for one's own situation and condition; (3) Reasoning, which involves the ability to engage in a reasoning process about the risks and benefits of participating in the research proposed versus alternatives to participation; and (4) Choice, or being able to choose whether or not to participate. No cognitive screening tests are appropriate to establish the residents' decision-making capacity (Moye et al., 2006). There also tend to be discrepancies between the clinician's opinion and family opinion of the resident's decisional capacity. Clinicians generally base their beliefs in the resident's ability to provide informed consent on the individual's cognitive status (Resnick et al., 2007). Family members may base their decisions about the individual's ability to provide informed consent on less clinical information. Physicians were actually noted to be the most lenient in their judgment of the incompetence of the resident, while family members were more stringent (Vellinga, et al., 2004).

One criterion for decision making, often presented with regard to informed consent, is the confirmation of the decision after a period of time during which the patient can consider the issues at hand. Unfortunately, we often do not have the luxury in our current health-care system to allow the individual, and the health-care team, the time needed to make informed decisions. Likewise, we do not always provide individuals with the necessary information to make these decisions. Ideally, a person making a care decision would have complete information about the full range of options and the risks and benefits associated with each option. The decision-making process would be structured to allow the individual (and perhaps the family) to identify which outcomes (from a large menu) they would like to achieve. In some cases there is insufficient evidence-based information to inform the individual, and in some situations health-care providers may withhold information to avoid upsetting older individuals and/or their families. Although different in nature from treatment-related decisions (eg, surgery), decisions about transitions to alternative levels of care require the same level of serious attention accorded to those about treatments. Alternative members of the health-care team, such as social workers or nurse case managers, may be the best at delineating the choices and implications of such moves and older individuals should be referred to these individuals as appropriate. Specific information that needs to be presented includes cost and cost-based alternatives, privacy issues, safety, social issues, and access to appropriate health care.

ADVANCE DIRECTIVES AND END-OF-LIFE CARE

It is important to distinguish between ADs and decisions or preferences at the end of life (Table 17-2). The former asks people to make decisions about how they believe they would wish to be cared for, were they in some hypothetical situation of severe impairment. People tend to exaggerate the fears of unknown states. (As Shakespeare observed in Macbeth, "Present fears are less than horrible imaginings.") The latter addresses much more real issues. Unfortunately, the debate on end-of-life care confuses these two quite distinct decisions.

Advance Directives

One way of trying to deal with the situation when the patient cannot express a preference is to encourage the development of ADs. The development of ADs allows older adults to indicate what they want to be done under certain circumstances. Federal law requires that all persons entering a hospital or a nursing home be offered the opportunity to indicate ADs. Too often, this exercise involves asking older persons about possible procedures they would want to have if the occasion arose. Done poorly, the experience can provoke unnecessary anxiety and lead to poor decisions that may be regretted later. The two most common forms of these ADs are living wills and durable powers of attorney. The former indicates in as much detail as possible what actions should or should not be undertaken in specific clinical circumstances. Some ADs state expressly the preferences of the patient in particular situations. Others offer general guidance from the patient, but leave the decision to the agent based on all the relevant information available at the time a decision must be made.

Living wills can range from being too vague or too specific, and a person's intentions and preferences change with circumstances (Ditto et al., 2006). Preferences were most stable for illness scenarios in which the individual was the least or the most seriously ill. Age, gender, education, and prior completion of an AD were all related to preference stability, and evidence indicated that declines in physical or psychological functioning resulted in decreased interest in life-sustaining treatment. Living wills most often address the issue of extraordinary actions to sustain life, focusing mainly on the question of resuscitation, hospitalization, use of life-sustaining therapies including parenteral and tube feeding, and even the use of antibiotics. They provide a means to indicate whether the patient prefers that heroic measures not be undertaken. Specific orders are better than vague statements. Under what conditions? What constitutes a heroic measure? Forgoing heroic measures based on a "do not resuscitate" (DNR) request is not the equivalent of providing no care when acute events happen, such as a fall, or when the individual is not responding to appropriate nonheroic measures. Ethical and

TABLE 17-2   DEFINITIONS OF TERMINOLOGY RELATED
             TO END-OF-LIFE CARE

TERM	DEFINITION
Advance health-care directive	A written instructional health-care directive and/or appointment of an agent, or a written refusal to appoint an agent or execute a direction
Living will	Also referred to as instructional health-care directive/preferences for care. The "living will" is a written directive describing preferences or goals for health care at the end of life
Agent	Is an individual designated in a legal document known as a power of attorney for health care to make a health-care decision for the individual granting the power to make such decisions
Advance care planning	The process of discussing, determining, and/or executing treatment directives and appointing a proxy decision maker
Capacity	An individual's ability to understand the significant benefits, risks, and alternatives to proposed health care and to make and communicate a health-care decision
Competency	Is a legal status imposed by the court
Guardian	A judicially appointed guardian or conservator having authority to make a health-care decision for an individual
Palliative care	Also referred to as "comfort care" and is a comprehensive approach to treating serious illness that focuses on the physical, psychological, and spiritual needs of the patient. The major focus of palliative care is to relieve the patient of suffering

practical considerations need to be addressed. At best, one may get a sense of a person's priorities and feelings about active, aggressive attempts to support and sustain life. Although there is a requirement that ADs be solicited whenever an older individual is admitted to a health-care institution, this is not the ideal time to expect the individual to make clear, thoughtful decisions. Ideally, the health-care provider has discussed AD and there has been time and thought given to the development of appropriate documents. The acute event requires only that these previously stated decisions be revisited to make sure the choices are consistent with the individual's current philosophy. The advantage of asking new residents or admissions about their AD is that it prompts the health-care provider to obtain this information and the older individual and/or family to make sure the appropriate forms have been completed. If it is more appropriate to postpone the discussion until the individual has adjusted to the new environment, systems should be in place to be sure the information is obtained at a later date. There are standard forms available on the web for patients and/or families to download and complete (ADs in Maryland; http://www.aetnacompassionatecareprogram.com/EOL/ihtEOL/ r.WSEOL000/st.36926/t.36985.html). Filling this out, however, may be disconcerting for some individuals. More than two-thirds of the states have some form of living will legislation, but the precise nature of those laws varies greatly in terms of what must be specified and under what conditions the delineated preferences can be followed. Individuals that spend part of the year in one state and part in another should be aware of the state laws with regard to living wills. If the states vary, they may need a different set of directives for when they reside in each of the states.

An alternative to the living will approach of prior specification is designating a proxy. A proxy is an individual authorized to act on the patient's behalf if that person is unable to communicate (ie, understand and express) his or her health-care preferences. This designation can be done by using a durable power of attorney, previously used to transfer control of property. States must specifically extend their durable power of attorney statutes to cover medical decisions. Under this approach, one can specify both the person one wishes to act as agent and the conditions under which such a proxy should be exercised. Table 17-3 shows the components of a durable power of attorney for health care.

With both the living will and the durable power of attorney, there is some potential for misuse. Decisions once made can be difficult to revoke. By the same token, physicians need to educate patients and proxies that a course of treatment, once started, need not always be continued. Sometimes a trial of a particular treatment may be attempted and later removed. There is currently no test of mental competence that allows one to change one's mind about a decision to not use life-support systems.

In the absence of any specification of actions or agents, someone must be identified to act for a person who is unable to act on his or her own behalf. There are legal procedures to accomplish this, which vary from state to state. In general,

TABLE 17-3   COMPONENTS OF A DURABLE POWER OF ATTORNEY
FOR HEALTH CARE*

Creation of durable power of attorney for health care
     Statement that gives intention and refers to statute(s) authorizing such

Designation of health-care agent
     Statement naming and facilitating access to (address, telephone number)
     agent; state laws will vary as to who may serve as agent—some states
     preclude providers of health care or employees of institutions where care
     is given; person designated as agent should have agreed to assume this
     role

General statement of authority granted
     Statement about circumstances under which the agent is granted power
     and indications of the power the agent will have in that event (usually a
     general statement about right to consent or refuse or withdraw consent
     for care, treatment, service or procedure, or release of information sub-
     ject to any specific provisions and limitations indicated)

Statement of desires, special provisions, and limitations
     Opportunity to indicate general preferences (eg, wish not to have life
     prolonged if burdens outweigh benefits; wish for life-sustaining treat-
     ment unless in coma that physicians believe to be irreversible, then no
     such efforts; wish for all possible efforts regardless of prognosis); oppor-
     tunity for specific types of things wanted done or not done and indica-
     tions for such actions

Signatures
     Individual dated signature
     Witnesses (better notarized): witnesses cannot be those named as agents,
     providers of health care, or employees of facilities giving such care

Conditions
     Form should have place where person signing indicates awareness of
     rights, including the right to revoke the document and the conditions
     under which the document comes into force; some states require a
     mandatory maximum period such a document can be valid without
     renewal

*Many state medical associations can provide a copy of a basic form of a durable power of
attorney for health care.

the two major classes of legally empowered agents are conservators and guardians. The latter usually have greater powers. A formal legal decision is needed to establish such a condition.

A critical question is: who is best qualified to assume that responsibility? Common wisdom suggests that it is the next of kin, but some argue that it should be the person most familiar with the patient's preferences, the person who can most closely estimate what the patient would have wanted. A rarely seen relative might know much less about the patient's wishes or lifestyle than might a close friend, clergyman, or even the attending physician. ADs are helpful ways for patients to give direction and simplify the decision-making process. For example, the children of a long-time marriage may be appointed to make decisions over a more recent spouse. Also, in a same-sex relationship an AD may be the only way in which a couple may be able to ensure who is the decision maker because the other may not have the rights of a "spouse." Where an AD does not appoint a proxy, the law may identify a hierarchy for the appointment of a proxy among candidates in particular degrees of relation.

The choice should rest on the level of knowledge possessed. Where there are multiple contenders for the role, the courts may have to decide who is best positioned to know the patient's preferences. This can become contentious. In cases where there is no one appropriate, the court may appoint a public guardian.

Agents, whether designated by durable power of attorney or chosen as the best available person, are vulnerable to pursuing their own interests rather than the patient's. At best, they must make inferences about the patient's wishes from their knowledge of the patient or the choice indicated in the durable power document. Surrogates' decisions may not be congruent with the wishes of the individuals they represent. They can be sincerely torn between acting in what they perceive to be the individual's wishes versus what may actually be their best interests in the given situation. The law typically imposes a standard of conduct on proxies appointed under ADs, proxies qualifying under applicable law, and guardians appointed by a court.

Substantial controversy surrounds end-of-life care with concerns around costs associated with implementation of medical futility. While care is never futile, medical interventions can be futile. Medical futility is described as proposed therapy that should not be performed because available data show that it will not improve the patient's medical condition. In some situations families and/or providers opt to engage in futile and expensive care (Bernat, 2005; Hariharan et al., 2003).

End-Of-Life Care

ADs provide a basis for making end-of-life decisions for those persons who are incapable of expressing their preferences at the time. Conversely, people are able to make their own decisions at the end of life. These individuals are faced with difficult choices that are based on current experience. In contrast to hypothetical imaginings of what it would be like to be in a given state, these people are experiencing that state or something quite close to it.

End-of-life decisions can be based on beliefs about both quantitative and qualitative futility. The former refers to an expectation that death is highly likely and that further efforts to postpone it are not likely to succeed. The latter addresses the quality of life if the patient survives. Will it be a life worth living? By the same token, health-care providers need to be cautious to avoid imposing decisions about another's quality of life, versus making a decision that care should not be ordered because it will not be effective, that is, it will not work.

The President's Council on Bioethics published a report entitled, Taking Care: Ethical Caregiving in our Aging Society (The President's Council on Biotethics, 2005). This report acknowledges the uniqueness of each case and helps health-care providers consider the relevant questions to facilitate decisions. These questions include:

1. What will happen if the patient is untreated?
2. Will nontreatment lead to increased suffering?
3. What are the possible indirect consequences of nontreatment?
4. What are the treatment options?
5. Are there reasonable alternative treatments?
6. Would "slowing down" a disease be a reasonable alternative to attempting cure?

Health-care providers may feel uncomfortable about encouraging patients/families/proxies to consider the option of saying no when we believe care is futile. It could be argued that this is the patient/family/proxy's right to decide. The ethics of medicine includes the principal of justice, which is geared toward maximizing benefits over harm and doing the greatest good for the greatest number. Utilizing health-care resources to provide a medical intervention that prolongs life but may worsen the quality of that life may not be the best decision for the community at large. Health-care providers have a duty to inform patients/families/proxies about the known anticipated outcomes of care, and when medically futile, palliative interventions should be considered so as to conserve resources for the entire community.

MOVING FROM DNR TO ACCEPTANCE OF NATURAL DEATH

The 1990 Patient Self Determination Act (PSDA) has encouraged health-care providers to ask patients about their AD and establish if the patient is a Do Not Resuscitate (DNR). There is a new trend emerging, however, for health-care providers to encourage patients to declare an Acceptance of Natural Death (AND) or decisions to receive palliative or comfort care when care is deemed medically futile. Increasingly, we may see these decisions on charts within all health-care settings.

Determining when further care is futile, however, is difficult. The American Medical Association (AMA) has outlined an approach to make this determination (American Medical Association, 1999). When further intervention to prolong the life of a patient becomes futile, health-care providers have an obligation to shift the intent of care toward comfort and closure. However, there are necessary value judgments involved in coming to the assessment of futility. These judgments must give consideration to patient or proxy assessments of worthwhile outcome. They should also take into account the perception of intent in treatment, which should not be to prolong the dying process without benefit to the patient or to others with legitimate interests. They may also take into account community and institutional standards, which in turn may have used physiological or functional outcome measures.

The decision to withdraw life support can be emotionally painful. Clinicians play a vital role in providing timely clinical and prognostic information, as well as emotional and social support to families. Moreover, a key principle of palliative care is the commitment and work of an interdisciplinary team in the management of patient symptoms at the end of life (Matzo and Sherman, 2004).

Managing the end of patient's life is a serious undertaking. In addition to facilitating decisions about the extent of heroic measures to be tried, much can be done to make that period as peaceful and unpleasant as possible. First-order issues involve the relief of unnecessary symptoms, such as pain, itching, nausea, and shortness of breath. Palliative care, which began with the hospice movement (see Chap. 15), has made great strides in bringing care not only into the hospital but also into patients' homes. Moreover, there is a growing science focusing on managing the symptoms that are commonly experienced at the end of life such as those shown in Table 17-4. In addition to avoiding inappropriate prolongation of dying, other end-of-life tasks include helping the patient to achieve a sense of control, relieving burdens, and strengthening relationships with loved ones.

THE HEALTH-CARE PROVIDER'S ROLE

The primary health-care provider may feel great pressure in facilitating end-of-life decisions. The provider is at once the patient's advocate, an agent of society, and a person in his or her own right. At times, the provider's preferences will differ from those of the patient or the patient's agent.

Most older individuals, along with their families, want to have input into end-of-life decisions. In some cases, however, the older individual may ask his or her health-care provider to make health-care related decisions. The provider must then decide how actively personal preferences should be voiced. Providers have

TABLE 17-4   GOALS OF CARE AND SYMPTOMS REQUIRING MANAGEMENT AT THE END OF LIFE

Be kept clean

Have a designated decision maker

Have caregivers with whom one feels comfortable and can trust

Know what to expect about one's physical condition at the end of life

Have caregivers who will listen and help manage physical and psychological symptoms

Maintain one's dignity

Have financial affairs in order

Have pain optimally managed

Maintain humor and integrate humor into care and end-of-life challenges

Have an opportunity to say goodbye to loved ones

Experience optimal control of shortness of breath

Experience optimal control of feelings of anxiety

Have appropriate individuals to discuss/express fears

Opportunities to resolve unfinished business with family or friends

Have opportunities for appropriate levels of physical touch

Have providers whom you know and who know you

Help older individuals feel reassured the family is prepared for their impending death

Assure the presence of family

Assure older individual that their end-of-life preferences are known to all providers

A plan in place for optimal death (eg, who will be at the bedside etc)

Provide opportunities for life review

an obligation to provide patients with a full set of information: the alternatives and the risks and benefits associated with each option, and to be sure that the patient appreciates that information. It is difficult to be fully objective in many instances.

Health-care providers may not accurately understand what the patient knows and believes about his or her end-of-life situation (DesHarnais et al., 2007). Improved communication is needed to optimize the transfer of information and assure patient understanding. Provider values may unconsciously distort the way options are portrayed; risks may be minimized or even overlooked. In addition, there are some providers who tend to think of themselves simply as conduits of information, whereas others believe strongly that their opinions should be counted. In an era of litigation, providers are increasingly sensitive to a need to provide all options, particularly those focused on interventions to treat an under-lying illness. At the same time, providers may offer their opinions and give their reasons. Frequently, this is done in the context of what the provider might do for his or her mother or family member. Situations may arise in which the provider disagrees with the decision of the patient or proxy for ethical reasons. This might occur, for example, if the treatment requested by a patient is believed to be futile, based on current research findings. These patients can be referred to another health-care provider, and/or resources such as the health-care facility's ethics committee, social services staff, or agencies who advocate for the older adults at the end of life can be contacted (Poncy, 2007). A recent court decision affirmed that "competent patients have the right to decline life-prolonging treatment, even if physicians disagree because of conscience or ethics."

A committee of the American College of Physicians and the American Society of Internal Medicine (Meisel, Snyder, and Quill, 2000) identified seven legal myths about end-of-life care that may prevent adequate care.

1. Forgoing life-sustaining treatment for patients without decision-making capacity requires evidence that this was the patient's actual wish.
2. Withholding or withdrawing artificial fluids and nutrition from terminally ill or permanently unconscious patients is illegal.
3. Risk-management personnel must be consulted before life-sustaining treatment can be terminated.
4. ADs must comply with specific forms, are not transferable across states, and govern all future treatment decisions; oral ADs are unenforceable.
5. If a physician prescribes or administers high doses of medication to relieve pain or discomfort in a terminally ill patient, which results in death, the physician will be criminally prosecuted.
6. When a terminally ill patient's suffering is overwhelming despite palliative care, and the patient requests a hastened death, there are no legally per-missible options to ease suffering.
7. The 1997 US Supreme Court decisions outlawed physician-assisted suicide.

SPECIAL PROBLEMS WITH NURSING HOME RESIDENTS

Nursing home residents present some unique challenges with regard to end-of-life decisions related to care. Older adults are usually admitted to nursing homes because of a reduced capacity to function either physically or mentally. Many suffer from some degree of cognitive impairment. Consequently, there may be some caregivers who assume that their quality of life is miserable and their lives have limited value.

Table 17-5 lists four areas where clinical decisions in treating long-term care patients may pose the greatest ethical dilemmas. As noted in Chap. 16, beyond the

TABLE 17-5   MAJOR TOPICS FOR CLINICAL ETHICAL DECISIONS
ABOUT NURSING HOME RESIDENTS

Resuscitation

Transfer to alternative levels of care (eg, nursing home, hospital, hospice)

Treatment of infections and other physical changes such as electrolyte
imbalance, fracture, or exacerbation of heart failure

Nutrition and hydration

Secondary prevention: screening interventions

---

usually considered question of resuscitation, the health-care provider faces difficult decisions in determining when it is appropriate to transfer a patient from a
nursing home to a hospital or when to intervene aggressively to treat changes in
physiologic status from fluid imbalance or infection. Perhaps one of the most perplexing areas is when to pursue heroic measures to maintain nutritional supports.

Artificial feeding decisions seem to arouse more controversy than other life-
sustaining treatment issues, especially when the individual has not clearly stated his
or her preferences. Recent research suggests that advance care planning, quality
palliative care training, and administrative support are necessary to assure that
resident preferences related to nutrition at the end of life are honored (Monturo
and Strumpf, 2007). Health-care providers must be diligent in working to preserve the patient's personhood. Essentially, nursing home residents should not
lose any of their rights as people just because they enter a nursing home. They
should be eligible to participate in a full range of activities and to make choices
about their lives and their health care. They should be the first ones consulted
about changes in their condition or therapy. Decisions about ADs take on special
meaning in the nursing home context because of the complex nature of the residents and the likelihood of survival being quite low, following interventions such
as cardiopulmonary resuscitation (CPR) (Shah, Fairbanks, and Lerner, 2007).
Because nursing home residents are vulnerable, special care is needed to protect
their rights. The general goal is to maximize the resident's autonomy in making
decisions about treatment. Several ombudsman groups have created a parallel set
of concerns in the form of a resident's bill of rights, which outlines the choices
that should be available and the protections that can be sought. Likewise legal aid
is available through projects such as the Bioethics Law Project (Poncy, 2007).
The goal of the Bioethics Law Project has been to serve as a bridge between the
medical and legal communities involved in end-of-life issues through education,
intervention, and advocacy.

One useful approach to help address ethical issues in long-term care facilities is to establish an ethics committee composed of persons within and outside the facility (Powers, 2003). Ethics committees are required in hospitals and long-term care facilities accredited by the Joint Commission on Accreditation of Healthcare Organizations (JCAHO). Most long-term care facilities, however, do not have JCAHO accreditation. Traditionally, the function of the Ethics Committee has been on case reviews, education of health-care providers, residents, and families and policy review as relevant to the committee. Such committees are especially useful when they operate in a proactive manner, exploring issues in advance rather than assessing actions already taken.

SPECIAL CASE OF DEMENTIA

The wishes of patients with dementia may be ignored or undervalued. It should be recognized that a diagnosis of dementia does not necessarily imply an inability to state preferences (Mezey et al., 2000). Because dementia effectively robs individuals of personality as well as memory, it can be very difficult to assess the quality of lives and hence the extent of effort appropriate to prolong them (Vollicer, 2007). The discussion related to AD is often done by the social worker in the facility (Lacey, 2006). Individuals identified to act as agents for older adults with cognitive impairment must struggle with the difficult issue of determining the quality of life for the individual, given the associated loss of self-awareness and ability to maintain relationships constitutes substantial suffering.

In addition to end-of-life ethical concerns with older adults with dementia, daily ethical issues can arise in the care of these individuals. These daily issues as associated with the common symptoms of dementia such as wandering, agitation, hitting, biting, disinhibited speech, or apathy and refusal of care. Wandering, either deliberate or aimless, can be intrusive for other residents and a significant clinical problem. Ethical issues arise when a resident with dementia invades the privacy and space of another resident, who does not consent to the visit. The balance between the autonomy of the individual who is wandering versus the greater good of the community must be resolved. Options that could be considered include such things as moving the resident who wanders or putting up a stop sign on the door to prevent entry. Alternatively, a resident with dementia may have significant apathy and may refuse to engage in any type of care activity, just wanting to lie in the bed. If allowed to make this decision, the individual will be at risk for pressure ulcers, deconditioned, increased risk of falls, and contractures and will ultimately require higher level nursing interventions and resources. The prevention of these problems would benefit not only the individual in terms of preventing pain and suffering but the community at large. Ethical choices need to be made to resolve the discrepancies between individual choice versus allowing harm to occur. In this situation, ongoing motivational interventions and capturing the individual at the opportune moment to engage him or her in activities would help to resolve the ethical dilemma.

POLICY ISSUES

Older people are prime targets for rationing efforts because they consume disproportionately large amounts of medical care and because they are seen as having already lived their lives. At a more subtle level, measures of program effectiveness tend to use something equivalent to the quality-adjusted life year (QALY). This term implies that valuable life must be lived free of dependency. Such proxies for program effectiveness incorporate ethical components subtly. Society has not established the base on which to put a value on life lived at some level of dependency. To assume that it has no value, as is implied by active life years, appears to contradict the very purpose for geriatrics, which treats primarily dependent older people. Many older people would actively challenge the tenet that disability implies an absence of quality of life. Severely disabled persons at various ages can continue to enjoy pleasant and productive lives. As advocates for their patients, geriatricians must be extremely vigilant to how such terms are used both in everyday speech and in analyses. It is important to bear in mind that any measure that uses life expectancy will tend to be biased against the elderly. One that relies on dependency as the primary outcome implies that those who are dependent no longer count; by such logic disability is equivalent to death. At a time when there is an effort to pit one generation against another, care must be taken to avoid setting the terms of the debate such that the outcome is inevitable.

The issue of futility of care and the impact the implementation of futile care interventions have on the individual as well as community in terms of resource use are critical. The avoidance of futile care, with the full understanding and acceptance of the older individual and his or her family is consistent with ethical mandates. Consequently, there has been a strong emphasis on ADs. A recent review of literature in this area (U.S. Department of Health and Human Services Assistant Secretary for Planning and Evaluation Office of Disability, 2007) recommends that we work to increase the number of individuals who have ADs, increase the availability of the ADs to health-care providers when they are needed, and increase adherence to established ADs on the part of health-care providers.

ADs have been shown to improve the quality of life at the end-of-life (Teno et al., 2007), although there is still a significant need to improve on symptom management. Unfortunately, the research suggests that even when ADs are executed, health-care providers are frequently unaware of them, ADs are not easily available to surrogates when needed, the ADs are too general and/or are inapplicable to clinical circumstances, and/or they are invoked late in the dying process or are at times overridden by providers and families (Fagerlin and Schneider, 2004b;

Lorenz et al., 2004). Medical care tends to be driven first and foremost by a patient's clinical circumstances. The patients' perceived quality of life and the wishes of family also affect clinical decisions at the end of life along with preferences expressed in ADs.

A main concern in the early days of ACP was whether discussions about end-of-life care and ADs would have a negative impact on patients. The evidence suggests that ACP is not distressing to patients and that intensive educational interventions are acceptable to patients, families, and physicians (eg, intensive ethics consults, facilitated family/provider conferences, palliative care consult teams, etc). There is, therefore, a need to increase advance care planning on the part of all adults, with a special focus on older individuals. Recommendations to increase awareness and involvement of patients and providers in completing ADs include the use of health information technology (HIT), social marketing, and policy initiatives.

HIT is being used increasing in the health-care arena and is anticipated to improve the quality of care and the efficiency with which it is provided. Use of HIT with regard to AD focuses on cueing providers to complete an AD with a new admission, for example, or as a way to improve accessibility by having the AD follow the patient electronically. Current examples of this include electronic records used in programs such as Evercare or the use of an implantable device that contains the individuals' AD such as that developed by VeriMed (VeriMed, 2007). Clearly, there will continue to be an increase in the development of such systems and ongoing evaluation is needed to determine if in fact that do improve completion of ADs and accessibility of these as needed across different sites of service.

Social marketing has also been recommended as a way to increase awareness of and completion of ADs. Social marketing is "the planning and implementation of programs designed to bring about social change using concepts from commercial marketing" (Social Marketing Institute, 2007). Included within social marketing is a focus on product, price, place, and promotion. Several programs have been implemented using a social marketing perspective including a Robert Wood Johnson funded program, Last Acts (Robert Wood Johnson Foundation, 2008)), a program to improve end-of-life care in Hawaii "Kokua Mau" (Braun, et al., 2005), and "Respecting Choices" which focused on education around AD (Respecting Choices, 2007).

Lastly, the role of policy and policy initiatives is critical to encourage the development and use of ADs. In 1991, the Patient Self-Determination Act (PSDA) was established. The Patient Self-Determination Act requires that most United States hospitals, nursing homes, hospice programs, home health agencies, and health maintenance organizations (HMOs) provide adults, at the time of inpatient admission or enrollment, information about their rights under state laws governing ADs, including: (1) the right to participate in and direct their own health-care decisions; (2) the right to accept or refuse medical or surgical treatment; (3) the right to prepare an AD; and (4) information on the provider's policies that govern the utilization of these rights. The act prohibits institutions from discriminating against a patient who does not have an AD. The PSDA further requires institutions to document patient information and provide ongoing community education on ADs. The law does not state, however, that an AD must be established.

The passage of the PSDA, unfortunately, has had minimal impact on increasing the numbers of individuals with ADs (Teno et al., 1997). At the state level, AD laws have similarly not been particularly effective and there are recommendations to relax requirements involved with completion of ADs, such as removing the requirement to have the AD be witnessed. Addition revisions include increasing the involvement of the proxy in decision making while the patient is still competent, requiring providers to record the name of the proxy, requiring providers to give written information to proxies about the health status of the patient, the development of a clearly delineated process of informed consent emphasizing the provider–proxy interaction, and changing state law so that there is a recognition of the authority and discretion of the proxies over the authority of the AD (U.S. Department of Health and Human Services Assistant Secretary for Planning and Evaluation Office of Disability, 2007). This final revision would help manage those situations in which the individual's living will, or specific preferences, is not consistent with what may be in his or her preferences at the time. For example, the individual may have indicated that he/she does not want intravenous hydration. In a self-limiting acute situation such as a gastrointestinal virus in which dehydration has occurred, it may be appropriate for the proxy to select to use short-term intravenous hydration to facilitate the return of the individual to his or her baseline status.

ETHICAL ISSUES CONCERNING CAREGIVERS

An important ethical issue closely linked to long-term care policy concerns the appropriate role of caregivers. Informal caregivers provide a significant amount of caregiving at the end of life with limited resources (Wolff et al., 2007). In Chap. 15, we noted the central role played by informal caregivers, who constitute the backbone of long-term care. For example, the Family Medical Leave Act asserts that an employee cannot be denied leave if the employee has a medically certified condition, or is caring for a covered individual who has a medically certified condition. The question then is, how much of such care should they be expected to provide? What is the nature of the obligation of one generation to another, or even to spouses and siblings from the same generation? A substantial portion of informal care is undoubtedly provided out of love and compassion. This approach works well when it is left up to the family to decide how much care they can give, but what happens when such care becomes mandated? Pressure to control public costs of long-term care could easily lead to demands to require care from families or to require that families pay directly for a certain amount of that care. Concerns have already been expressed about the possibility that older persons are manipulating their assets to become unfairly eligible for Medicaid coverage, or that younger generations gain control over elders' assets to ensure that funds are left to the next generation through the use of public funding to care for indigents. Although there is little substantiation for these claims of divestiture, advertisements for seminars on how to do it create an image of exploitation. Federal law plays a role in issues surrounding divestiture of assets to qualify for public assistance. Policies focused on familial responsibility would undoubtedly create a new demand for private long-term care insurance, because preservation of older persons' assets primarily benefits the heirs.

There has been significant press around the cost of care in the last year of life. Specifically, in the last year of life combined Medicare and Medicaid spending for dually eligible beneficiaries was more than $40,000 per beneficiary (Liu, Wiener, and Niefeld, 2006) . There is, however, evidence to support that the use of hospice and palliative care not only improves quality of life for individuals but also decreases costs (Brumley et al., 2007). Organizations such as the Veteran's Administration has demonstrated that by increasing access to services such as hospice there is increased use of these choices among veterans (Edes, Shreve, and Casarett, 2007). Conversely, it is possible that with continued emphasis on hospice and hospice services, for example, cost savings around end of life may actually result in new economic pressures on health-care systems (Payne et al., 2007). Similarly, coordinated care services have demonstrated increased completion of ADs and decreased costs of care among individuals with advanced illness (Engelhardt et al., 2006). It is anticipated that these types of programs and services will continue to increase. The benefit of this is twofold: options for palliative or hospice give patients a choice that is not simply one of care/treatment versus the converse which is believed by some patients and families to mean no care.

SUMMARY

Ethical issues around care of older people are played out at all levels. Policy issues largely address questions of access and coverage, but these can be influenced by an individual clinician's beliefs about what elements of care are "appropriate" for older people. These beliefs, in turn, can reflect stereotypes. Microethical issues occur at the bedside when decisions about initiating or continuing treatment are made.

These decisions, too, are based on beliefs about appropriateness, including who should have the ultimate word about how much and what kind of care is rendered. Some of these decisions are couched as ethical issues because the requisite facts are not known. When there is evidence of efficacy or futility, the discussion changes and decisions can be made on more substantial facts. Often, other factors than age are much better predictors of who will likely benefit from a given type of treatment. Great care must be taken to avoid couching rationing decisions as ethical dilemmas. Measures that discount older or frail people will inevitably lead to decisions against treating older persons.

Elderly patients should not lose their rights to full consideration of options and participation in the decisions that affect their care. The principles of autonomy and beneficence, which form a central part of the ethics of medicine in general, are strained with dependent older persons because the temptation toward paternalism is greater in the presence of the tendency to infantilize frail elderly patients, especially when they cannot readily communicate. Concerns about how to make decisions for persons unable to express their own preferences are often couched in terms of fear of litigation, but the growing body of experience suggests that carefully pursued efforts to establish agency and act accordingly will not put health-care providers or institutions at great risk of lawsuits. Rather, there is a risk of litigation if the wishes of the patient are not followed. Finally, it is important to recognize that the life of dependent older persons, especially those in nursing homes, is composed of many little incidents. The daily loss of dignity, privacy, and self-respect may be too readily ignored or may need to be balanced through negotiation based on the needs of the entire community. To be truly the patient's advocate, the health-care provider must be vigilant to these small but critical ethical insults and work toward optimal solutions for the good of all.

Clinicians should bear in mind that ethics is not a "slang" term without a particular meaning or that it simply reflects a set of general principles. Rather, state law may set out ethical standards with particularity. Moreover, clinicians can be effective advocates for patients, both while they are competent and after they are no longer authorized to act for themselves, based on both helping to facilitate ADs and making the various clinical findings that are relevant concerning capacity, levels of care needed, and whether the particular care will be clinically effective or, instead, simply futile. Knowledge of the distinctions between types of ADs, how others may act as proxy, and the availability of ethics committees are all important tools. While physicians do not dictate care, they have not been reduced to passive participants in the process. By understanding both the clinical situation and choices and the ethical and legal context that exists at a particular time, clinicians are empowered to act in an ethical way, in the best interest of patients.

References

Bernat JL. Medical futility: definition, determination, and disputes in critical care. *Neurocrit Care*. 2005;2(2):198-205.

Braun KL, Zir A, Crocker J, et al. Kokua Mau: a statewide effort to improve end-of life care. *J Palliat Med*. 2005;8(2):313-323.

Brumley R, Enguidanos S, Jamison P, et al. Increased satisfaction with care and lower costs: results of a randomized trial of in-home palliative care. *J Am Geriatr Soc.* 2007;55(7):993-1000.

Catt S, Blanchard M, Addington-Hall J, et al. Older adults' attitudes to death, palliative treatment and hospice care. *Palliat Medi.* 2005;19(5):402-410.

DesHarnais S, Carter RE, Hennessy W, et al. Lack of concordance between physician and patient: reports on end-of-life care discussions. *J Palliat Med.* 2007;10(3): 728-740.

Ditto PH, Jacobson JA, Smucker WD, et al. Context changes choices: a prospective study of the effects of hospitalization on life-sustaining treatment preferences. *Med Decis Making.* 2006;26(4):313-322.

Edes T, Shreve S, and Casarett D. Increasing access and quality in Department of Veterans Affairs care at the end of life: a lesson in change. *J Am Geriatr Soc.* 2007;55(10): 1645-1649.

Emanuel LL, and Emanuel EJ. The Medical Directive. A new comprehensive advance care document. *JAMA.* 1989;22:3288-3293.

Engelhardt JB, McClive-Reed KP, Toseland RW, et al. Effects of a program for coordinated care of advanced illness on patients, surrogates, and healthcare costs: a randomized trial. *Am J Manag Care.* 2006;12(2):93-100.

Fagerlin A, and Schneider CE. Enough. The failure of the living will. *Hastings Cent Rep.* 2004a;34(2):30-42.

Fagerlin A, and Schneider CE. Enough. The failure of the living will. *Hastings Cent Rep.* 2004b;34(2):30-42.

Hariharan S, Moseley HS, Kumar AY, et al. Futility-of-care decisions in the treatment of moribund intensive care patients in a developing country.*Can J Anaesth.* 2003;50(8):847-852.

Lacey D. End-of-life decision making for nursing home residents with dementia: a survey of nursing home social services staff. *Health Soc Work.* 2006;31(3):189-199.

Liu K, Wiener JM, and Niefeld MR. End of life Medicare and Medicaid expenditures for dually eligible beneficiaries. *Health Care Financ Rev.* 2006;27(4):95-110.

Lorenz K, Lynn J, Morton SC, et al. End-of-Life Care and Outcomes. Available at: http://www.ncbi.nlm.nih.gov/books/bv.fcgi?rid=hstat1a.chapter.77852/. Last accessed July 2008.

Matzo ML, and Sherman DW. *Gerontologic Palliative Care Nursing.* Philadelphia, PA: Mosby; 2004.

Meisel A, Snyder L, and Quill T. Seven legal barriers to end-of-life care: myths, realities, and grains of truth. *JAMA.* 2000;284:2495-2501.

Mezey MD, Mitty EL, Bottrell MM, et al. Advance directives: older adults with dementia. *Clin Geriatr Med.* 2000 May;16(2):255-68.

Monturo CA, and Strumpf NE. Advance directives at end-of-life: nursing home resident preferences for artificial nutrition. *J Am Med Dir Assoc.* 2007;8(4):224-228.

Moye J, Gurrera RJ, Karel MJ, et al. Empirical advances in the assessment of the capacity to consent to medical treatment: clinical implications and research needs. *Clin Psychol Rev.* 2006 Dec;26(8):1054-77.

Payne G, Laporte A, Deber R, et al. Counting backward to health care's future: using time-to-death modeling to identify changes in end-of-life morbidity and the impact of aging on health care expenditures. *Milbank Q.* 2007;85(2):213-257.

Poncy MR. Bioethics Law Project. 2007. [Electronic Version] from http://www.whcoa. gov/about/policy/meetings/Sept_2005/MarniePoncy.doc.

Powers BA. *Nursing Home Ethics.* New York, NY: Springer Publishing Company; 2003.

Puchalski CM, Zhong Z, Jacobs MM, et al. Patients who want their family and physician to make resuscitation decisions for them: observations from SUPPORT and HELP. Study to Understand Prognoses and Preferences for Outcomes and Risks of Treatment. Hospitalized Elderly Longitudinal Project. *J Am Geriatr Soc.* 2000;48(5):S84-S90.

Resnick B, and Andrews C. End-of-life treatment preferences among older adults: a nurse practitioner initiated intervention. *J Am Acad Nurse Pract.* 2002;14(11):517-522.

Resnick B, Gruber-Baldini AL, Pretzer-Aboff I, et al. Reliability and validity of the evaluation to sign consent measure. *Gerontologist.* 2007;47(1):69-77.

Respecting Choices. [Electronic Version] 2007 from http://www.respectingpatientchoices. org.au/background/about-us.html. Last accessed July 2008.

Robert Wood Johnson Foundation's (RWJF) Last Acts(r) campaign for improving end-of-life care. Available at: http://www.rwjf.org/reports/npreports/eol.htm. Last accessed July, 2008.

Shah MN, Fairbanks RJ, and Lerner EB. Cardiac arrests in skilled nursing facilities: continuing room for improvement? *J Am Med Dir Assoc.* 2007;8(3):27-31.

Social Marketing Institute. Social Marketing [Electronic Version]. From http://www. social-marketing.org/sm.html. Accessed Mar 22, 2007.

Teno J, Lynn J, Wenger N, et al. Advance directives for seriously ill hospitalized patients: effectiveness with the patient self-determination act and the SUPPORT intervention. SUPPORT Investigators. Study to Understand Prognoses and Preferences for Outcomes and Risks of Treatment. *J Am Geriatr Soc.* 1997;45(4):500-507.

Teno JM, Gruneir A, Schwartz Z, et al. Association between advance directives and quality of end-of-life care: a national study. *J Am Geriatr Soc.* 2007;55(2):189-194.

The President's Council on Bioethics. Taking care: ethical caregiving in our aging society. [Electronic Version]; 2005. Retrieved September, 2007 from www.bioethics.gov.

U.S. Department of Health and Human Services Assistant Secretary for Planning and Evaluation Office of Disability Aging and Long-Term Care Policy. Literature review on advance directives [Electronic Version]; 2007. Available at: http://aspe.hhs.gov/daltcp/reports/2007/advdirlr.htm. Last accessed July, 2008.

Vellinga A, Smit JH, van Leeuwen E, et al. Instruments to assess decision-making capacity: an overview. *Int Psychogeriatr.* 2004;16(4):397-419.

VeriMed. VeriMed patient identification [Electronic Version]; 2007. From http://www. verimedinfo.com/.

Wolff JL, Dy SM, Frick KD, et al. End-of-life care: findings from a national survey of informal caregivers. *Arch Intern Med.* 2007;167(1):40-46.

Web-Based References (Last Accessed July 2008.)

Review on Advance Directives. Available at: aspe.hhs.gov/daltcp/reports/04alcom.pdf.

Advance Directives in Maryland. [Electronic Version]. From www.aetnacompassionate-careprogram.com/i/E/EOLSalesMDrev.pdf.

Aging with Dignity: Five Wishes. Available at: http://www.agingwithdignity.org/5wishes.html; 2007.

American Medical Association. Decisions around futility of care at end-of-life. [Electronic Version]; 1999. From http://www.ama-assn.org/ama/pub/category/2830.html.

State-specific Advance Directives Online available at:

www.LegacyWriter.com.

www.CaringInfo.org.

SELECTED INTERNET RESOURCES ON GERIATRICS

ORGANIZATIONS

Administration on Aging	www.aoa.gov/
AgeNet Eldercare Network	www.aplaceformom.com/
Alzheimer's Association	www.alz.org/
Alzheimer's Disease Education & Referral Center	www.nia.nih.gov/alzheimers
American Academy of Pain Medicine	www.painmed.org
American Association of Homes and Services for the Aging	www.aahsa.org
American Association of Retired Persons	www.aarp.org/
American Geriatrics Society	www.americangeriatrics.org/
American Geriatrics Society Foundation for Health in Aging	www.healthinaging.org/
American Health Care Association	www.ahca.org/
American Medical Directors Association	www.amda.com/
American Pain Foundation	www.painfoundation.org/
American Pain Society	www.ampainsoc.org/
American Parkinson Disease Association	www.apdaparkinson.org/
American Society on Aging	www.asaging.org/

American Society of Consultant Pharmacists	www.ascp.com/
Arthritis Foundation	www.arthritis.org/
Centers for Disease Control and Prevention	www.cdc.gov/
Center to Advance Palliative Care	www.capc.org
Gerontological Society of America	www.geron.org/
Medicare	www.medicare.gov/
National Association of Area Agencies on Aging (N4A)	www.n4a.org
National Association for Continence	www.nafc.org/
National Association of Directors of Nursing Administration/ Long Term Care	www.nadona.org/
National Association of Nutrition and Aging Services Programs	www.nanasp.org
National Council on the Aging	www.ncoa.org
National Institute on Aging	www.nih.gov/nia
National Parkinson Foundation	www.parkinson.org/

CLINICAL TOPICS—FOR PROFESSIONALS

Alzheimer Disease

| "Progress Report on Alzheimer's Disease 2004-2005" | www.nia.nih.gov/Alzheimers/ Publications/ADProgress2004_2005 |

Hearing Impairment

| American Academy of Audiology | www.audiology.org |
| Clinical Advisory: NIDCD/VA Clinical Trial Finding Can Benefit Millions with Hearing Loss | www.nlm.nih.gov/databases/ alerts/hearing.html |

Hearing Loss   www.merck.com/mmpe/sec08/
                                     ch085/ch085a.html

Low Vision
American Academy of   www.aao.org/
  Ophthalmology
American Glaucoma Society   www.glaucomaweb.org/
Macular Degeneration Foundation   www.eyesight.org
Foundation Fighting Blindness   www.maculardegeneration.org
Macular Degeneration Network   www.macular-degeneration.org
Macular Degeneration Partnership   www.macd.net

Medications
American Society of Consultant   www.ascp.com/
  Pharmacists

Pain Management
"The Management of Chronic   www.americangeriatrics.org/
  Pain in Older Persons"   products/chronic_pain.pdf
"Treatment of Pain at the   www.ampainsoc.org/advocacy/
  End of Life"   treatment.htm
American Society for Pain   www.aspmn.org
  Management Nursing

Parkinson Disease
American Parkinson Disease   www.apdaparkinson.org/
  Association–Free brochures for
  patients and caregivers

Urinary Incontinence
National Association for Continence   www.nafc.org/

CLINICAL TOPICS—FOR PATIENTS

Alzheimer Disease

"Alzheimer's Disease Fact Sheet"   www.nia.nih.gov/Alzheimers/
Publications/adfact.htm

Depression

"Depression in Older Adults"   www.nmha.org/ccd/support/older.cfm
Depression and Bipolar   www.ndmda.org/
Support Alliance

General

A Consumer's Guide to Nursing   www.ahca.org/forms/
Facilities   consumer_request.html
American Geriatrics Society   www.healthinaging.org/
Foundation for Health in Aging
Five Wishes   www.agingwithdignity.org/
5wishes.html
Nursing Home Compare   www.medicare.gov/
nhcompare/home.asp
"Nursing Home Checklist"   www.nursing-homes.aplaceformom.com/
articles/nursing-home-checklist/
Health Care & Elder Care   www.nolo.com/resource.cfm/

Hearing Impairment

Healthy Hearing   www.healthyhearing.com
Hearing Aid Help   www.hearingaidhelp.com/
Hearing Loss   www.quickfactscenter.com/
qfcArticle.cfm?topic=17

Low Vision

American Macular Degeneration   www.macular.org/
Foundation
Facts about Age-Related Macular   www.nei.nih.gov/health/maculardegen/
Degeneration   armd_facts.htm

"Learn about Glaucoma"   www.glaucoma.org/learn/
Macular Degeneration Foundation   www.eyesight.org
Foundation Fighting Blindness   www.maculardegeneration.org
Macular Degeneration Network   www.macular-degeneration.org
Macular Degeneration Partnership   www.macd.net

Medications

ASCP's Prescription for Quality   www.ascp.com/medicarerx/upload/
Care" Preventing Medication-   quality.pdf
Related Problems Among Older
Americans

"Top Ten Dangerous Drug   www.scoup.net/M3Project/topten/
Interactions in Long-Term Care"

Pain Management

Pain (PDQ): Supportive Care-Patients   www.cancernet.nci.nih.gov/

Parkinson Disease

"NINDS Parkinson's Disease   www.ninds.nih.gov/
Information Page"   health_and_medical/disorders/
                                       parkinsons_disease.htm

"Parkinson's Disease—Hope   www.ninds.nih.gov/
Through Research"   health_and_medical/ pubs/
                                       parkinson_disease_htr.htm

INDEX

Note: Page numbers followed by "*t*" indicate tables; page numbers followed by "*f*" indicate figures.